Edwin Lankester

Our food

A series of lectures delivered at the South Kensington Museum

Edwin Lankester

Our food

A series of lectures delivered at the South Kensington Museum

ISBN/EAN: 9783337201418

Printed in Europe, USA, Canada, Australia, Japan

Cover: Foto ©Andreas Hilbeck / pixelio.de

More available books at **www.hansebooks.com**

OUR FOOD:

A SERIES OF LECTURES DELIVERED AT THE
SOUTH KENSINGTON MUSEUM.

BY

E. LANKESTER, M.D., F.R.S.

SUPERINTENDENT OF THE ANIMAL PRODUCTS AND COLLECTIONS.

𝕿𝖍𝖎𝖗𝖉 𝕰𝖉𝖎𝖙𝖎𝖔𝖓.

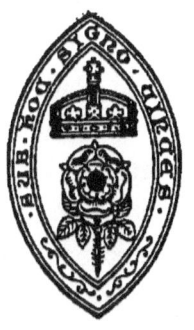

LONDON
HARDWICKE & BOGUE, 192 PICCADILLY.
1876.

PREFACE.

A WORD in explanation of the history of these Lectures seems necessary. The substance of them formed a part of my course on Materia Medica and Therapeutics, at the St. George's School of Medicine, and of a course on the Vegetable Kingdom, in relation to the Life of Man, at the Royal Institution of Great Britain. The form they now assume depended on my appointment to the scientific superintendence of the Food Collection at the South Kensington Museum.

Feeling that our great public museums ought to be connected with oral teaching, in order that they might become the means of educating and elevating the people, I obtained the permission of the Committee of Council on Education to deliver courses of Lectures, for the purpose of supplying instruction in connection with the Food Collection. These Lectures were well attended, and I had every reason to be satisfied with their success. Under these circumstances, I agreed to a proposal of the Publisher of this volume to correct reports of them by a short-hand writer. The six first were thus published, when it was considered desirable that my public instructions at the Museum should be discontinued. As only a part of the Lectures had been delivered when their publication commenced, I was obliged to complete the

Course by writing out the remainder from my notes. The last six will, on this account perhaps, be found less conversational and familiar; but, I hope, not less instructive.

These attempts at popular instruction have been produced at a very low price, in the hope that they may contribute in some measure to advance the study of those laws by which life and health are secured, and without a knowledge of which man can never realize the highest objects of his existence.

8, SAVILE ROW,
August, 1861.

CONTENTS OF FIRST COURSE.

ON WATER :—

Relation of Water to Life—Rain Water—River Water—Spring Water—Nature of Pure Water—Tests for Pure Water—Danger of Impure Water .... *Page* 3

ON SALT :—

The Mineral Substances of Food—Their Nature and Sources—Different kinds of Minerals in various Foods—Importance of Mineral Substances in Food 33

ON HEAT-GIVING FOODS :—

Nature of Animal Heat—Heat-giving bodies—Sources of Starch—Its connection with Sugar—Sources of Sugar—Kinds of Sugar 61

ON OIL, BUTTER, AND FAT :—

Action of Starch and Sugar as Heat-givers—Different action of Oils, Fats, and Butters—Vegetable Oils—Olive and Almond Oil—Animal Oils—Butter, Fat, Suet, Lard 91

ON FLESH-FORMING FOOD :—

Vegetable Albumen, Fibrine, and Caseine—Wheat, Barley, Oats, Rye, Maize, Beans, Peas, Lentils 119

ON ANIMAL FOOD :—

Milk, the Type of all Food—Composition of Animal Food—Beef, Mutton, Pork, Venison, Fowl, Fish 149

CONTENTS OF SECOND COURSE.

ON ALCOHOL.
Process of Fermentation—Production of Alcohol—Action of Alcohol on the Human Body—Effects of Alcohol on the Stomach, the Blood, the Heart, and the Nervous System .... *Page* 179

ON WINES, SPIRITS, AND BEER.
The Manufacture of Beer — Nature of Malt — Hops— History of the Grape—Composition of Wines—Bouquet of Wines—Distilled Spirits: Brandy, Rum, Gin, Whisky 213

ON CONDIMENTS AND SPICES.
Nature of Condiments and Spices—Artificial Manufacture of Volatile Oils — Condiments: Pepper, Mustard, Horseradish, Onions, Spices, Cinnamon, Cloves, Nutmegs and Mace, Ginger—Flavours: Oil of Bitter Almonds, Vanilla, Lemon Peel 253

ON TEA.
Action of Theine on the Nervous System—Early History of Tea—Culture of Tea—Action of Tea on the System —How to make Tea 291

ON COFFEE AND CHOCOLATE.
Use of warm Beverages—Salep—Introduction of Coffee —Establishment of Coffee-shops — Substitutes for Tea and Coffee — Paraguay Tea — Chicory — Cocoa and Chocolate—Action on the System 321

ON TOBACCO.
Distinctions between Food, Medicines, and Poisons— Action of Narcotics—History of the Introduction of Tobacco—Composition of Tobacco and Tobacco Smoke —Other Narcotics—Opium—Hemp—Coca—Henbane —Stramonium—Conclusion 353

FIRST COURSE.

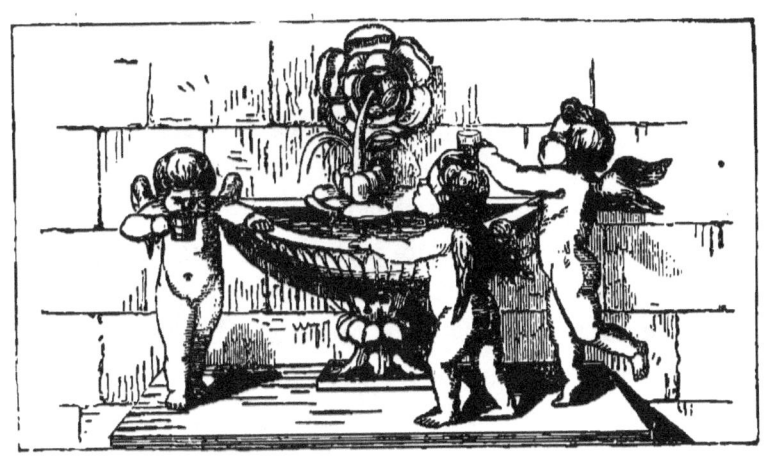

ON WATER.

THE object I have in view in this course of Lectures is to bring under notice the principal forms of those subtances of which we partake, from day to day, under the name of Food; by means of which we live, and without which we should die. The life of man is like a fire. Just as the fire must have fuel in order that it may burn, so we must have food in order that we may live; and the analogy is in many respects quite correct; for we find that man really produces in his body a certain amount of heat, just as the fire does, and the result of the combustion of the materials of his food is the same as the result of burning fuel in a fire. Man, in fact, exists in consequence of the physical and chemical changes that go on in his body as the result of taking food.

One of the most important results of the taking of food is that the human body, which is destroyed from day to day by the processes and the wear and tear of life, is kept up and maintained at a given bulk. Thus, we find, if we take, for instance, a man weighing 154 lbs., that he would lose in the course of a day from three to four pounds of matter by the various vital processes of his body. Now this matter must be supplied in order that he remain the same. Then, again, man's body is maintained at a given temperature. If we take a thermometer, and put it under the tongue, and compare it with the atmospheric temperature, there is usually a difference. The thermometer will stand at 98° in the human body, whatever may be the external temperature; and this is the result of a certain quantity of food being consumed in the system. Our food, then, first nourishes the body; and, secondly, maintains its heat. We shall find, however, that although these are the principal processes that go on, they are attended with others connected with the suppply of food. I have here drawn up a table, as a kind of classification of food.

CLASSIFICATION OF FOOD.

CLASS I.—*ALIMENTARY OR NECESSARY FOOD*.

Group 1.—MINERAL:—
  Water; Salt; Ashes of Plants and Animals.

Group 2.—CARBONACEOUS—FORCE AND HEAT-GIVING:—
  Starch; Sugar; Fat.

Group 3.—NITROGENOUS OR NUTRITIOUS—FLESH-FORMING:—Albumen; Fibrine; Caseine.

CLASS II.—*MEDICINAL OR AUXILIARY FOOD.*

Group 4.—STIMULANTS:—Alcohol; Volatile Oils.

Group 5.—NEUROTICS:—Alkaloids.

Group 6.—NARCOTICS:—Tobacco; Hemp; Opium.

CLASS III.—*ACCESSORY FOOD.*

Group 7.—Cellulose; Gum; Gelatine.

You will see that food is divided into two great groups;—into that which is *necessary* from day to day, and without which we could not live, and that which acts rather as a medicine or as an *auxiliary*. There is also a third group, which may be regarded as *accessory* foods. Taking the first group of dietetical substances, we come to water. We cannot do without water; we must drink; and thus it becomes a necessary of life. Most of the other substances in this group are necessarily taken from day to day. Then, in the auxiliary group you will see spirits, wine, and beer: they are not absolutely necessary to life; many persons live without them. Then we have tea, coffee, and cocoa—they are auxiliaries; and so on with the other substances mentioned in this part of our table. I call these substances medicinal, because they act on the system as medicines. We take alcohol as food, just as we administer sal volatile, camphor, and other drugs as medicines. Medicine and food are more allied to each other than most persons think; and medicines are constantly administered from a dietetical point of view.

In the present course of six lectures, I propose to treat of the group of the alimentary, or necessary substances of our food. I have divided these groups into seven, and you will see the first group is more nearly allied to the third than to the second; but taking the first, we find that water constitutes the basis of all the beverages we take from day to day. When we take beer, we take a large quantity of water; when we take tea or coffee, we take water. Then there are certain mineral substances which are necessary to form the fabric of our bodies. If we take an animal body and analyze it, we find that there are certain incombustible matters in that body—ashes as we call them. These constitute our mineral food. Then there is the group, consisting of substances taken for the purpose of giving force and maintaining animal heat—such as starch and sugar; they are necessary, inasmuch as they act upon the animal system by coming in contact with the oxygen of the air, and give out heat; so we call them combustible. These substances will supply us with material for our first four lectures. We then come to the nutritious group, which constitutes the flesh-forming substances of our food. These are necessary for forming the muscles and nerves of our body.

I now commence with water. Water, in many respects, more closely resembles nutritive food than it does force-giving food; that is to say, it more closely approaches, in its relation to the human system, the character of flesh than it does the character of starch or sugar; and for this reason, that it combines with the tissues of the body, and forms a necessary part of its structure.

I have made a calculation that a human body

weighing 154 lbs. contains 111 lbs. of water. You see, then, how necessary water is. If you reduce the size of the man, you reduce the quantity of water; and you will find that water enters into the composition of all our food.

Before speaking more particularly of water, I will call your attention, in the first place, to its composition: it is not my province to dwell on the elementary composition of food any further than it throws a light on its action. Water, then, is composed of two gases, one called oxygen, and another called hydrogen; and we can easily decompose water so as to demonstrate its composition. If you take a piece of potassium, which is a metal so malleable that you can cut it with a knife, and put it into water, it has such an affinity for the oxygen of the water, that when combined with it, it inflames. On putting it into water, the metal actually appears to take fire, and is converted into common potash. The hydrogen gas of the water is liberated, and it is this gas which burns during the decomposition of the water. This is a beautiful chemical experiment, and demonstrates the composition of water. But there are many other ways of doing this. If we take a little alcohol, or anything which contains hydrogen, and burn it in atmospheric air, under a glass vessel, we shall find that we produce water; so that we can easily by household experiments demonstrate the composition of water.

I now come to speak of water in relation to the life of plants and animals. Both animals and plants require it; and no animal, and no plant, exists without certain quantities of water. Sometimes it is so large in quantity, that it constitutes the great mass of the animal or plant. Thus, if we take some plants that grow in water, we find that they are formed of from 90 to 95 per cent. of water; and many of the little animals contained in water, if we take them and expose them to heat, so as to evaporate their water, almost entirely disappear. Even solid timber contains as much as 30 per cent. of water. Plants will not live without water: if we refrain from watering them, they die. The water passes in at their roots and up their stems and into their leaves, and the sun dries them, and evaporates their moisture. The water taken up by plants contains their food,—carbonic acid gas and ammonia. These two substances pass into the plant with the water, and out of these things we have manufactured in the system of the plant all our vegetable food. Carbonic acid gas, ammonia, and water, then, are the food of plants. They contain the four elements, carbon, oxygen, hydrogen, and nitrogen; and of these the food of man principally consists.

I told you just now that a human body weighing 154 lbs. contains 111 lbs. of water; but there are some animals in the lower scale which contain larger quantities than this. Thus Professor Owen tells us he took a jelly-fish, and found it weighed 2 lbs., and when dried in the sun, its solid parts weighed only 16 grains; so that you see there were 2 lbs. of water organized by 16 grains of solid matter. If we examine the tissues of animals, we shall find that they contain large quantities of water. This water, which is contained in animals, just the same as in plants, is constantly liable to evaporation. If you take a piece of blotting-paper, and roll it up, and put the other end in water, you will find the water will be gradually drawn up, and get into the dry end, which you may cut into strips, so as to resemble the expanded leaves of a plant. In this way, water finds its way to the leaves and flowers of plants, and the heat of the atmosphere causes the water to evaporate from the expanded surface of the plant, in the same way as in the blotting-paper: the mass is constantly losing its moisture, and water must therefore be supplied.

Water is contained in our solid food, and we thus get it entirely independent of our supplying it in a liquid form. I will here call your attention to the table of constituents of food,* and I shall constantly have occasion to refer to it.

This table contains a list of the chief articles of our food, and the cross lines indicate 100 parts, which you may read as grains, pounds, or hundred-weights. If you look at it, you will see the various chemical constituents of food are marked in different ways: thus we have flesh-formers marked in one way, heat-givers in another, and so on. Now, then, if you add together the lines which indicate the flesh-formers, the heat-givers, and the mineral matters, all the rest of any one of these articles of food will be water. Let us take, for instance, potatoes:—The flesh-forming matter in potatoes weighs 2 lbs. in the 100,—there is a figure in the third column to indicate this fact; the heat-giving matters weigh 23 lbs., and the mineral matters weigh 1 lb.; so that we get 26 lbs.

* This table is given opposite the first page.

of solid matter—all the rest in the 100 parts, that is to say 74 parts, is water. When you purchase 100 lbs. of potatoes, you do not purchase 100 lbs. of solid material, but 74 lbs. of water. Now I will draw your attention to the great importance of understanding the fact that certain forms of solid food contain but very little water, and that other forms contain a great deal. Thus, for instance, those who live chiefly on potatoes, as the Irish peasantry, require but very little water in their ordinary diet. A very curious fact illustrative of this, took place during the famine in Ireland in 1847. It was all at once discovered that Ireland, in the midst of her famine, was beginning to consume a larger quantity of what might be regarded as the luxuries of diet, such as sugar, tea, coffee, chocolate, and the like. The explanation is this:—When the potatoes became diseased, the peasantry ate corn, maize, Indian meal, and rice in their place, and therefore lost a quantity of water, to which they had been accustomed in their potatoes; and then it was they took tea and coffee, to which they had not been accustomed before; and there can be no doubt these were consumed in larger quantities for the purpose of supplying the necessary water to the system.

From this table you may also calculate the quantities of water in a pound of any kind of food. The quantity of water in a pound of potatoes is about twelve ounces, and this is not got rid of by cooking. Let us now look at the quantity in rice: instead of having twelve ounces, as in the potato, you have but two ounces and an eighth. There is barley, which contains but two ounces of water in sixteen of barley; and in beans there are but two ounces of water in the pound. With regard to the other cereal and leguminous foods, they have very much the same quantity of water. But there are the cabbage, the parsnip, the turnip, and the carrot, with larger quantities of water than the potato; thus accounting for the comparative inutility of carrots, cabbages, and potatoes as compared with beans, peas, and other materials with which animals are fed. Then with regard to the beverages which we take, such as tea and coffee, we find that the greater portion is water. Even with regard to beer, taking table beer, which, by the bye, is much the best for ordinary drinking, it contains not more than half an ounce of alcohol in a pint, and the rest is water; while the strong pale ales and stout contain two ounces of alcohol, the rest being water. Taking the French wines, very few of them contain more than two ounces of alcohol in a pint of twenty ounces. Even our ports and sherries, brandied as they are, contain as much as twelve or fourteen ounces of water in the pint.

Now the action of water in our food is very important. There would be no carrying of food into the system but for the agency of water. It dissolves everything that we take; and nothing that we take as food can become nutriment that is not dissolved in water. It would not do to test that by taking things and putting them into water, and seeing whether they dissolve, and rejecting them as food according to that circumstance; because food undergoes a considerable change in the stomach. It undergoes a change, to begin with, in our mouth. One of the great objects of that change is to render things soluble which had been before insoluble in water. Starch, which we cannot dissolve in water out of the stomach, is dissolved in water directly it gets into the mouth, for the starch is changed by the saliva into sugar, and that which would lie unchanged in water for months, is so changed by the saliva of the mouth and the gastric juice of the stomach, that it is speedily dissolved. Then, where we are taking considerable quantities of dry food, it becomes absolutely necessary that we should add a certain quantity of water, so that this dry food should become dissolved. Such things as oats, barley, wheat, rice, maize, and the other articles of diet in our table containing little water, must have water added, in order that their starch, fat, and gluten may be dissolved and enter into the system.

Having indicated the necessity of water, let me call your attention to the sources of water as drunk ordinarily for the purposes of diet. People are generally very indifferent about water; and perhaps it arises from the fact that boiling it before we make tea or beer, makes us independent of the impurities of water in its natural condition. At the same time, I do not think it is wise to be dependent for the water needed by the system on beverages containing a variety of foreign ingredients; and for this reason : that the water gets its soluble powers interfered with by having things in solution. Thus a pint of beer will not dissolve so much of the starch or digested meat as water. So with regard to the food which is digesting; it is sometimes better that we should pour upon it cold pure water than hot water containing a variety of substances in solution. I am not advocating the giving up of tea, coffee, beer, or wine, but the necessity of taking a portion of the water we daily consume as pure as it can be had.

Now there are many sources of water. The first great source is the ocean, which collects all the water from the earth; and this water contains so large a quantity of salt, that none of us can drink it. The shining sun, however, bears down upon the ocean's surface, and its heating rays penetrating the water, combine, as it were, with it, and raise it up. The atmosphere, like a sponge, absorbs the vaporous water, carrying it from the Equator to the Arctic and the Antarctic regions; thus distributing it north and south. It then condenses in the form of rain and of snow, when, sinking into the earth and pouring down its mountain-sides, it forms springs and rivulets, entering the ocean again in the form of rivers; and now man catches it in tubs or cisterns, in its progress in the rivers, or digs down into the earth, and catches it as it passes along beneath his feet. Thus we have rain-water, river-water, and spring or well-water.

I need not dwell on sea-water; but it is a very interesting fact to know, that by a process invented by my ingenious friend Dr. Normandy, sea-water may be distilled and rendered perfectly pure and fit for human use.

With regard to rain-water, there is no doubt that it is one of the purest waters that we have, arising from the fact that it is the first condensed *water* after it has passed from the ocean into the atmosphere; but its use is liable to the objection, that, where it runs down the sides of houses into cisterns, it passes through an atmosphere frequently contaminated with sulphurous acid and ammonia; and the unconsumed carbon of chimneys, of which we have so constantly unpleasant reminders in large towns. Still, where rain-water can be collected in the open country, there is no doubt that it is the purest form of water. It is, however, on spring and river-water that we are more dependent; and to the spring and well-waters I would more especially call your attention.

There are two kinds of well-waters, or spring-waters, which are consumed in London, as well as most other parts of the world; and those are the surface-well waters and the deep-well waters. In London, we dig down deep into the chalk and get water from below the London clay; this is deep-well water. If you glance at this diagram (Fig. 2), you will see how this is.

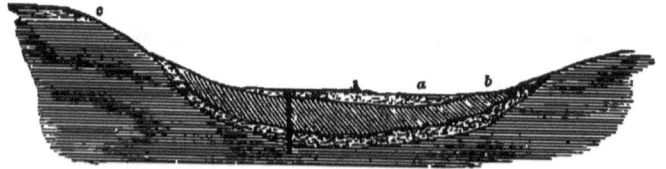

Fig. 2.—Diagram of London Basin.

a. *Gravel.*   b. *Clay.*   c. *Chalk.*

Here we have represented a section of the valley in which London is situated: it is formed in the chalk. London is, in fact, situated in a basin of chalk. Above the chalk is a deposit, varying in thickness, branching off to the side of the basin, as you see of London clay; above this clay is a layer of gravel. Now the water passing through or under this gravel, gradually accumulates on the clay; so that if you dig 20 feet or 25 feet in any of the gravelly districts of London, you get plenty of water; this is called surface-well water; but, if you want to get pure water, you must dig deeper than the clay; you must go through the clay down to the chalk. Wells dug down to the chalk are called Artesian wells. I shall have to speak of these waters again when I speak of the constituents of water; but I may just say here, that persons suppose it is a matter of indifference whether they obtain their water from surface-wells or from deep wells. This, however, is not the fact; for, although surface-well water is frequently clearer, cooler, and more sparkling than deep-well water, it is always liable to suspicion. The sparkling of these waters arises from the carbonic acid gas they contain; and in nine cases out of ten that carbonic acid is derived from the decomposition of animal and vegetable matters. Their cooling taste is no less indicative of their impure origin, as it arises from the formation of salts, which could only occur from the decomposition of organic matter.

The situation of these wells, especially in London, explains the origin of these impure matters. The water that supplies the surface-wells of London is derived from the rain which falls upon the surface of the land, and which percolates through the gravel, and accumulates upon the clay. Now this gravel contains all the soakage of London filth; through it run all the drains and sewers of London, and its whole surface is riddled with innumerable cesspools. Here is the source of the organic matter of surface-well waters, and also the cause of their coolness, their sparkling, and their popularity. In most small towns there is a public pump, and, when this is near the churchyard, it is said to be always popular. The character of the water is no doubt owing to the same causes as that of London surface-wells, the remains of humanity in the churchyard supply the nitrates and carbonic acid of the water.

From this kind of impurity the water of deep wells in London, and of wells cut into rocks which bring their water from a distance from towns, are entirely free. They frequently contain inorganic salts in abundance, but they do not contain organic matters; hence, for drinking purposes, they are very preferable to the waters of surface-wells. A great number of these wells exist in London. There is one attached to almost every brewery in London, and other manufacturers, who need pure water for their operations, sink these wells.

If you require ocular demonstration of the impurity of surface-well water, let me draw your attention to a series of these waters in the South Kensington Museum, where you will observe that the effect of time and exposure upon the surface-well water has been to organize their dissolved organic matters, and the bottles exhibit a variety of forms of plants which have been thus developed.

Then we come to river-water. The great distinguishing feature of river-water is, that, being exposed to the air, it becomes the medium of life to both plants and animals. We have not only fish, and snails, and reeds and pond-weeds growing in river water, but we have innumerable forms of microscopic animals and plants. Even after this water is filtered, and supplied to towns, as in the case of the Thames to London, these microscopic creations abound. Here we have a drawing,

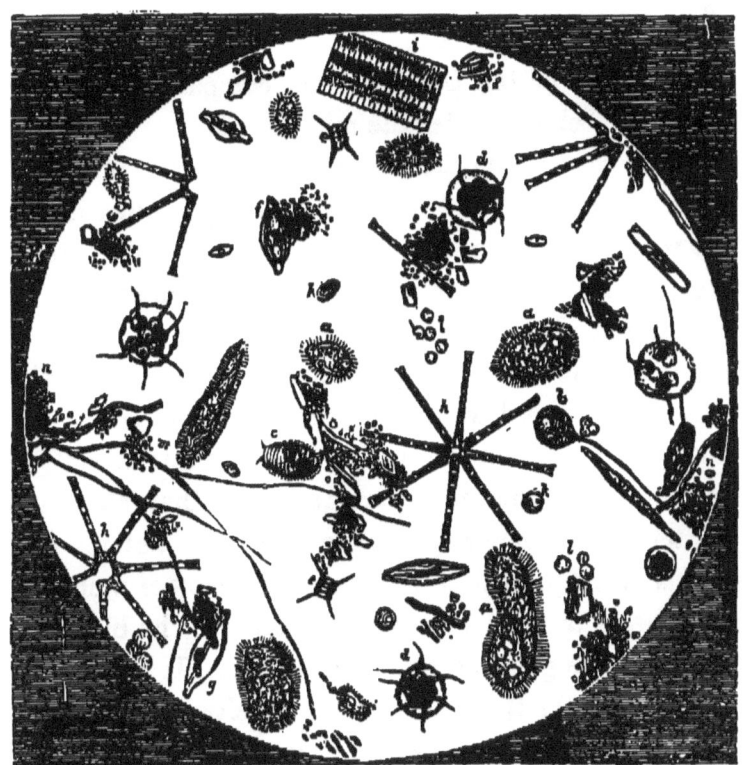

Fig. 3.—*Water from Grand Junction Company (from Cistern).*

a. *Paramæcia*, 2 species.
b. *Vorticella convallaria.*
c. *Coleps hirtus.*
d. *Pandorina Morum.*
e. *Scenedesmus quadricauda.*
f. *Navicula umphisbæna.*
g. ———— *sphærophora.*
h. *Asterionella formosa.*
i. *Fragilaria capucina.*
k. *Brown active sporules.*
l. *Stationary Green sporules.*
m. *Threads of slender Fungus.*
n. *Organic and Earthy Matter.*

copied from one published by Dr. Hassall, representing some of the interesting microscopical objects which are supplied in the river-water. The filtration is improved since this drawing was made, but there is still enough of them supplied to render the Thames water, as supplied by any of the London water companies, a highly interesting object under the microscope.

There is also another source of impurity in river-water: our lands and farms are highly manured, and the water passing over them carries the constituents of the manure to the river; and the river-waters are to that extent objectionable.

I will now draw your attention generally to the contents of these waters, and endeavour to show you the action of what are called their "impurities." I do not know that it is correct to say that all saline matter is an impurity; our own blood contains 420 grains of saline matter in a gallon. Now if a physiologist were to say this was an impurity in the blood, he would be laughed at for his assertion. If water contains saline matters, it is the necessity of the thing, and, in small quantities, these impurities have never been proved to do any harm. By analysis, however, we can come to the conclusion whether these things are in quantities likely to be injurious. We may have more saline matter in the blood than 420 grains to the gallon; then it would be an impurity. We must therefore recollect how this word impurity is used. There are two kinds of substances in water which are generally called impurities:—the first consists of saline substances, as common salt, carbonate of soda, and sulphate of lime: these are called saline impurities. Sometimes these saline substances are found in so large quantities as to render the waters medicinal, as in the waters of Cheltenham, Leamington, Harrowgate, and many other places. Such waters are called "mineral." They are remarkable for the permanence of their constituents, and many of them have been known in this country to possess the same constituents for hundreds of years. The most generally useful of these waters, are those which contain iron, and are called "chalybeate," as the waters of Harrowgate and Tunbridge Wells. Some of these contain larger quantities of sulphuretted hydrogen than our foulest sewer-waters, and yet are drunk medicinally; such are the waters of Askern, Harrowgate, Moffat, and Gillesland. That these waters may be drunk with impunity, should be a hint to those who imagine that sulphuretted hydrogen is in itself a dangerous gas. The fact is, it is not so; and in drains and sewers, and decomposing animal and vegetable compounds, it is not the cause of danger, but a sign of danger. The springs of Epsom are charged with sulphate of magnesia; hence we call this substance Epsom salts. Other substances, more or less injurious in their action upon the human system, are contained in mineral springs, and are prescribed according to the special need of those who seek their aid as medicines.

Now I will call your attention to those substances which occur more or less in all our drinking-waters. There are, in the first place, certain gases contained in water, which I will just mention, and there are two which more especially characterize waters:—First, there is carbonic acid gas. This gas is found in a variety of substances in nature. Thus, it is found in carbonate of ammonia, and by pouring a little acid of any kind upon this substance, we are able to liberate the carbonic acid. If you take a piece of chalk and expose it to the action of any acid, you will produce a bubbling, which is the carbonic acid gas escaping. Now this gas has certain properties by which we recognize its presence anywhere; for instance, if you put a lighted match into it, it immediately extinguishes the light; if you put a little clear lime-water into a jar containing it, the water becomes turbid. Now this gas accumulates in such quantities in some waters, that they are called mineral on account of its existence: such are the waters of Carlsbad and Seltzer. Soda-water, as it is called, is an imitation of these waters. Spring-waters frequently contain from 12 to 20 cubic inches of carbonic acid gas to the gallon. It is not contained in so large a quantity in river-waters as in well-waters; for when water is exposed to the atmosphere, it flies off.

Then there is sulphuretted hydrogen gas, of which I spoke just now. It is not contained in waters ordinarily drunk. It is, however, formed under two circumstances:—First, it occurs in certain mineral springs, and here it arises apparently from the decomposition of sulphides, which exist in the rocks through which the water flows. In the next place, it exists in waters where animal and vegetable matters are allowed to remain in contact with the salts called sulphates. This is a very curious subject, and one in which many years ago I took a good deal of interest. It was asserted that sulphuretted hydrogen produced yellow fever, and that it had been found to exist in the water of the sea off the coast of Africa. The late Professor Daniell examined specimens of water brought from the delta of the Niger, and found that it contained large quantities of sulphuretted hydrogen. At that time I had been experimenting on the production of sulphuretted hydrogen by the decomposition of sulphates in contact with organic matter. My object was to account for the presence of sulphuretted hydrogen in waters, for which there was no evident origin but the sulphur of the neutral sulphates.* I found that the sulphates of all the metals which formed soluble sulphides produced sulphuretted hydrogen, and I pointed out the probability of this decomposition having occurred in Professor Daniell's specimens; thus accounting for the sulphuretted hydrogen they contained. This turned out quite correct; for neither the water of the Niger nor the sea off the coast of Africa, has been proved to contain any sulphuretted hydrogen when examined on the spot.

The water of the Thames contains a certain amount of sulphates, and these becoming decomposed, contribute to a considerable extent to produce the disgusting smell of the Thames, as well as of the ditches it overflows on its banks. If you neglect to empty the water-bottle which you employ for cleansing the mouth in the morning, especially in the summer, in London, you will find that in the course of a few days it will smell of sulphuretted hydrogen.

Waters containing sulphuretted hydrogen give rise to a peculiar growth of both plants and animals. There is a minute plant, a conferva, which flourishes only in waters containing sulphuretted hydrogen. I have observed this plant in most of the sulphureous springs of Great Britain; it is snowy-white in appearance,

* History of Askern and its Mineral Springs. By E. Lankester, M.D. London: Churchill. 1841.

and wherever sulphureous waters exist, they may be detected by the presence of this curious plant. In some stages of its growth, it assumes a beautiful pink colour, and the snow-white and pink deposits of this plant have given rise to much speculation amongst writers on these waters.

I now come to speak of the saline ingredients of waters. The most common of these matters is carbonate of lime, or common chalk. Carbonate of lime alone is insoluble in water, but it is dissolved when water contains carbonic acid. If you take a piece of chalk and put it into a bottle of soda-water, you will dissolve a certain quantity of it, and you will see that it is in this way that water may be rendered impure, or rather, may be made to take up a very considerable quantity of carbonate of lime. We have seen how waters get their carbonic acid; how waters thus charged with this gas passing over a soil containing chalk or limestone, will dissolve the carbonate of lime. It is natural for waters in chalk districts to take up as much chalk as their carbonic acid will dissolve; and, when waters are highly charged with carbonic acid, they will dissolve large quantities of carbonate of lime. Thus it is that many of our surface-wells contain as large quantities of chalk as those which come out of a chalk rock. This is always a suspicious circumstance; and when waters contain much carbonate of lime, and do not come from a chalk rock, you may depend on it there is something wrong about their antecedents.

Carbonate of lime thus dissolved in carbonic acid may be easily detected by the addition of lime-water. The lime unites with the carbonic acid, which holds the carbonate of lime in solution, and forms with it a fresh portion of carbonate of lime; and as this salt is insoluble in water, it falls down in the form of a white powder; and not only the carbonate of lime that is formed, but that which was held in solution is deposited also; and thus the water loses all its carbonate of lime. Now this is the philosophy of Dr. Clark's process for softening hard water. He adds lime to it, and the water is deprived of its hardening ingredient, the carbonate of lime. Dr. Clark's process not only renders the water much softer for washing and cooking purposes, but, whilst the carbonate of lime is falling, it entangles, as it were, the organic matters, and renders it much purer for drinking purposes. Great objections have been urged against Dr. Clark's process; but my conviction is, that all hard waters are improved by it; and, although it has been extensively employed, I am unacquainted with a single drawback to its employment.

There is another salt of lime found in water,—sulphate of lime. This may be easily detected by nitrate of baryta. The sulphuric acid unites with the baryta and forms an insoluble precipitate. Wherever there is any considerable quantity of sulphate of lime, we can easily detect it by the agency of the nitrate of baryta. Again, if we want to know whether our sulphate is of lime or not, we must add a solution of oxalic acid or oxalate of ammonia, which will throw down the lime. By these tests we may judge of the quantity of sulphuric acid approximatively; but, in order to get a knowledge of the exact quantity of these substances, we must collect the precipitates and weigh them.

Another substance of some importance in water is the chloride of sodium, or common salt, which can only be accounted for in our surface-well waters by the fact of the salt being constantly used by man in cooking, &c., and thus passing into the drains and sewers, is washed into the wells. When we find this substance in waters, we should be careful of using them dietetically. The best test for chloride of sodium is nitrate of silver. It throws down the chloride in the form of a chloride of silver. It is a creamy-looking precipitate, at first white, and gradually becomes bluish-black by the agency of light. It is, in fact, one of the salts used by the photographer to produce his pictures on paper.

I might continue these illustrations, but I hope I have shown you sufficient to indicate that a very little chemistry will enable an intelligent person to detect whether water contains large quantities of the more common impurities of water.

There is another method of extracting approximatively the quantity of saline impurities in water. If we take a quantity of water and boil it in an evaporating basin, the water will at last entirely disappear, and the inorganic matters will be left at the bottom of the vessel. By taking two or three waters, and thus treating them, we can judge, within a little, of their relative amount of impurity. We may judge also to some extent, by this test, of the quantity of organic matters present in water; for, according as these are present, will the precipitate be of a dark and dirty colour.

You must not suppose, however, that the saline impurities I have mentioned are all that are to be found

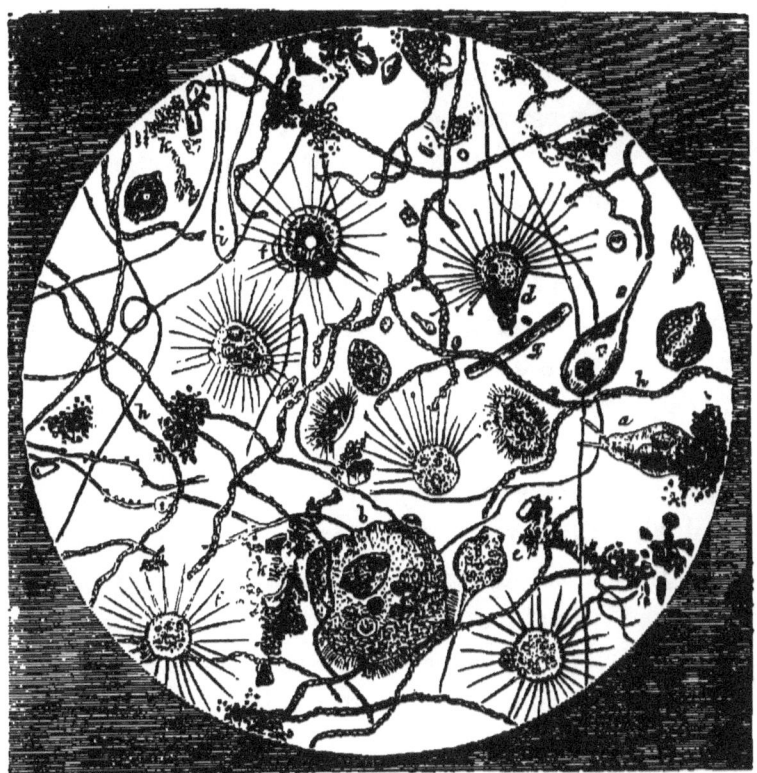

Fig. 4.—*From Water of Well at Sandgate (on Mr. George's premises).*

a. *Rotifer.*
b. *Bursaria?*
c. *Paramæcium.*
d. *Acineta tuberosa?*
e. *Vorticella.*
f. *Actinophrys Sol.*
g. *Filament of Conferva.*
h. *Stems of Anthophysa?*
i. *Slender Fungus.*
k. *Earthy and Organic matter.*

in water. There is chloride of calcium, which sometimes occurs in such large quantities as to produce very disastrous results on the system. Iron frequently occurs in such quantities as to flavour the water which contains it, and when taken in large quantities, it seems to act injuriously on the system. Nitrates occur as the result of the decomposition of animal and vegetable matter, and sometimes in sufficient quantities to act in a depressing manner on the system. The soluble phosphates have also all been found in surface-wells, and evidently come from decaying animals or animal refuse of one kind or another.

I now come to speak more particularly of the organic constituents of water. These are of two kinds—*living* and *dead*. The living are sometimes contained in water in very large quantities. I do not know that the living things are so objectionable as the dead. I believe it to be a much more healthy practice to swallow oysters while alive than to wait until they are nearly putrid; and that is just the difference between swallowing living and dead animal matter in water. There are two sorts of living things in water—plants and animals. I have before drawn your attention to the forms of plants and animals in Thames water. Fig. 4 is a drawing of the living organic constituents of a well-water that was known to have produced disease; and Fig. 5 is another drawing of the living creatures which inhabit sewer-water. Of course, these things are all microscopic.

Although fish, snails, and shrimps live in water, I need not warn you against these, as everybody can avoid them if he choose. Now, if you look at the contents of the two last waters I have mentioned, you will find amongst the plant-like bodies certain filamentous bits, which are really half-developed forms of some low fungus. I do not know if these are themselves poisonous, but I do know that when present they indicate that a water is dangerous. In 1854 I was requested by the Vestry of the Parish of St. James, Westminster, to examine the water from the pump in

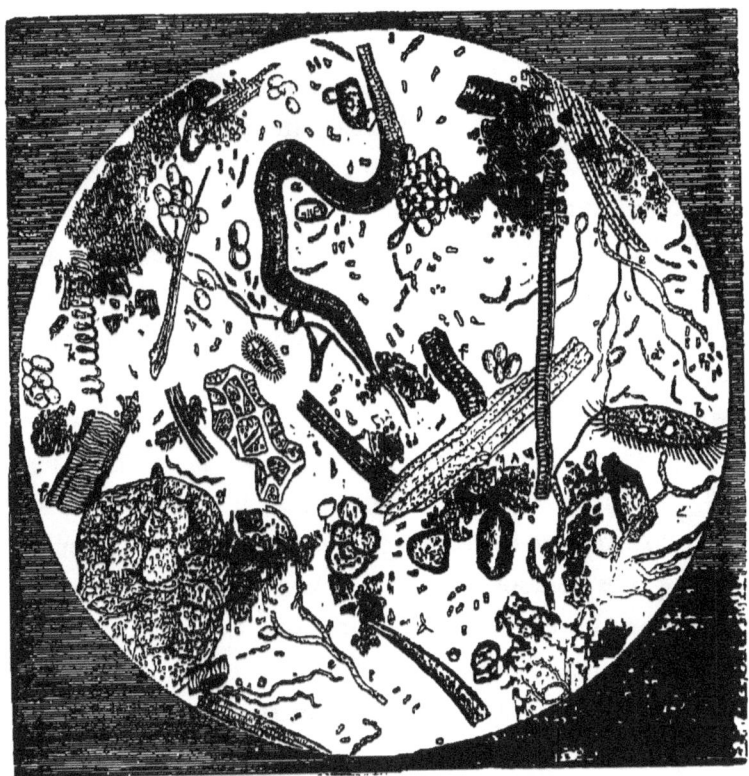

Fig. 5.—*Sewer Water (taken from the Sewer in Silver Street).*

a. *Anguillula fluviatilis.*
b. *Oxytricha.*
c. *Paramæcium.*
d. *Vibriones.*
e. *Filaments of Slender Fungus.*
f. *Fragments of Muscular Fibre.*
g. *Cells of Potato.*
h. *Starch granules of Wheat.*
i. *Hairs and integuments of Wheat.*
k. *Spiral Vessels.*
l. *Dead and Decaying Organic matter, as dotted ducts, hair of animal, grit, and débris.*

Broad Street, Golden Square. The cholera had broken out there, and killed five hundred people in less than a week, and the late Dr. Snow had accused the pump of doing all this mischief. Now I detected nothing remarkable in that water but the filaments of a fungus.

(Fig. 6). It was a very curious fungus, and interested me so much, that I published an account of it.* Its discovery in the water led to an investigation of the condition of the well, and then it was discovered that the well had for some time been in communication with the cesspool of an adjoining house, and subject to periodical overflows of its contents. I have since seen these flocculent fungi in impure water, and you will easily recognize them in the organic contents of the well-water and sewer-water in the illustrations (*h*, Fig. 4; *e*, Fig. 5). These fungi-form filaments are accompanied with sombre, ugly-looking animalcules, which are seldom found in pure water (*b*, Fig. 5). There is also an ill-favoured-looking little worm, much smaller than a thread-worm, and belonging to the same family of animals, which constantly presents itself in impure waters (*a*, Fig. 5). These things live in water containing decomposing animal and vegetable matter; and it is this matter which is injurious. So that, although the living creatures themselves are not injurious, the water they live in is.

With regard to the dead organic matter, which, by its existence and decomposition, gives life to the living structures, it is of two kinds. Either it is in the form of disintegrated, insoluble matters, or it is dissolved in the water. The first you can discover by the aid of the microscope. Thus, if you look again at the drawing of the contents of sewer-water, you will find portions of dead plants and animals. In Fig. 5 you have a fibre from the muscle of some animal, and there

---

* Quarterly Journal of Microscopical Science, vol. iv.

are other odds and ends of organic matters there. These organic matters, when fresh, are not injurious, nor are they injurious when they are entirely decomposed and have entered into new compounds; but it is while in a

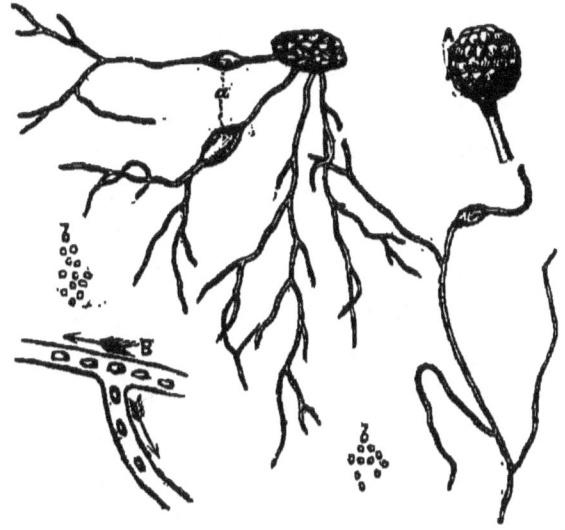

Fig. 6.—Mycellium of Fungus.
a. *Enlargements seen on larger branches.* A. *Spore-case of same fungus.*
B. *Moving particles passing through the branches.* b. *Moving particles.*

state of change that they act injuriously. They act as ferments, and communicate the state they are in to other bodies with which they come in contact. A curious instance of this tendency of organic matter in water to act as a ferment was related to me by Dr. Dauglish, the patentee of the new process for making aërated bread. This bread is made without fermentation, and for the purpose of preventing some of the bad effects of fermentation on bread; but, during the last summer, it was found that this bread underwent a change similar to that of fermented bread. Dr. Dauglish suspected it might be owing to the organic matter from the Thames water supplied to the bakery, and had his suspicions confirmed by the fact, that when the water was boiled and filtered before it was used for making the bread, no unusual change was observed. The existence of these organic matters can be best tested by the aid of the microscope.

But organic matters may be dissolved in water, and then they cannot be found by the microscope. The chemist estimates these by the quantity of nitrogen which he obtains from the deposit of water which has been evaporated; but it is very difficult to estimate this form of impurity. I have found the permanganates of potash and soda a very good rough test for ascertaining the presence of this dissolved matter. Permanganic acid and the permanganates contain large quantities of oxygen; and, when they are brought in contact with organic matters, they lose their oxygen and become changed in colour. If you take permanganate of soda, which is sold in the shops under the name of Condy's Disinfecting Fluid, and put it into pure water, it produces first a deep violet, and afterwards a beautiful permanent red colour. If the water, however, contains organic matters, the red colour soon disappears, and, in proportion to the quantity of organic matter, will be its decolorizing agency. Now if you take a series of waters of different degrees of impurity, you will find that the water which has least impurity retains the most colour. I have tried this in so many instances with a perfectly successful result, that I can confidently recommend it as a test for ascertaining the relative quantities of impurity in water. The same test has been applied by Dr. Angus

Smith for ascertaining the organic impurity of the atmosphere; and by this means he has arrived at some very interesting results. It should, however, be recollected that many other impurities besides those of organic origin may exist in the atmosphere and act upon the permanganate. This is the case, for instance, with sulphurous acid, which is constantly present in an atmosphere where coal and coal-gas are burned.

Before leaving the subject of organic impurities, I would call your attention to the fact that it appears to be through their agency that water acts on lead. You know it is a common practice to store water in leaden cisterns, to serve it in leaden pipes; and in this way the water acts upon the lead, and deposits certain quantities of it; and those who drink it suffer as the result. The theory of this action, according to Dr. Medlock, is that the nitrogen of the organic matter becomes oxidized, and converted into nitrous acid, which attacking the lead, forms a nitrite of lead. This is decomposed, and, by yielding up its oxide of lead to carbonic acid, forms an insoluble carbonate of lead, leaving the nitrous acid free to act on further portions of lead. Whether this theory be the true one or not, I will not undertake to say, but it certainly does explain the somewhat anomalous cases of the action of water on lead. Thus water containing small quantities of carbonates—from ten to twenty grains in the gallon, will not act on lead, although they contain organic matter. This is the case with Thames water. Distilled water, that is water once distilled, will act on lead: this arises from the fact that it mostly contains organic matter. I was surprised to find, when first using the permanganate test, that it was always decolorized by distilled water. But if you re-distil water with hydrated potash, and then expose it to the action of lead, you will find that it will take up no lead. At Manchester and Liverpool, the inhabitants are supplied with water remarkable for its freedom from saline impurities; but it has organic matter enough to act on lead. In a recent visit to these cities I had the opportunity of ascertaining this fact in the laboratory of Dr. Edwards, of Liverpool, and Dr. Crace Calvert, of Manchester. The fact is, such is the tendency of water to act on lead, and so deleterious are the effects of this agent on the system, that I have no hesitation in recommending the entire abolition of lead in the manufacture of cisterns and pipes for the service of water for the drinking-supply of towns.*

There are many other important relations of water to man to which I could not even incidentally advert: I have endeavoured to direct your attention to it from a dietetical point of view; but I trust you will have seen how deep an interest every community has in understanding the physical and chemical properties of a substance on which not only our material progress and manufacturing greatness, but our comfort, health, and very existence depend.

* In preference to lead pipes, I can unhesitatingly recommend the lead-incased block-tin pipes, which cannot be acted upon by any kind of water.

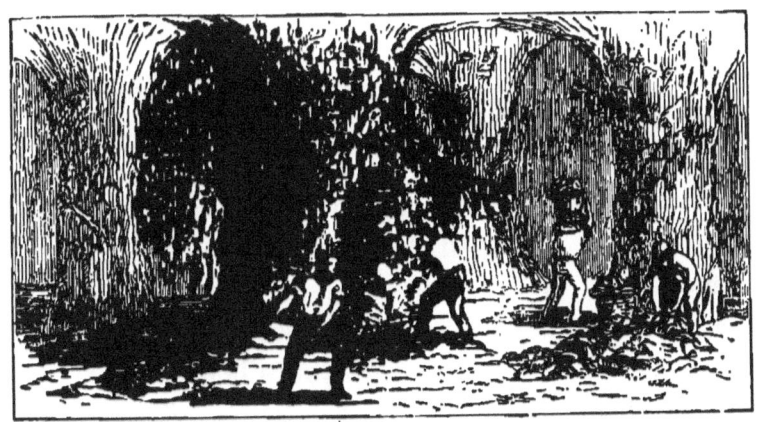

Fig. 1.—*Salt Mine.*

ON SALT AND MINERAL FOOD.

In this lecture I wish to bring before you what I have called the mineral substances of food; and sometimes these substances are called mineral food.

The table of constituents of food indicates these mineral matters of our food, and to which people, generally speaking, attach very little importance. Persons who prepare our food—cooks in the kitchen, ladies who superintend cooks, and order dinners for large families, and people who consume food from day to day, never think of asking whether food contains the right proportions of these ingredients to secure health. Yet, without these, babies get rickets, young ladies acquire crooked spines, fathers get gouty, and mothers have palpitations; and they do not, however, think of ascribing these things to the food which has deprived them of the proper constituents of their blood. I think I can show you that this subject is a matter of great importance. I will call your attention to the table again. You will find there the mineral matters marked in by little cross lines, so that you see in cheese there are 3 lbs. in the hundred; and so, if you cast your eye down the table, you will see they are in small quantities in different substances. Now let me call attention to the flesh-forming and heat or force forming materials of our food. If you give flesh-forming materials, as caseine alone, to a dog, he will die. Then take butter, which is a heat-giving material. If you feed a dog on that he will die, as though you gave him nothing. Then let us take cooked meat, with nitrogenous and fatty matter, 35 lbs. in the hundred, squeeze out of it the mineral matter, and give it to the dog, and he still dies. No matter, you may mix the caseine, and fat, and starch, and sugar, and yet the dog dies unless you give him the mineral substances about which I wish to speak more particularly in this lecture. I believe it can be proved that those who have acted upon the supposition that the flesh-forming and heat-giving materials were the only things necessary for them, and have neglected attending to these mineral constituents, have suffered in their health. Hence I have put them prominently forward, and I shall endeavour to-day to show you where you can get them, and avoid the danger of neglecting them altogether.

Now let me draw your attention to the composition of the human body. Suppose we taken a human being weighing 154 lbs., and submit him to analysis, we should find that we should obtain 111 lbs. of water; and the next thing that would come off would be carbonic acid gas, and then there would be ammonia and sulphuretted hydrogen, and phosphoretted hydrogen, and gases of that sort: at last we should get a quantity of ashes. Now, in the water, we have oxygen and hydrogen; and in the carbonic acid gas, carbon and oxygen; and in the ammonia, nitrogen and hydrogen. In the ashes which are left, you get a variety of mineral substances,—salts, as they are called. We get phosphate of lime, carbonate of lime, fluoride of calcium, chloride of sodium, chloride of potassium, sulphate of soda, carbonate of soda, phosphate of soda, sulphate of potash, peroxide of iron, phosphate of potash, phosphate of magnesia, and silica. These are the things about which I shall have to talk to you to-day—these ashes which are left, and without which we cannot live. Now if you will persist in having only refined sugar, and the whitest flour, rejecting the bran; if you will persist in rejecting the salt, and avoiding the liquor that meat is boiled in, you may get albumen and fibrine, but none of these other substances; and then the first attack of fever or cold may prove fatal. Four men shall be travelling outside an omnibus,—one may get acute inflammation of the lungs, another bronchitis, and the other two shall come off free. Was it the riding outside of the omnibus that caused the two to fall ill? No, it was the state of their blood. They had lived somehow irregularly; somehow their bodies had been deprived of their proper constituents. So you may find half a dozen children, all exposed to the contagion of scarlet fever;—two take it; one dies, and the other four are free: but the two that have caught it have lived in such a way that their blood has readily taken in the contagion; and the one that has died has got into a condition which has produced death. Hence the importance of attending to these subjects thoroughly; not getting a little knowledge of them, but a knowledge of what is necessary to the feeding of children and the feeding of men. If we do not attend to these things, we shall, somehow or other, suffer.

Now I shall take up these constituents as I have mentioned them, and which is very much according to their importance. You cannot expect me to go into an exhaustive chemical analysis of this subject, and I may just say that chemical science is not in a condition to do so. Neither the chemist nor the physiologist has gone into the phenomena of the action of these substances in our system.

The first substance I shall take up is chloride of sodium, common salt. This is the only substance which we take directly from the mineral kingdom. All the other salts we get through plants or animals. But salt is a substance which we take direct from nature, and thus we satisfy the cravings of our system for this substance. Now this salt is composed of two elements—of chlorine, a gas, and of sodium, a metal. Chlorine is a most suffocating and even dangerous gas to experiment with. Sodium is a metal so easily oxidised in the air, that we are obliged to keep it in naphtha, and when we throw it into warm water it takes fire just as potassium does. Now we may well wonder that these two substances, so energetic and even dangerous when separated, should be so benignant and beneficial when united. Chlorine is not only a suffocating gas, but, like oxygen, it is a supporter of combustion, and has very powerful affinities. It can be easily separated from common salt by mixing it with peroxide of manganese, and pouring on them a little sulphuric acid. The greenish fumes that arise are chlorine. On account of its energetic chemical action it is used as a disinfectant, a deodoriser, and a bleaching agent. It is used by the paper maker and the calico-printer for the purposes of bleaching. It acts upon colouring matter by decomposing it and uniting with the hydrogen it contains, forming hydrochloric acid. In this way it acts as a deodoriser. Most of the disagreeable smells given off by decaying animal and vegetable matter depend on compounds of hydrogen, and the chlorine, uniting with this substance, destroys them. This is the substance, then, which, combining with sodium, forms common salt.

Salt determines the life and forms of both plants and animals in the ocean. Withdraw the salt from the ocean, and you will have none of the life which now exists there. Herrings, mackerel, codfish, and all the forms of fish that we get out of the sea, would retire, and we should have in their stead the fish of our rivers, such as roach, carp, dace, and bream. Instead of the seaweeds, we should have the plants of our fresh waters, the valsineria, the potamogetons, the anacharis, and the water-lilies. In this you will see how this salt influences life and the forms of life. We get it for our own use from the sea, and from those deposits of salt which the sea has left in the bowels of the earth. When obtained from the sea, the sea water is evaporated, and contains from 16 to 1,800 grains of salt to the gallon of water. But the sea in former times has formed bays, and those bays have been gradually silted up, and the sea has retired from the bay, and the bay now becomes a lake, and this lake is a salt lake. We have many such salt lakes; they are numerous in the Crimea. The Dead Sea is a great salt lake. You will see by this diagram how these changes take place.

If the lake thus cut off from the sea receives but little fresh water from rain or rivers, the water will go on evaporating till the lake becomes excessively salt; and this is the case with many salt lakes. It is especially the case with the Dead Sea, where the water is so dense from the salt it contains, that it is said a human body will not sink in it. Such lakes eventually get dried up, leaving the salt at the bottom, which gets covered up by some insoluble material; the whole goes again under the sea, and, rising as dry ground, we dig into the earth and find the lake has become a salt-mine. Such mines are found in the new red sandstone of Cheshire, on the continent of Europe, and other parts of the world. The salt obtained in these districts is frequently in a state of solution, and is pumped from wells which are called "Brine Springs."

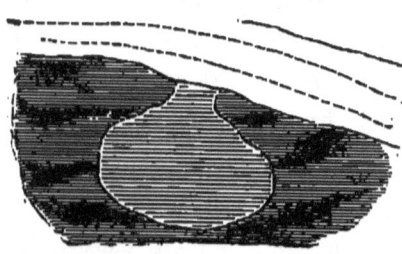

Fig. 2.
The sea. Lake formed from bay.

Now, not only do animals that live in the sea require salt, but we find that all animals require it. We find, for instance, in the great salt lakes and salt bogs of Kentucky, that there is a certain district there which is salt, called the Big Bone Lick, from the existence in it of the bones of gigantic animals who have died there. These animals, that lived in America before man, were attracted by the salt, and in seeking it there have perished in the swamp, and left their great bones behind them. Now, not only do these large animals require salt, but man requires it. It is so necessary to him, that to tax his salt is one of the surest sources of income to a government. A part of the British revenue in India is still raised on salt.

Now, the question comes as to how this salt acts upon the system? The quantities of the various saline matters entering into the composition of a human body weighing eleven stone, I have calculated is as follows:—

	lbs.	oz.	grs.
1. *Phosphate of Lime*, forming the principal part of the earthy matter of the bones	5	13	0
2. *Carbonate of Lime* also entering into the composition of bone	1	0	0
3. *Fluoride of Calcium*, found in the bones	0	3	0
4. *Chloride of Sodium*, common salt	0	3	376
5. *Sulphate of Soda*	0	1	170
6. *Carbonate of Soda*	0	1	72
7. *Phosphate of Soda*	0	0	400
8. *Sulphate of Potash*	0	0	400
9. *Peroxide of Iron*	0	0	150
10. *Chloride of Potassium*	0	0	12
11. *Phosphate of Potash*	0	0	100
12. *Phosphate of Magnesia*	0	0	75
13. *Silica*	0	0	3

The quantity of salt contained is not much, but still it is more than any other mineral constituent of the human body, except phosphate and carbonate of lime. When we take these away, we have only left about ten ounces more of these ashes, or mineral matters, and of these ten ounces, the chloride of sodium, or salt, is three ounces and three quarters. Now the question is, where this salt exists. If you take the muscles or the nerves of animals, you do not find that they contain salt; but if you take the blood of animals, you will find that it contains salt. I do not wish to produce upon your minds any disagreeable reflection, but those of you who have tasted your own blood, must recollect that it tastes salt, and we find three drachms of salt in a gallon of human blood, and that is the quantity nearly in all animals. It is not found in the muscles, in the nerves, or in the bones, or other tissues, but it exists only in the blood. You can easily prove this by taking a little blood, allowing the red particles to coagulate, and then placing a few drops on a piece of glass. If you hold this over the flame of a spirit lamp, so as to evaporate the water, you will have a number of crystalline bodies formed, amongst which the crystals of salt will be most prominent.

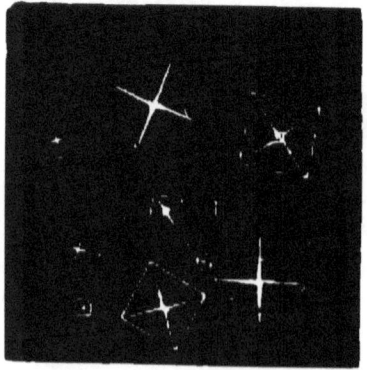

Fig. 3.—*Crystals of Salt.*

Now, it may be asked, of what good is the salt? You may be sure that it does good. There are some people who are foolish enough to believe that man has been wrong in all ages, and that salt has done harm. A medical man wrote a book to show that salt was the forbidden fruit that was eaten in the garden of Eden. He died not very long ago, and as I understand, a victim to his folly. There are some people who have no hesitation in rejecting the practices of their fellow-creatures—there are some who insist upon living upon vegetables—and I saw a book the other day, written by a person who said he never knew what health was until he lived entirely on animal diet.

Let us, then, inquire a little into the probable uses of salt in our system.

If we take a vessel, and divide it into two parts by an animal membrane such as exists in our own body, and then put salt and water on one side, and spring water on the other side, so that they may both stand at the same level, in the course of time we shall find that the spring water will go down, and the salt water will rise up and flow over.

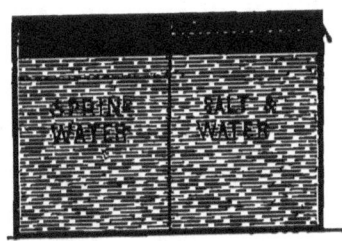

Fig. 4.

The pure water in fact passes through the membrane, but the salt water will not. Now, this is precisely the relation of the blood to the membranes of the stomach. It is a solution of salt; and if we place in our stomachs pure water, it will pass through the membranes of the stomach just in the same way that it passes through the membrane in the vessel. This, then, appears to be one of the important functions performed by salt. It facilitates the absorption of water into the system. This will also account for the thirst produced by taking excessive quantities of salt, or salted food of any kind.

Another action of salt to which some physiologists have attached importance is, that it supplies to the system a certain quantity of chlorine which is necessary to the perfection of some of the vital processes. Thus during digestion a fluid is thrown out from the stomach, called gastric juice. This fluid contains free hydrochloric acid, and the chlorine of this compound could be only furnished by the salt taken with the food.

Then salt appears to facilitate certain changes in the system which are beneficial to health, which are difficult to explain exactly. The nature of these changes is indicated by such an experiment as the following: A number of oxen were taken by a great French chemist and experimentalist; he fed one set of them with salt, and another set of the same weight without salt. For a short time there appeared no difference; but at the end of a month the cattle that had the salt were sleek and well favoured, while the others had rough coats, and looked less comfortable, and so it went on for two years; and at the end of that time there was no doubt that the healthier animals were those which had the salt. There seemed to be some improvement in the quality of the blood going on by the action of the salt. The practice of placing pieces of rock-salt in meadows for horses, cows, and sheep to lick, is quite common in this country. It is also well known that marshes which have been overflowed by salt water give an improved appearance to the stock which grazes on them.

If you take a very small quantity of hydrochloric acid and salt and put it into water, and then add to it a portion of the white of egg, and expose it to a temperature of 98°, the egg begins to dissolve; but if you put it into water without the salt it does not dissolve. From this experiment, you see there is this first action of salt in assisting digestion; you may see from this the propriety of adding small quantities of salt to our food. There are some persons who, from a morbid fancy, will not take it; such persons are preserved from danger by the cook, who puts it into puddings and cooked meats, and the baker, who puts it into the bread.

Such, in fact, appears to be the importance of salt in the blood, that a special provision actually exists, for maintaining, within certain limits, of course, the quantity of salt at a given point. For we find that if we feed our animals either on food containing a large quantity or only a small quantity of salt, that the quantity of salt in the blood remains the same, any excess being thrown off from the system. Of course, a long-continued abstinence from salt in food will lead to a diminution in the blood and ultimately to disease.

The history of the use of salt is interesting. The Jews used it in their sacrifices. The Arabs put it on the table as a mark of hospitality. The Abyssinian gentleman carries a piece in his pocket, and takes it out and offers it to a friend to lick as a mark of respect and esteem, which is a process you may not approve. Then the Hindoos swear by their salt, and many of you may recollect that during the late war in Hindostan, the sepoy was reminded of his having sworn by his salt to serve the queen of England. Then, again, it was formerly a mark of distinction in England. In olden times, persons who sat above the salt were higher in dignity than those who sat below it.

Besides being an article of our diet, salt is interesting to us on account of its power of preserving both animal and vegetable food from decomposition. We salt beef, pork, herrings, and other animals, also beans, peas, and various articles of vegetable food, which we are enabled to keep for a great length of time by its agency. It should, however, be recollected in these cases that the salt takes the place of other mineral matters which exist in the fresh food, and which we ought to know the system cannot be deprived of for any length of time without the risk of danger.

The next thing of which I will speak, is the phosphate of lime, which forms the principal part of the earthy matter of the bones. Of this I calculate, that there are 5 lb. 13 oz. in a human being weighing eleven stone. It is a crystalline body, and assumes the appearance of Fig. 5 under the microscope. Now this phosphate of lime must be a very important thing, or it would not occur in such large quantities. I draw your attention to it in the first place, as constituting the earthy matter of bone. If we suppose that there are

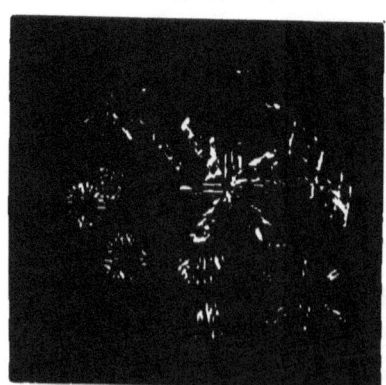

Fig. 5.—*Phosphate of Lime.*

5 lb. 13 oz. in the system, at least 4½ or 5 lbs. of that will be contained in the skeleton, in the solid part of the bones of the human body. I shall have occasion again to refer to the composition of bone; but bone contains about 40 per cent. of gelatine, 50 per cent. of phosphate of lime, and 9 per cent. of chalk or carbonate of lime, and 1 per cent. of fluoride of calcium, which is also known as Derbyshire Spar and Blue John. Now, phosphate of lime is so called from being composed of phosphoric acid and calcium. Calcium is a metal, which lies at the base of lime; calcium and oxygen form lime. If you take a piece of chalk and burn it, you know carbonic acid gas is driven off, and quick lime is left. This oxide of calcium combines with phosphoric acid in order to form phosphate of lime. We get phosphorus for chemical purposes from bones.* Phosphorus is a very interesting substance on account of its highly inflammable nature. We make lucifer matches from phosphorus. These matches would not take fire but for the presence of a little phosphorus in the matter at the end. If you take a piece of phosphorus and place it on a plate, and bring a lighted match near it, you will see how rapidly it takes fire. The phosphorus combines with the oxygen of the air, and beautiful white fumes of phosphoric acid are the result. It is strange to see these elements, so terrible when out of our body, all converted to our use when in the body.

Now, I should give you a very wrong idea of the importance of this phosphate of lime, and especially of

---

* See Lecture on Bone, in the Course on the Uses of Animals.

this phosphoric acid which is contained in it, if I left you to suppose that the only important thing was its existence in relation to the lime in the bones; for the fact is, we find phosphoric acid in the blood, in the liver, and in the lungs, in a free condition. It is introduced into the system as phosphate of lime; and, perhaps, as phosphate of soda, or phosphate of potash. At any rate, from whatever source it comes, during the changes that go on in the system, we find phosphoric acid playing a very active part. Now, that is an important thing to recollect, because we may be taking a diet which excludes the phosphate, or taking a diet in which it abounds. If we have it in too large a quantity, we are sure to suffer. No sort of medicine that I know of will in any way correct this; and if you are not taking a food which will supply the phosphate of lime, no kind of medicine that I know of will supply its absence.

Now, how do we get these phosphates? I have shown you that phosphate of lime is the most important, but there are phosphates generally in the system. We find not only phosphate of lime, but we find phosphate of soda, phosphate of potash, and even phosphate of magnesia in the system; and thus, you see, there are other phosphates besides the phosphate of lime. How do we get them? There are two sources of phosphates in our food. The first great source is the cereal plants, and the second is animal food. When I say cereal plants, I mean all those which belong to the natural family of grasses eaten by man. Wheat is the most important to us; but barley, oats, rye, rice, maize, all contain phosphates. Animals, you know, eat grasses of various kinds, and from this source they obtain their phosphates, and when we eat the blood, the nerves, and the muscles of animals, we get our phosphates at second-hand, as it were. It is with wheaten bread and flour that we get the largest quantity. A very interesting question has arisen out of our recent knowledge of these facts, and that is, What is the cheapest way of supplying these phosphates to the human body? The food which contains them in the largest quantity is the cereal grasses, but these grasses must get the phosphates before they can supply them to us. Now, it was long ago pointed out, by the great German chemist, Liebig, that one of the great drawbacks on the growth of wheat, and other grain crops, was the want of phosphates in the soil; and that one of the great hindrances to the development of animals, and of man, was the want of phosphates in the food which they take. He also pointed out that we might supply this phosphate of lime, not merely by the agency of animal and vegetable manure, but by the means of what are called "artificial manures." Amongst the sources of phosphate of lime, as bones, he pointed out that the so-called "coprolites," the petrified dung of the extinct Saurian reptiles of the Liassic period was capable of supplying enormous quantities of this material. The experiment was tried and found to answer, and now these remains of former generations of animals are not only obtained from the Lias, but from the Wealden, the Green Sand of Cambridgeshire, and the Red Crag of Suffolk, and are used as manures. The phosphate itself is insoluble, but if we pour sulphuric acid on it we render it soluble, and fit it to become the food of plants. These facts becoming known, have led to further researches, and to further discoveries of this phosphate of lime. It exists in a mineral which is called Apatite, and this is now obtained in large quantities from Sweden, and various other parts of the world, for the purpose of being converted into superphosphate, which is manufactured in the same way from the apatite as from the coprolite, and the superphosphate is now generally sold as a manure. Thus, you see, this phosphate of lime is supplied artificially to the plant, and from the plant we receive it into the system. There is one question which I will just mention here, which is of some practical importance. In nature we have no superphosphate manufactory. There is no Mr. Laws, our great superphosphate manufacturer, to supply sulphuric acid to the phosphates in the forests of Brazils and the backwoods of America. How is it, then, that plants in nature get a supply of phosphate of lime, if this substance is insoluble? The explanation will give you an idea how it is that certain substances, which as well as phosphate of lime are insoluble in pure water, get into our systems. I told you in my last lecture that carbonate of lime is soluble in carbonic acid gas and water, and so is phosphate of lime, and when the water comes down upon the earth which contains this phosphate it is charged with carbonic acid and the phosphate is dissolved, and then the plant can take it up. In the same way, if we take carbonic acid gas into our stomach, or mix it with our food, the solution of the phosphate is facilitated. This is probably the reason that we prefer water with carbonic acid gas in it, and why we consume those waters which imitate the natural waters of Seltzer—as soda water and water acidulated in gazogenes. It may be, too, that this constitutes the ground of the preference given to bottled beer, which contains a considerable quantity of carbonic acid gas, and champagne also, which owes its sparkling qualities to the carbonic acid gas it contains.

Before I leave this subject, let me call your attention to an interesting feature in the history of this phosphate of lime. Liebig has shown that it is highly probable that one of the causes that led to the destruction of the great cities of antiquity was the difficulty of obtaining a supply of food for their inhabitants. As they went on increasing, the soils in the immediate vicinity became exhausted of the phosphate, and, at last, refused to grow food at all. As the means of transit were not so perfect as they are now, men found it easier to go to places where the virgin soil produced abundance of food, than to bring the food to their cities. Hence the migrations of peoples, and the desolation of once busy cities. In America this process is going on every day. When a district is exhausted of its mineral food, the farmer finds it easier to transport his whole family and possessions to the backwoods, where there is a virgin soil, than to send to a distance for his manures to fertilise his land. It has been, then, a most providential event for Europe the discovery of these artificial manures, for we have been consuming our own food, the phosphates of our soil; and instead of returning them to the land, throwing them into the sea. But even these artificial sources may fail, and then, unless we have learned the art of recovering the phosphates we have used for our life, it will be our turn to share the fate of the cities of antiquity, and men will point to the ruins of our cities, as we now do to those of Babylon, and Tyre, and Sidon.

I now come to speak of the salts of potash, which, although small in quantity, appear to be very important. The basis of these salts is the metal potassium. Although a metal, it is so light that it floats on water, and it has so strong an affinity for oxygen, that it combines with it, giving out heat and light even when placed on water. It is on this account that we are obliged to keep it in naphtha. It is a beautiful experiment to put the potassium on water; it inflames and runs about the water, and at the same time the hydrogen gas is given off in an inflammable state from the water. Now this substance is at the base of what we call common potash. Just as we find sodium in plants that grow in the sea, we find potassium in plants that grow away from the sea. Land-plants contain large quantities of potash, hence its name, from the fact that wood which is used for boiling the pot leaves these ashes, and hence they are called pot-ashes. The potash, or oxide of potassium, in these ashes is combined with carbonic acid; for, during the burning of the wood, its carbon combines with the oxygen of the air, and thus the carbonic acid is formed which unites with the potash. If you pour sulphuric acid on the potashes of the shops, you will expel the carbonic acid and procure a sulphate of potash. So you see the carbonate of potash is not found in the plants any more than carbonate of soda in sea-weed; it is formed by combustion.

There are some plants which are called potash plants, and I call your attention to them, because I do not know a more practical point than that certain plants evidently contain potash, and that the exclusion of these from diet is a very bad thing. Potatoes, for instance, contain potash. Now I do not know whether any of you have speculated upon the reason why Europe should have seized with such avidity upon that plant which is foreign to its shores; but there are philosophical writers who trace the cessation of plague and other epidemic visitations to the use of the potato. When we come to compare the potato with wheat and the cereal grains, we find it contains not so much starch as rice, or wheat, or barley, and very little nutritive matter. It seems then, looking at it from this point of view, as if it was a matter of very little importance whether we eat potatoes or not, as long as we got flesh-forming and heat-giving substances from other sources; but here are these ashes, one pound in a hundred pounds, and what are they principally? Why, salts of potash. It is not much to be sure—about a drachm in the pound—but that quantity seems in some measure explanatory of its influence on the health of the populations of Europe.

The salts of potash are found in other vegetables, as asparagus, radishes, turnips, carrots, and parsnips. Those who exclude these things from their diet are running the hazard of injuring themselves. It is even best not to throw away the water in which these things are boiled. Soups should be made of the water, and people should be encouraged to take them. Watercresses, lettuce, chicory, endive, and such plants, contain potash, and may be eaten with advantage as salads; and when they cannot be got fresh, they may be dried and used in soups. My friend Dr. Noad, at my suggestion, made several analyses of the water in which vegetables were boiled, and he found that the water, after boiling 1 lb. of potatoes, contained 17 grains of carbonate of potash, and the water in which cabbages were boiled contained 21 grains of sulphate of potash; and he found the same salt in the water in which carrots were boiled; and if he had gone through the whole range of these potash-plants, I believe he would have found undoubted evidence of the existence of the salts of potash. I do not, however, think that by taking the potash in its crystallized or dissolved form that it would act so favourably. I therefore would not advise you to substitute carbonate of potash from the doctor's shop, for the potatoes, cabbages, watercresses, and those things. I believe that sometimes, medicinally, potash may save a man's life. Now let us inquire how it is probable the potash acts.

If you put it in contact with certain substances, and expose them to the air, they will be oxidized. If, for instance, you bring potash in contact with tannic acid and expose it to the air, the tannic acid will be oxidized, which it would not be if the potash had not been present. That would appear to be one of the ways in which potash acts in the system. It assists the oxidating processes that are always going on there.

Then if you give men food containing chloride of sodium, to the exclusion of the salts of potash, you generate a disease which more than decimated the navies of Europe up to the end of the last century.

This disease is scurvy. That disease broke out with great intensity during the potato famine, and although the people were supplied with rice and other things, the disease went on,—thus showing that the potash arrests certain changes that go on in the body, and without which the blood is broken up, the bones become soft, and men can hardly use their muscles, or exercise their brains.

It was about the year 1780 that Sir Gilbert Blane discovered that lemon juice would cure scurvy, and not only cure it, but, if taken daily, would prevent scurvy on board ship. Since that time no ship goes out for a long voyage without lemon juice or lime juice on board. You all heard the sad story of the *Tasmania* transport-ship the other day, that brought our Indian heroes home half-starved and scorbutic. The worst part of that story was, that the lime juice was not lime juice at all, but sulphuric acid and water. It is not the acidity that is wanted, but it is the combination of an organic acid with potash that is required. We are indebted to my friend Dr. Garrod for having pointed out this relation of scurvy to potash. Practically, it is of very great importance to know that, unless men are fed with fresh vegetable diet, that contains potash salts, or with lemon or lime juice, they get scurvy.

Bread contains phosphate of lime and less potash, than the potato, and bread alone will produce scurvy. Now-a-days potatoes, cabbages, turnips, and carrots are pressed into a small space, and can be carried about everywhere with their potash in them, and wherever scurvy arises there must have been gross ignorance of the facts which I have brought before you.

I come now to the carbonate of lime. Well, this is an important thing,—not so important, perhaps, as the other two; but when I tell you that we have got 1 lb. of it in 154 lbs., you will see that there is quite a sufficient quantity to make it of importance, and I could not say that phosphate of lime would make up for carbonate of lime. The higher animals require phosphate of lime, the lower animals require carbonate of lime— which is chalk. This substance constitutes the chief bulk of the coral animals, and of the shells of the various forms of shell fish.* Now, we can get it from the same sources as these animals—we can get it from the water that we drink. I pointed out to you in the last lecture that nearly all the water we got from wells in London contained carbonate of lime. We may, then, get our carbonate of lime from the water we drink, but there are a number of plants which we eat that contain considerable quantities of carbonate of lime. Beans and peas contain it, and most leguminous plants, which all grow best in a chalk soil. When we take it in the form of the water which we drink, then we take it already dissolved in the carbonic acid of the water. There is, however, no doubt that carbonate of lime is deposited in the system, independent of our taking it in this form. When it

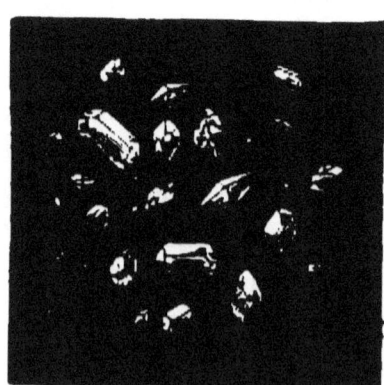

Fig. 6.—Carbonate of Lime.

* See Lecture on Bone in Course on Uses of Animals.

exists in the fluids of the body it may be easily crystallised, and then it assumes the forms at Fig. 6.

The next thing to which I call your attention is iron. It exists only in very small quantities. There is not more than 150 grains in the human body weighing 154 lbs. Iron, however, does not exist in its pure form in the blood. It is combined with oxygen, forming an oxide of iron. Although small quantities seem to be necessary to the health of our body, we meet with persons with pale faces, and bloodless lips, and pearly whites of their eyes—all indicative of the want of iron. We do not administer medicines in homœopathic quantities in this case, but we give iron, and give it in sufficient doses, and they recover their good looks, and the roses which had been lost begin to bloom again, and all from the iron getting into their blood. The French are in the habit of performing the process of incremation on their dead friends; that is to say, instead of burying them, they burn them, which is a much more wholesome process. The Romans burned their dead, and collected their ashes in an urn, which they kept as a memorial; but the Frenchmen do better than this: they would not be Frenchmen unless they could improve upon the old Roman plan. The French, after burning their friends, take the ashes and extract the iron, and convert it into a mourning ring, which they wear in memory of their dead friends. Here, then, we have a very conclusive proof that iron really exists in the human body.

There is a popular notion that iron is good for the system, and some persons, every time their beer is brought to table, thrust the red-hot poker into it.

Others go and drink from the water in which the blacksmith puts his iron, and that is not a bad thing. Others, again, sprinkle their bread and butter with iron filings at breakfast, and there is no objection to these practices if persons require iron.

The other substances are perhaps not so material. There is silica, which exists only in a very small quantity in the human body. It is distributed to the hair and the nails, but it is found more especially in the enamel of the teeth. The teeth have all of them a coating of enamel, which is formed of a certain quantity of silica, so that it seems to be necessary to the comfort and welfare of man. The silica assumes the crystalline form as seen in Fig. 7.

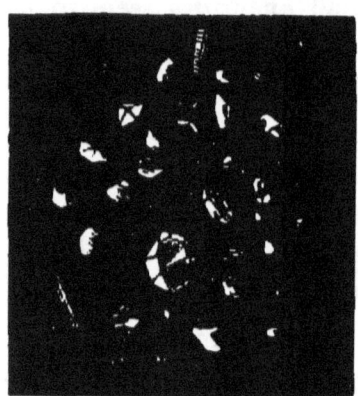

Fig. 7.—*Silica.*

In the list of substances found in the human body mention is made of magnesia. This is an earth like lime. It has for its basis a metal called magnesium. Of its properties as a medicine a good deal is known. Sulphate of magnesia is Epsom salts, but of its relation to the human body as a necessary constituent little is known. In certain diseases of the body it becomes remarkably manifest. It undoubtedly plays an important part in some of the functions of the body, and is a constituent, like the others I have previously mentioned, necessary for its welfare. It is found in the ashes of all our common edible plants in the proportion of 5 to 10 per cent., but in much smaller quantities in the human body.

I will now draw your attention to two or three constituents of the body which are probably only accidental.

Manganese exists in the soil of Scotland. It is taken up by the oat plant, and thus conveyed into the blood of the Scotch, who feed on porridge, and Scotchmen are said to have manganese in their blood.

If there is not enough iron in the blood, many of the metals will supply its place. Even mercury will supply its place for a time, and this will explain perhaps how it is that blue pill acts as a tonic. Copper has been found in human blood, but this is evidently accidental. It appears that, as we are in the habit of eating pickles, and these pickles contain copper, which is added to them to make them green and inviting to the eye, we thus introduce copper into our blood.

Then there is the beautiful substance iodine, which exists as a solid body at ordinary atmospheric temperature, but rises into the atmosphere as a gas at an increased temperature. It exists in sea water with chloride of bromine, and thus it appears that it occasionally enters into the human system, and it has been found in small quantities in the human breath, and there has been a dispute as to whether it is an essential element of the human body.

It has been recently asserted that this iodine exists in the bodies of Frenchmen, but not in the bodies of the Genevese, and it has been supposed that this accounts for the fact that the Genevese have *goitre*, whilst the French do not have it. This swelling of the glands in the neck is frequently cured by iodine, and it is supposed that the presence of a certain quantity in the system prevents its occurrence. This disease is common among the Swiss Alps and the Pyrenees. Iodine has also been found in watercresses, especially those watercresses which grow near the sea. I have, however, recently examined watercresses sold in London, but have not been able to detect iodine.

Before concluding, I should wish to enforce a practical point or two to which I have before alluded. I have shown you that in cooking, especially in boiling food, you are very likely to get rid of some of these mineral constituents of your food. In cooking, therefore, care should be taken not to throw away the water in which animal and vegetable food has been cooked. Of course, I must leave it to each individual cook to carry out this suggestion in his own particular way. But it is even possible for cooking so to change the constituents of our food, that they may not convey to the system the elements in those forms in which they are most fitted for the nutrition of our bodies. Under these circumstances, it appears to me a practice in accordance with sound theory as well as experience, for persons to eat certain quantities of uncooked food every day. I do not say uncooked meat, although the universal practice of eating live oysters, and the occasional sucking of uncooked eggs, might be quoted as a precedent; but I do say uncooked fruit and vegetables. The daily consumption of a few ounces of uncooked fruit, as pears, apples, oranges, grapes, &c., and where these cannot be got, the various plants eaten as salads is, I believe, essential to the diet of those who would maintain their health in perfect integrity.

As some people are so little used to eating salads, and may be glad to know something of these plants, I will conclude this lecture by referring to a few of the more common forms.

First, there is the Lettuce (*Lactuca sativa*). This plant is a cultivated variety of the wild lettuce, *Lactuca virosa*. It contains in its juice an active principle, which in large quantities exercises a narcotic influence on the human system. The Water-cress (*Nasturtium officinale*). This plant grows wild in ditches and damp places in this country, and is also extensively cultivated in the neighbourhood of London. It contains a large quantity of mineral matter, and in some districts is found to contain iodine. The Endive (*Cichorium Endivia*). This plant is probably a variety of the common chicory (*Cichorium Intybus*). It is cultivated extensively on the continent, and its blanched leaves are eaten as a salad. It can be obtained in the winter. It has a slightly bitter taste and acts as a tonic on the system. Celery is the *Apium graveolens*. When wild, this plant contains an acrid principle, which is poisonous, but by culture its stalks are blanched, and it then becomes an agreeable and valuable article of food. The Garden Cress is the *Lepidium sativum*. This plant is not a native of Great Britain, but it is easily cultivated, and extensively used as an early spring salad. The seeds are sown with those of mustard (*Sinapis nigra* and *Sinapis alba*), and the young plants are both eaten together under the name of "mustard and cress." Red Beet, the *Beta vulgaris* of botanists. There are two varieties of this plant used as salad. First, a variety called *la Carde*, which has a small root and large leaves; the latter are eaten in the same way as lettuce. The other variety is called *Betterave*, in which the roots are largely developed. The roots are boiled and sliced, and eaten with vinegar, oil, pepper, and salt, as other salads. The Radish is the *Raphanus Raphanistrum*. The roots of this plant are eaten uncooked, and, like the family to which they belong, contain a subacrid oil, which gives them an agreeable flavour. They are less digestible than many other plants eaten as salad. Lamb's Lettuce or Corn-salad is the *Valerianella olitoria*. This plant is a native of Great Britain, and is often cultivated for use as a salad. The leaves for this purpose should be cut young, or they will have a disagreeable bitter taste. The common Sorrel is the *Rumex acetosa*. The acid taste of this plant depends on the presence of oxalic acid. It is much used as a salad in France. The common Dandelion is the *Leontodon Taraxacum*. This plant, though very common in England, is not much used as a salad. It has, however, when young, the flavour and properties of lettuce, and is extensively employed as a salad on the continent.

Many other plants have been used as salads in this country, and I might enlarge the list by telling you of foreign plants easily cultivated, or British wild plants, which might be consumed with advantage in the form of salad, but these must suffice for the present.

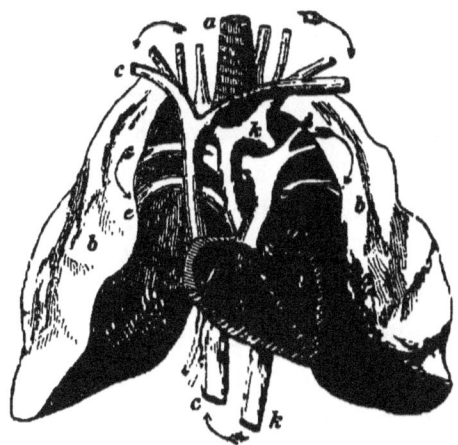

Fig. 1.—*Heart and Lungs.*

- a. *The trachea.*
- b b. *The lungs.*
- c c. *Veins going to heart.*
- d. *Pulmonary artery going to lungs and terminating in*
- e. *Pulmonary vein going to left side of heart.*
- f. *Right auricle of heart.*
- g. *Left auricle of heart.*
- h. *Right ventricle of heart.*
- i. *Left ventricle of heart.*
- k k. *Arteries carrying blood from heart, and terminating in the veins c e.*

HEAT AND FORCE-GIVING FOODS.

I HAVE now to call your attention to the group of foods called Carbonaceous. We have spoken first of Water, and then of the Saline or Mineral substances in food; and now we have left two groups of substances: the first called Combustible, from the fact of their being burned in the system; and Carbonaceous, from the fact of their containing large quantities of carbon or charcoal. The next group is called Nitrogenous, because it contains nitrogen—or Nutritious, because the substances it embraces form the tissues of the body.

First, then, of the force-giving—combustible or carbonaceous—foods. Before speaking of them in detail, I would call your attention to the fact, that the heat which we have in the body is precisely the same as the heat which exists independently of the body: it has the same nature, and the same properties, and is measured by the same instruments, and produces exactly the same results; therefore, although we call the heat of the body animal heat, it is not at all different from the ordinary heat of a fire-place or lamp. Now, the ordinary heat that we find given out by a fire, or candle, or lamp, is the result of the union of carbon and hydrogen with oxygen gas—the oxygen of the atmosphere. The burning of a spirit-lamp will illustrate this fact as well as anything else. Spirits of wine is composed of carbon, hydrogen, and a little oxygen; the oxygen is not enough, however, to interfere with the burning of the carbon and hydrogen. The hydrogen produces heat, and the carbon produces the colour of the flame, and supplies the principal material of the combustion; and we have two things, water and carbonic acid gas, coming off as the result of the union of the hydrogen and carbon with the oxygen of the atmosphere. If you take a cold glass and hold over the burning spirit-lamp, you can collect a vapour, which is the vapour of water. If you cover it over with a bottle, you will find that as the oxygen is withdrawn the lamp will go out. If you now take a little lime water and put into the bottle, the lime water, when it comes in contact with the carbonic acid gas, forms chalk, which, being an insoluble substance, will fall to the bottom as a white precipitate. Thus, then, we find that ordinary combustion, attended by heat, is the result of the union of carbon and hydrogen with oxygen gas, and that the substances formed during this combustion are carbonic acid gas and water. In the great majority of cases where heat is produced upon the surface of the earth, we find that it is the result of precisely the same process—the union of oxygen with carbon, and with hydrogen.

Now, there are some cases in which animal and vegetable matters are exposed to the action of the oxygen of the atmosphere, and the result of the union of the oxygen with the carbon of the animal and vegetable matters is just the same as in the case of the lamp, but in these latter cases there is no light given out. Light does not appear until a burning substance attains a temperature of 700° or 800°. When oxygen unites with carbon and hydrogen at a temperature lower than this, no light is given out, but heat is generated. Thus, if you put a quantity of decaying vegetable matter in a heap in your garden, you get heat developed, which your gardener uses for his cucumber frames; and it is an extraordinary fact, that the instincts of some animals have guided them to this method of developing heat. There is in the Zoological Gardens a bird called the Brush Turkey, an inhabitant of Australia, which does not make an ordinary comfortable nest, but heaps together the leaves of the forest in a great mass; she then deposits her eggs in the midst, and having covered them up with leaves, she watches around the heap of leaves till they give out a sufficient quantity of heat to hatch the eggs: then when the young ones are hatched, she assists them out of their leafy cradle.

This is a very curious instance of an animal availing

itself of artificial arrangements for the purpose of the production of heat. Then occasionally we find vegetable matter catching fire. When cotton is heaped together, especially if it is damp, it frequently catches fire. This spontaneous combustion, arising from the oxidation of decomposing vegetable matter, is a frequent cause of fire. Then we find this oxidation goes on in living plants. There has been a variety of experiments performed, which prove that, at certain seasons, the plant has a temperature higher than the atmosphere. This is especially the case with the plants which belong to the same family as those commonly known to us as "Lords and Ladies," the *Arum maculatum*. This plant, if you put the bulb of the thermometer within its flower-leaf at the time of opening its flower, will show you that the temperature is much higher than at any other time. During this process there is a true oxidation of the plant going on, and thus you have heat. Mr. Lowe, of Highfield House, near Nottingham, has performed a very large number of experiments with a very delicate thermometer, and has always found that the opening of flowers was attended with an increase of heat. Then we find this to be the case with animals: the animal body of the higher animals especially is constantly warmer than the surrounding atmosphere, and there is no doubt that the whole of the mammalia and birds have fixed temperatures—a temperature which never changes during life and health. Those animals, however, which have imperfect hearts, do not maintain the same temperature—these are called cold-blooded, as crabs, lobsters, fishes, and reptiles. Man has a fixed temperature under all circumstances: whether living under the tropical sun of India, America, or Africa, or at the Poles, we find that his temperature is the same, and that temperature is always 98°. There is no departure from this, except in the case of disease. Wherever human beings have been submitted to the test for temperature, it has always been 98°, and it is easily proved by placing the bulb of a thermometer under the tongue, or in some covered part of the body. Of course, the hand is exposed to the atmosphere, and you cannot get it from the hand, and so with the face; but the covered parts of the body give 98°. If you look at the common Fahrenheit's thermometer, which is constantly employed in this country to measure temperatures, you will find that water freezes at a temperature of 32°, and that blood heat is marked as 98°. I would especially recommend to your attention the study of this useful instrument. It should be a household instrument, and every one should be acquainted with the nature of the facts it registers. You will recollect this, that the temperature of 98° in the human body must be maintained from sources quite independent of the external atmosphere. If a man is submitted to a low temperature in the Arctic regions, as many of our travellers in those climates have been, and still maintains a temperature of 98°, it becomes a necessary conclusion that this must be kept up from sources independent of the external atmosphere. Now, this is supplied by the food which we take—by the heat-giving food—of which I have now to speak. I have not time to enter fully into the question of how that temperature is maintained, but it is very curious, that whilst we pass from regions where the temperature is 40° below the freezing point to regions where the temperature rises to above the natural heat of man, to observe that that temperature of 98° is maintained in all cases. Now, the cause of this is the structure of the skin. The skin is covered over the body in such a way that, by causing the evaporation of water, it keeps the body constantly at the same temperature. If you take a tea-kettle, and cover it with a wet cloth, by sprinkling cold water over the cloth you may keep the temperature of the kettle at a fixed point, because the water in passing from its liquid to its vaporous condition takes up and absorbs a large quantity of heat, and carries it off. So that when we are exposed to warm climates and warm temperatures, when the body does not require the large quantity of heat that the heat-giving food that we have taken in gives off, then the skin throws off that fluid which we call perspiration, and thus the temperature is kept down in warm climates. It is the skin, then, that regulates the temperature of the body.

We now come to consider the parts of the body by which this effect is produced. Our food is first taken into the mouth, where it undergoes important changes. It is first masticated with the teeth, and then there is poured into it the secretion called saliva. This is called insalivation. This process is attended by the conversion of the starch of our food into sugar, and other important changes. The food is then carried into the stomach, where it meets with the gastric juice, and is converted into chyme. Chyle is formed on the external surface of the chyme, and taken up by the little projecting bodies called villi, and from these transferred to the lacteals, which eventually empty the chyle into the blood. The blood then is the great receptacle of all our available food. Let us now trace it to the blood. It passes along the veins to the right side of the heart; for the heart is double, and has two sides. It first goes to the right side of the heart, into the cavity which is called the right auricle, and passes out of this into another cavity, called the right ventricle. (See Fig. 1, at the beginning of this lecture.) These cavities contract so that the blood cannot return into the veins, because of the valves which prevent it,— it must go forward; and now, when these cavities contract, let us see where it goes to. It goes on to the left side of the heart, but it first passes through the lungs. They form two masses, which lie on each side of the chest; the blood passes into them along the pulmonary arteries; and now, when in the lungs, we find that these organs are so constructed that the blood may be exposed to the largest possible surface. The air-tubes of the lungs terminate in cells, the blood-vessels are distributed on the walls of these cells, and whilst there, the blood is exposed to the action of the atmosphere. Every time we breathe we take in a quantity of air from the atmosphere, the atmosphere containing 21 parts of oxygen gas, and 79 of nitrogen. Every time we inspire, the air passes down the trachea, or windpipe, which we can easily see in our throats, and passes on through smaller tubes to the lungs, and then to the minute air-cells. It is here, then, that the oxygen gas of the atmosphere meets the blood which has come from the right side of the heart, and there is a wonderful arrangement made by which the oxygen of the air actually penetrates through the blood-vessels, so that the little blood globules receive the oxygen from the outside of the vessels. There is no direct exposure of the blood to the air, but there is a membrane lying between the blood and the atmosphere, and it is through that membrane that the air penetrates. It is one of the wonderful physical properties of this membrane that when moist, it has the power of absorbing the oxygen of the air. The blood has been brought from the right side of the heart, of a blue or black colour; but no sooner has the oxygen penetrated these blood-vessels, than it becomes bright red. It then passes back to the left side of the heart by means of the pulmonary veins.

These vessels empty themselves into the left auricle, and this contracting, sends the blood into the left ventricle, which sends the blood into the great aorta, which, in the end, distributes the blood into all parts of the system, the arteries beating regularly with every pulse of the heart. The arteries pass from the aorta into all the limbs: they pass down the arm beating until we come to the artery in which the doctor feels the pulse. The arteries all terminate in little tubes which are called capillary vessels; and it is in these minute vessels that the union of the oxygen of the air with the carbon of the blood takes place, by which the animal heat is produced. These minute vessels are distributed to every part of the body; and we find that the oxygen passes apparently out of these vessels—these capillary vessels—into the tissues, into the muscles, and into the nerves; and whilst we are living, whilst we are thinking, whilst we are acting, whilst we are performing the various functions of life, we are doing it under the agency of this life-giving oxygen. The oxygen and carbon are united; and, just as a lamp has no light unless it burns, so we have no life unless we burn. This burning gives force to the muscles, and there is no force in the body without heat. You know how a candle goes out if we put something over it: so it would be with any one of us. If I were to put you under a jar for three minutes you would die, irrecoverably die, as if you were drowned. We hang a man up by a rope for five minutes, and thus cut off the oxygen, and destroy his life; and that is the way we judicially dispose of our great criminals.

Now, the oxygen has united with carbon and heated the whole body, and it results in carbonic acid gas; and just as the oxygen is lost we find carbonic acid is formed, and takes its place. The blood now prepares to return. It passes into the veins, and returns back to the heart: it runs up the legs and arms, and down the jugular vein, and comes to the right side of the heart once more. In this course, however, it does not go from the stomach and bowels direct to the heart; the veins from these parts join to form a great vessel, called the portal vein, which terminates in the liver. Here it is distributed to a number of little secreting sacs, or cells, which set to work to separate from the blood it contains two products—the bile and a sugar-forming substance. The bile is carried to the gall-bladder, from whence it is carried to meet the food as it passes along the bowels; whilst the sugar-forming substance is carried into the blood to be disposed of there.

Let us now follow the blood once more to the lungs. It goes to the lungs charged with carbonic acid gas;

it delivers up the carbonic acid gas at the moment that it takes in the oxygen. The carbonic acid gas goes out of our lungs every time we expire. The passage of the oxygen into the blood, and the carbonic acid out of the blood, may be represented by the accompanying rude diagram.

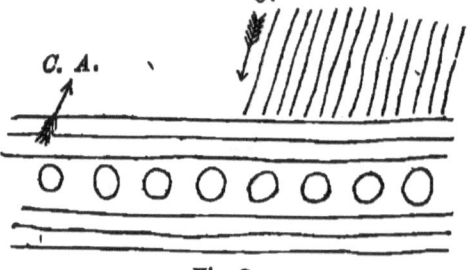

Fig. 2.

That we throw out carbonic acid gas from our lungs can be easily proved, by taking a bottle of water, then inverting it in a basin of water, and filling it with air from the lungs by blowing into it with a bent tube. Carefully cork the bottle while the mouth of it remains immersed, now take the bottle out of the water, and having previously lighted a small piece of candle, uncork the bottle, and place the candle in it, when the light will be extinguished for want of oxygen to support combustion. And if you pour in some lime water you will get the characteristic deposit of carbonate of lime.

The properties of this carbonic gas are worthy of our consideration. It is the product of combustion. It is a gas that will not support combustion. When a lighted candle or lamp is plunged into it, it goes out. Just as the lamp goes out in an atmosphere of carbonic acid gas, so we go out; and just as a lamp burns slowly in an atmosphere charged with carbonic acid gas, so we burn sluggishly in an atmosphere charged with carbonic acid gas: changes do not go on in our system which ought to go on. This shows the necessity of getting rid of the carbonic acid gas of our lungs from our houses, from our sitting-rooms, and from our places of assembly, but, above all things, of getting rid of it from our keeping-rooms and sleeping-rooms, where we spend the larger portion of our time. I believe there is evidence to show that the want of pure air, and the retention of carbonic acid gas in the air we breathe, is one of the greatest sources of that most terrible and afflicting disease, consumption of the lungs. The want of a due supply of fresh air, and the retention of this carbonic acid gas in the house, and the lungs, are the great sources of this disease. I have not time here to dwell on the evidence, but it is a point of great practical importance, in which every one here is interested. Care should be always taken, and the means secured for letting fresh air into rooms and carrying off the heated and poisonous carbonic acid gas.

I come now to speak of the fuel for the maintenance of animal heat and force. That fuel is our food, and it is to the nature of that food, or some portion of it, to which I wish now to call your attention.

There are several substances which are capable of acting in this way, and their chemical history has been studied with much attention. I shall speak of them under the names of starch, sugar, and fat.

There are various forms of starch, sugars, and fats, and I shall have incidentally to allude to these, but they are sufficiently obvious in all their forms to be easily understood. The insipidity of starch, the sweetness of sugar, and the insolubility of fat, are sufficient to characterise them. Every child knows the difference between bread, butter, and sugar.

First, then, with regard to starch. In the first place, I would impress upon you the fact that starch is not merely the thing which is used for domestic purposes for starching linen and so on, but that it is a substance which is universally present in plants, and that there is very little of our vegetable food that does not contain a larger or smaller quantity of it. Starch as it exists in plants is found to assume a granular form; but these granules are so small that they cannot be seen with the naked eye. In order to make out their existence and structure you must use the higher powers of the microscope.

These granules present a variety of form, according to the plants from whence they are derived; but they are so definite, that the source of any particular form of starch may be determined by the aid of the microscope. Mostly the granules are single, as in the case of potato and wheat starch, but occasionally they are united together, forming compound granules. Under the microscope they frequently present a little dark spot, which is called the hilum or nucleus. With polarized light they exhibit a coloured cross, which render them amusing and instructive in the application of polarised light to the microscope. When we come to study them more closely, we find that these starch granules appear to be composed of bags containing the true starchy or amylaceous matter of the starch. When they are submitted to sulphuric acid or heat they expand, and it is in this way that we ascertain that there is a delicate bag on the outside. These granules when chemically analysed, are also found to contain a little flint or silica, also a little potash, and there is a very small quantity of nitrogenous matter which cannot be got rid of; but these things do not constitute one per cent. of the starch of any of the plants with which we are acquainted, so that for dietetical purposes we may regard starch as a definite chemical compound. Starch is insoluble in water, and it is upon the knowledge of this fact that the process for separating starch from the cells in which it is contained is founded. If I take a potato, for instance, and scrape it, and put a little of the scraping into water, I shall find that a portion of the potato will fall to the bottom, but the starch will be suspended in the water. If I now pour off the water which contains the starch, and let it stand, the starch will sink to the bottom of the water in the course of time, and I can then dry it and collect it. Thus starch, you see, is diffusible in water, but not soluble in it; that is the difference between it and the cellulose which forms the cell in which it is contained.

If you look at a section of a potato under the microscope (Fig. 3), you will see that it consists of a series of cells of various forms, and in those cells you have the starch granules. Now, these cells are composed of a substance which is analogous to the wood of which tables and chairs are composed. It is in fact the wall of the cell,

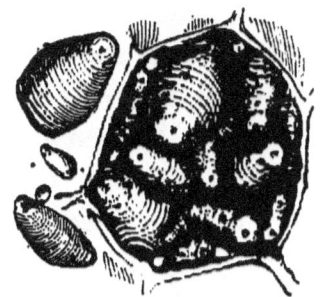

Fig. 3.—Granules of Potato Starch in cells.

and the cell-walls of the plants are always composed

of this matter. It is called cellulose or lignine. This substance is always present in our vegetable food. If you take any plant you will find that there is a quantity of what is called woody fibre in it; of that woody fibre there is the eighth of an ounce in a pound of potatoes, and this cellulose we find in wheaten flour and all the ordinary preparations of vegetable food. It is not, however, a thing which is digested or which acts as food. It is one of those substances which are, as it were, accessory to the real food. It is not to be rejected in all cases; it may sometimes disagree by its indigestibility, but it is not always advisable to reject this cellulose. I can illustrate this by the practice of feeding horses with beans and peas. These articles of food agree better with the horse when they are mixed with chaff or chopped straw. The effect of the indigestible substance is to render that which is digestible more easily appropriated.

I now come to speak more particularly of the chemical properties of starch. In the first place, starch is coloured blue by iodine. If you make a solution of iodine with iodide of potassium, and add a drop to any form of starch, it becomes blue directly. I do not know anything else which is coloured so deeply blue as starch by the agency of iodine. So that we thus have the means of detecting its presence very easily. Not only can we detect it thus in food, but we can also detect it by the aid of the microscope. In structures of doubtful character we add iodine, and the presence of the starch is immediately indicated. Now starch is composed of carbon, or charcoal, and water. I have before spoken of carbon entering into the composition of alcohol. Carbon is found in all vegetable and animal matters, and when the carbon is left after burning, we call it charcoal. The composition, then, of starch is this:—Carbon, 12 atoms; hydrogen and oxygen in the proportions in which those elements form water, 10 atoms. Now, if we calculate then the quantity of carbon and the quantity of water contained in starch, we shall find that every 162 lbs. of starch contain 72 lbs. of charcoal. Here, then, is the source of its heating power. When we eat starch in sago pudding, arrowroot, or whatever form we are taking it, we take just so much fuel; and just as we heap charcoal on a fire, so we add starch to our body to keep up our animal fire, and carbonic acid gas is the result. However, you must not imagine that we could live on charcoal, or that charcoal is good for dinner or for breakfast. The fact is, carbon in its pure form cannot be digested, and before you can consume it, you must digest it. Hence the necessity of finding something which will enable you to transfer the charcoal into the blood and tissues of your body. Even starch itself is not digestible; that is, it is not soluble in water, therefore it can never as starch get into the blood. There is never any in the blood. The fact is that starch, before it is used in the system, is converted into sugar, and unless the starch of our bread and our puddings is converted into sugar, it is not converted into blood at all. One of the curious properties of starch is, that when you submit it to the action of any nitrogenous or fermentable substance, it will be converted from starch into sugar. Such substances are called ferments. You know, when we want to change sugar into alcohol, we add a ferment. If we want to convert starch into sugar, and the sugar into carbonic acid in making bread, we add a ferment. The change which the starch undergoes is, that the 12 atoms of carbon get combined with 12 atoms of water instead of 10 atoms; and sugar is only a little more water chemically combined with starch.

Sugar can be artificially produced from starch, and wherever we have starch, in the vegetable kingdom, we have sugar. There is sugar in potatoes. It is also contained in rice. In sweet potatoes and carrots there are large quantities of sugar; also in turnips. Now, man is provided within his mouth with substances for converting starch into sugar. Underneath the lower jaws, are glands which produce salivine, or ptyaline. This ptyaline has the power of converting starch into sugar. The moment you take the starch into the mouth, and the saliva mixes with it, it is converted into this soluble sugar, and that is the way that the starch finds its way into the system.

There is one more property of starch that needs to be noted, and that is, the power it possesses of combining with water at a high temperature, and forming a thick gelatinous mass. This appears to depend on the bursting of the little starch bags, and the chemical union of the starch with the water. It is in this way that the soft liquid mixtures of starch become converted, by boiling or baking, into consistent puddings. There would, in fact, be no pudding making, were it not for this property of starch.

Before proceeding to speak of sugar, I will point out some of the sources of starch. One of the purest and most costly forms of starch consumed as diet, is arrowroot. This substance is obtained both from the New and Old worlds, and is sold as East Indian and West Indian arrowroot. It is the produce of a plant known by the name of *Maranta arundinacea* (Fig. 4). The arrowroot is procured from its large root-stocks, which are first bruised, and the starch is floated out as I mentioned just now. Under the microscope, the granules of arrowroot have a very definite appearance, so that you can easily distinguish them (Fig. 5).

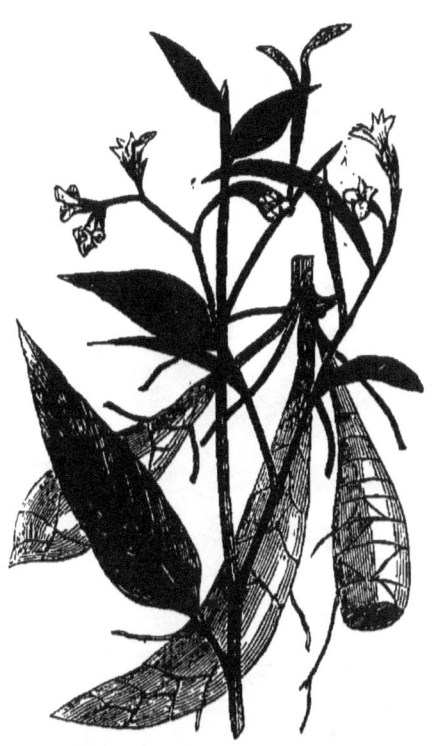

Fig. 4.—Maranta arundinacea.
(Arrowroot.)

There is another arrowroot sold

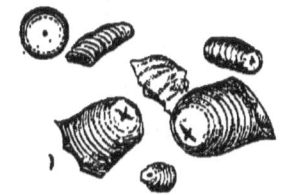 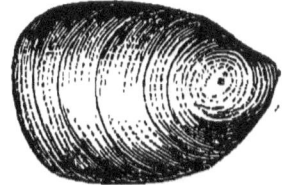

Fig. 5.—Granules of Arrowroot.   *Fig. 6.—Tous les Mois Granules.*

in the shops, by the name of *Tous les Mois*. It is the produce of a plant called *Canna edulis*, closely allied to the last. The starch granules of this root are much larger than the last (Fig. 6). Another form of starch is sago. There are several kinds of sago sold in the markets. That which is commonly used in England is brought from the islands of the Indian Archipelago, and is the produce of the sago palm, the *Sagus lævis* of botanists (Fig. 7). Other species of palm yield sago.

It assumes the appearance of little balls, from the way in which it is prepared.

The only other form of starch used for dietetical purposes is tapioca. This substance is procured from a plant which grows in British Guiana, and is known to botanists by the name of *Jatropha* or *Janipha Manihot*.

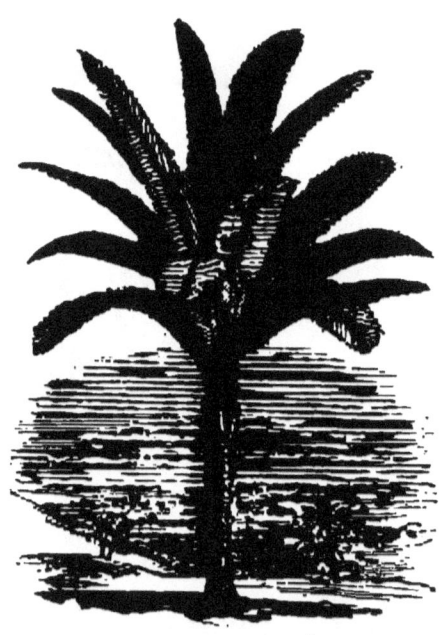

Fig. 7.—*Sagus lævis* (Sago).

The tapioca is prepared from the root of the plant, which, curiously enough, contains hydrocyanic acid; and it is said that the native Indians poison their arrows from the juice of the root, before they commence preparing the tapioca. The native cassava is also prepared from the same plant (Fig. 8). The granules of tapioca starch are smaller than those of arrowroot

(Fig. 9). Starch is separated from rice, and from maize, for dietetical purposes.

The granules of rice starch are irregular, and very minute (Fig. 10). Rice starch is sold for purposes in the arts and manufactures, as well as of diet. A beautiful preparation of rice starch has been recently introduced to the public, by Messrs. Coleman of Norwich. Starch is also obtained from the Indian maize. The gluten and the husk are separated, and the pure starch thus prepared is sold under the name of Corn Flour, and is dietetically superior to arrowroot, and yet is sold at a much lower price. The form of the granule of maize starch

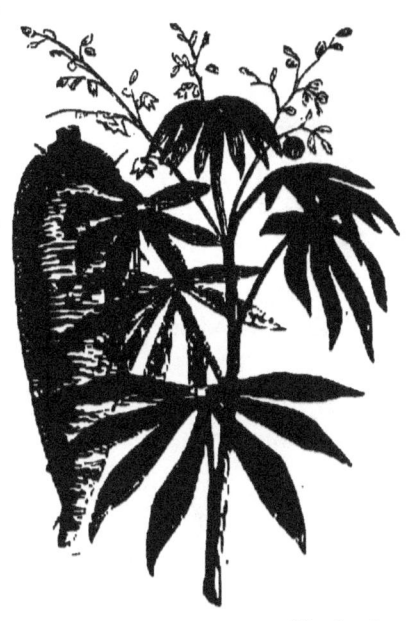

Fig. 8—*Janipha manihot* (*Tapioca*).

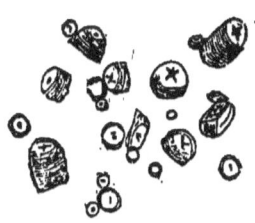

Fig. 9.—*Tapioca Granules.*

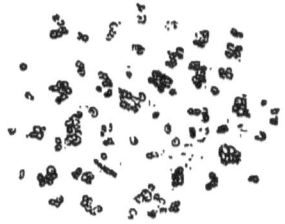

Fig. 10.—*Rice Granules.*

is very characteristic (Fig. 11). Where starches are properly prepared it is difficult to tell the difference by taste alone between them and the finest arrowroot.

Then we have starch in the various kinds of vegetable food which contain other things. Wheat flour contains starch and gluten. The starch of wheat is often separated for commercial purposes; the granules vary much in size (Fig. 12). The starch of the oat resembles that of wheat, but it is smaller, and the nucleus presents a stellate form (Fig. 13).

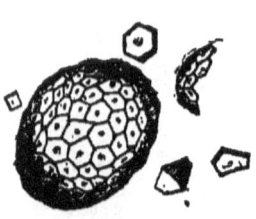

Fig. 11.
Indian-corn Granules.

The quantities of starch vary much in different kinds of vegetable food. Some foods contain starch and little

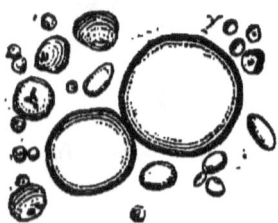

Fig. 12.—Wheat Starch.

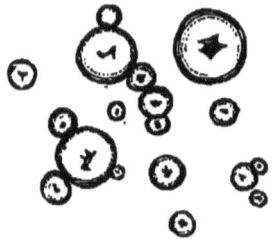

Fig. 13.—Oat Starch.

else; this is the case with the potato and rice. I therefore recommend that such things should never be eaten as substantial articles of diet, but as additions to food containing a larger amount of flesh-forming materials. It must always be recollected that starch is not a flesh-forming substance. Therefore if we give arrowroot, sago, or tapioca, or potatoes, or rice, we are giving food that contains little or no flesh-forming matter at all, and feebleness and disease must be the result of such a diet.

There are some other forms of starchy food to which I must draw your attention.

Salep or saloop consists principally of starch, and is prepared from the roots of the common male orchis (*Orchis mascula*). When it is boiled it forms an agreeable article of diet, and was commonly used in this country before the introduction of tea and coffee. Sassafras chips were frequently introduced into the decoction for the purpose of giving it a flavour. The roots of the *Orchis maculata* also yield an inferior kind of salep. Although now almost entirely disused in this country, it is still employed in Turkey and the East.

Starch differs in its physical and chemical properties according to the plants from which it is obtained. Thus inuline is a form of starch obtained from the elecampane (*Inula Helenium*), a plant not uncommon in this country.

Lichen starch or lichenine is found in lichens and in algæ. This starch has the same power of thickening water at a high temperature as arrowroot, sago, and tapioca. The gelatinous character of the liquid thus obtained has led to the erroneous supposition that it is nutritious, and to the use of lichens and sea-weeds as articles of diet.

One of the plants of this kind, which has been used most extensively, and is still largely employed, is the Iceland moss (*Cetraria Islandica*). It belongs to the family of lichens, and is a native of the northern parts of the world. This and other lichens probably contain other dietetical secretions besides starch, as we find they are capable of supporting animal life. The rein-deer moss (*Cenomyce rangeferina*) is an instance of this. In the northern parts of the world, as well as in mountainous districts, this lichen grows in great abundance, and during the winter season is the principal support of the rein-deer. In spite of the extreme cold to which it is subjected, this plant grows with vigour, and the rein-deer, in order to obtain it as food, is obliged to remove with its nose the snow with which it is sometimes covered for many feet. The cup moss (*Cenomyce pyxidata*) of our own moors belongs to the same genus as the rein-deer moss, and is also used as an article of diet in the same way as the Iceland moss. The *Tripe de Roche* is another of these lichens which has been used as an article of diet. It has a melancholy interest attached to it, as it has so often formed the chief article of vegetable diet to our Arctic navigators. Two species of lichens, the *Gyrophora proboscidea* and *G. erosa* afford the *Tripe de Roche*. Although they are said to be nutritious, they are described as having bitter, nauseous, and even purgative properties.

Amongst the sea-weeds (*Algæ*) which have been used as articles of diet, none is better known than the *Chrondrus crispus*, which, under the name of Carragen moss, Irish moss, and Pearl moss, has been for a long time used in Europe. It is recommended as a medicine, but it has no bitter principle, and is probably less tonic than the lichen. This and other sea-weeds have been occasionally had recourse to by the poor inhabitants of the sea-shores of Europe, more especially Ireland, when the ordinary corn or potato crop has failed. They contain, however, but little nutritious matter, and persons soon famish who live upon nothing else. There are certain forms of sea-weed which are often eaten as an addition to other kinds of food. There is in all of them a certain flavour of the sea, arising, probably, from the saline matter they contain, which renders them very objectionable to some persons as articles of food, and which will, probably, always form an objection to their general use.

Now I come to speak of sugar. I have told you that starch is converted into sugar, and you will not be surprised, therefore, to find sugar present in the same places that we find starch; and if you look at the analysis of vegetable food containing starch you will find that they all contain sugar. Sugar is found in wheat, and barley, and oats; in lentils, beans, and peas. In some cases we find large quantities of sugar where we find no starch. Take, for instance, the carrot and the sweet potato. Now, sugar is soluble in water, and we find sugar more generally contained in the juices or the sap of the plant than in any other form. It also has the remarkable property of fermentation. Thus carbon, and hydrogen, and oxygen, are capable of being converted into that substance which we know by the name of alcohol; and it is during the process of the decomposition of sugar that this alcohol is produced. Therefore, you see, we can make alcohol from starch, but we must first convert the starch into sugar. Of this matter we shall speak in a subsequent part of our lectures.

The general chemical composition of sugar is the same as starch. Sugar, like starch, contains carbon as its principal ingredient, and you can demonstrate this by a very pretty experiment. If you take a strong solution of sugar, and add to it about the same quantity of sulphuric acid, you will decompose the sugar; and the carbon, in the form of charcoal, is set free. It is in this way you can demonstrate the presence of the charcoal; and in this way that very useful material which we call blacking is manufactured. The shining blacking is the sugared charcoal. In this way you can prove that the starch is composed of the same material as sugar, because we can convert the starch into the sugar.

Let us now direct our attention to the history of the plant in relation to sugar. During the germination of plants sugar occurs in great quantities. If we take any seeds and throw them into the ground, the little embryo in the interior begins to grow, and this process is called germination. There is a large quantity of starch surrounding the embryo, and when it begins to grow this starch is converted into sugar. Sugar is as necessary for young plants as it is for young children, and the starch must be converted into sugar in order that they may grow. Now, this process is carried on on a very large scale in the process of malting. The maltster takes the seed of barley, immerses it in water, causes the young plant to germinate, and then he roasts the young plant, seizes the sugar which was created for its use, and converts it into beer.

Then, again, we find the stems of plants, at certain seasons of the year, contain large quantities of sugar; thus the whole of the grasses, including wheat, barley, oats, rye, rice, and maize, contain sugar in their stems just as they are about to flower; and it is just at this season of the year that the sugar-cane contains its sugar, which is used almost exclusively for man as an article of diet. But we need not confine ourselves at all to the sugar-cane. Why we get sugar from nothing else arises out of our fiscal system: revenue being obtained from it, and sugar is not allowed to be produced in this country; and, consequently, we are obliged to eat the sugar of the sugar-cane, or go without. In China they obtain sugar from the sugar Sorgho, the *Sorghum saccharatum;* which, like the sugar-cane, belongs to the family of grasses, and is cultivated in the north of China for the sugar it contains. Sugar has been obtained from this plant in France, and it flourishes in England. Then the maize, the plant which yields Indian corn, has been cultivated in America and Mexico, for the purpose of obtaining sugar; and when Cortes conquered Mexico, he found the natives cultivating the maize, and crushing it for sugar. The *Cocos nucifera*, or cocoa-nut palm, grows abundantly in the island of Ceylon, and is a principal source of sugar to the natives. They have a class of men, a caste, whose occupation it is to ascend these

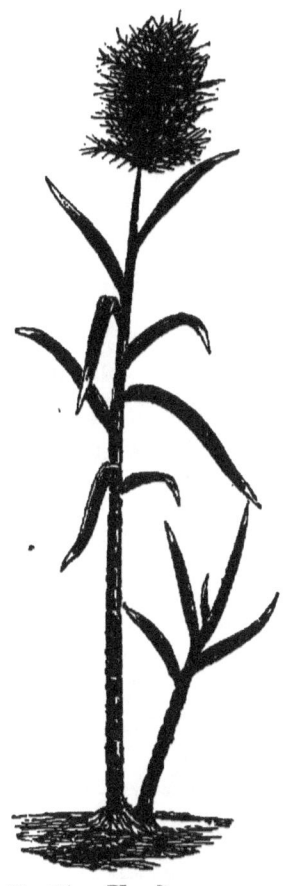

Fig. 14.—*The Sugar-cane.*
(*Saccharum officinarum.*)

trees, and putting over the cut blossoms of the tree a calabash, they catch the exuding juice, which is a daily article of diet in Ceylon. They call it toddy, and the men who draw it are called toddy-drawers.

Again, at the budding season of the plant the sap contains sugar. The common osier has it; and boys, after peeling osier twigs, put them into their mouths to taste the sugar. The birch, too, in England and Scotland, is tapped for its sugar. The sap is converted, in Scotland, into an effervescing wine, which is said by those who drink it to be as good as champagne. In America, the sugar maple (*Acer saccharinum*) contains so large a quantity of sugar that much of the sugar consumed in the United States is obtained from it. Then plants contain sugar in their roots. The beet, the carrot, and the turnip all contain sugar. When the first Napoleon Bonaparte pursued his "continental system," as it was called, he excluded cane-sugar from the French markets, and they set to work to supply the loss, and adopted a process invented by the Germans for the extraction of sugar from the beetroot. This manufacture was protected for many years in France, but now that the trade is free the beet sugar-makers are enabled to compete with the manufacturers of sugar from the sugar-cane.

Another source of sugar in our food, is the fruit which we eat. The fig, the pear, the apple, the orange, and the great majority of our fruits would be unacceptable to us but for their sugar.

Although sugar is always sweet, and we call everything that is sweet sugar, yet there are various kinds of sugar. Sugar exists in animals as well as plants.

Milk contains sugar, which is separated and sold under the name of milk sugar. The liver contains a sugar-making principle, and we can by digesting the livers of animals in water, obtain large quantities of sugar, called liver sugar. Thus we have several kinds of sugar, and, perhaps, it will be as well just to recapitulate. First, the cane sugar, which is composed of carbon 12, hydrogen 10, and oxygen 10. This cane sugar is unfermentable, and incapable of being converted into alcohol as simple cane sugar. Cane sugar is found in the stems of plants, and in all those cases where it is procured before the flowering of plants, and in the roots of plants, so that the beet-root sugar, and the ordinary sugar that we eat from day to day is cane sugar. But the sugar from fruit is different. It is uncrystallizable, and thus differs from cane sugar. This fruit sugar is almost identical with another sugar, which, because it is formed out of starch, is called starch sugar. Now fruit sugar and starch sugar are both known to chemists by the name of glucose, or grape sugar. Fruit sugar or glucose is fermentable. The cane sugar is called *sucrose*, and the sugar obtained from fruit *fructose*, and the starch sugar *glucose*. Milk sugar is called *lactose*, whilst liver sugar, I suppose, may be called *hepatose*. Our ordinary sugar is sucrose. All these sugars, with the exception of sucrose, are fermentable, and easily decomposed. If you take a little of this starch sugar, and put it into a test tube, and mix it with a little sulphate of copper, and put in some potash, you throw down a blue precipitate. Now the property of the glucose is to decompose this oxide of copper, and convert it from the blue oxide into a yellow oxide, and you will see that this will take place when you heat it; and in this way you have a proof that glucose exists in the mixture. I told you just now that the liver contained a quantity of sugar. I may say that I believe it has been demonstrated that the liver does not contain sugar itself, but it contains a matter which is so easily converted into sugar, that the instant you expose it to the air it becomes changed into sugar, and this matter is contained in the blood. This sugar-forming substance may, however, be collected from the liver, and, under the name of glycogene, has been separately exhibited. We do not yet know exactly from what this substance in the liver is formed in the food, but there seems to be little doubt, from observations made when the hepatose presents itself in disease in abundance in the blood, that cane sugar and starch mainly contribute to its production.

Although I have not had time to dwell on it, I need hardly impress on you what an interesting chapter in the physiology of life this discovery of sugar in the liver has opened up. We are evidently on the verge of discovering the causes of those remarkable morbid states of the system which have been known so long, in which the blood is poisoned by an immense accumulation of sugar. The sugar, then, surcharging the blood, has been evidently produced for the purposes of combustion and oxidation, the failure of which has caused its accumulation in the blood, and its elimination in an undecomposed form.

The ultimate action of all forms of sugar in the system is the same. We have seen that starch can only be absorbed as it is converted into sugar. The advantage, then, of sugar over starch, as an article of diet, appears to lie in the facility with which it can be absorbed into the blood. It is supplied to the young of all the higher forms of mammalia in their mother's milk, and its sweetness seems adapted to the instinctive tastes of children, who may always, with advantage, be allowed a free use of it in their food. At the same time what is good for children may not be so advantageous for fathers and mothers. Sugar readily enters into decomposition, forms other compounds, especially lactic acid, and sets in operation other dangerous changes in the food. Hence the dyspeptic, the gouty, the rheumatic, and the corpulent must be warned against it. Those who take alcoholic beverages need but little of it, whilst the teetotaller may be allowed its unrestricted use.

I have just a few concluding remarks to make on substances resembling starch and sugar, and which enter into our daily food, although it is very doubtful if they act on the system in the same way as starch and sugar.

Dextrine is formed in plants whilst starch is passing into the composition of sugar. Like sugar it is soluble in water, but not sweet. It is obtained from barley whilst being malted.

Gum may be regarded as fixed dextrine; it is soluble in water, but is incapable of being converted into sugar, and has no sweet taste. Although gum enters largely into some kinds of food, it does not enter the blood, or act as an aliment. It may be therefore properly regarded as an accessory food. Sugar is added to it, and it is used in the manufacture of lozenges. These are flavoured with various substances, as in the case of the *Pâté de Jujubes*.

Liquorice is found in many plants, but it is separated from the juice of the Liquorice Plant (*Glycyrrhiza glabra*). Like gum it is soluble in water, and has the sweet taste of sugar. It differs from sugar in not being fermentable. It is obtained from the root of the Liquorice Plant in the form of an extract, and comes to this country in solid sticks, which are sold under the name of "Spanish Juice." This is boiled down and refined, and sold under the name of "refined or pipe liquorice." The liquorice plant is cultivated extensively at Pontefract or Pomfret, in Yorkshire, and a manufacture of the liquorice is carried on in that town. The liquorice is made into cakes, which are called "Pomfret cakes." Liquorice, like gum, does not act as an aliment in the system.

Manna is another sweet substance, soluble in hot water, but not capable of fermentation. It is obtained for medicinal purposes from a species of ash, the *Fraxinus Ornus*. Several other plants yield manna, and it is used in some countries as an article of diet. Its value is, however, doubtful. This substance has sometimes been supposed to be the "manna" of Scripture, but the putrescent nature of that substance, and the absence of dietetical properties in the substance in question, renders this supposition exceedingly doubtful.

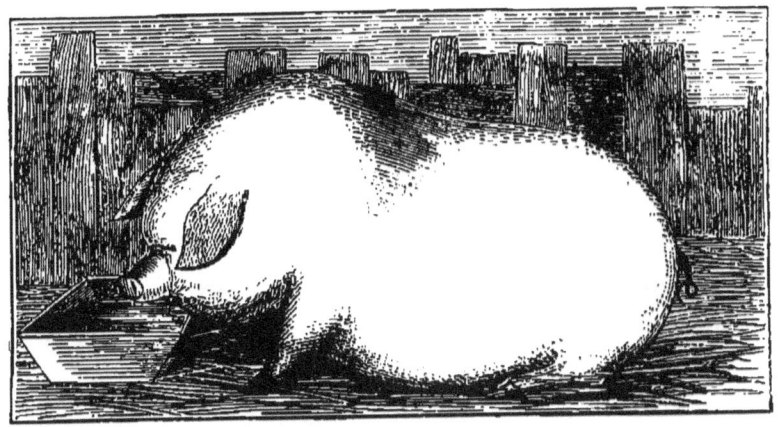

Fig. 1.

ON OIL, BUTTER, AND FAT.

In this lecture I shall continue my observations on that class of foods which are now known by the name of heat or force-giving.

This group may very well be divided into—first, those which contain starch and sugar, of which I have already spoken; and, secondly, those which contain oil or fat.

There is a great difference in the chemical composition of oils and fats, as compared with starch and sugar, which can be easily made apparent.

Taking, then, the composition of starch and sugar as carbon 12, hydrogen 10, and oxygen 10, which would express generally the composition of starch and sugar; or, taking the real weights, carbon 72, hydrogen 10, and oxygen 80, the quantity of carbon in starch and sugar would be nearly half their whole weight.

Now, if we take oil, we shall find the difference is very great. Taking all those substances which are indicated by the term oil, which are called fats, butters, lards, suets, greases, and tallows, their composition will be this—carbon 11, hydrogen 10, and oxygen 1. Thus you see, in the starch and the sugar, the hydrogen and the oxygen are just in the proportions in which those two elements form water; but if we take the fat and the oils, you will find a large quantity of the hydrogen to spare, and very little oxygen in these bodies at all. Oxygen, then, is not in the proportion in which it forms water with hydrogen, so that you see in an oil or fat, instead of having only half the bulk, as in the case of the carbon of starch and sugar, you have actually nearly the whole mass for combustion, 66 of carbon and 10 of hydrogen out of the 77 parts of oily matter. Now, this is a practical point of importance, for where you are substituting fat for starch or sugar, there you ought to substitute a very much less quantity. The proportion of the combustible elements in fat, as compared with starch and sugar, is as $2\frac{1}{2}$ to 1, so that you ought to take as a substitute for 1 pound of butter, $2\frac{1}{2}$ pounds of starch or sugar. It must, however, be recollected that sugar is more easily taken up into the system, and more available than starch.

Now, this oily matter, of which we have to speak, is used not only as an article of diet, but it is extensively employed in the arts.* I would remind you that

* See Lecture on Soap, in Uses of Animals.

ON OIL, BUTTER, AND FAT.

we use it for combustion. Until the introduction of gas it was the only substance that could be generally used for illumination. Then we use it, also, for diminishing friction. The power which oil has of diminishing friction is very great, and this physical property is of the greatest consequence to us as a manufacturing nation. We send to all parts of the world for oil to diminish the friction of our machinery, which would, in fact, fly on fire if it were not for oil in some form. This oily matter is also used for the manufacture of soap. Let me, then, first speak generally of the nature of oleaginous matter. I have said that all these matters which we call suets, fats, butters, tallows, or grease, have this general formula :—84 lbs. of any one of them would contain 66 lbs. of charcoal, 10 lbs. of hydrogen, and 8 lbs. of oxygen. Now, these substances, although they contain carbon and hydrogen, do not present themselves to us as simple compounds of carbon and hydrogen; and, though we know a good deal of their chemistry, we have undoubtedly much to learn, for carbon and hydrogen may unite in many proportions. One of carbon will unite with 1 of hydrogen, or with 2 of hydrogen, or with 3 of hydrogen, or with 4 of hydrogen, and so on, and yet constitute something different every combination. And again, you may take 2 of carbon and 1 of hydrogen, or 2 of carbon and 3 of hydrogen, or 3 of carbon and 1 of hydrogen, or 2 of hydrogen, and so on through an innumerable series of substances, and amongst them you will find the base of alcohol or ethyl, which consists of 4 atoms of carbon and 5 of hydrogen. Then, again, formyle, which is the substance which forms the base of chloroform, is 2 of carbon and 1 of hydrogen. Such compounds are almost innumerable, and show you what powerful chemical properties these two elements possess.

Now, if we take olive-oil and put it out into the winter's cold, you will find that it separates into two parts, and one sinks to the bottom and the other floats on the top.

All fats and oils contain one or both of these substances, the one solid and the other liquid; the one is called stearine, and the other oleine. Sometimes we have another substance mixed with fat and oils. Thus, if you take human fat or goose fat, and their composition is the same, you would get, instead of the stearine, a substance called margarine. It differs so little from stearine, that we need not speak of it as a separate substance, for there is only a little more oxygen in margarine, which makes the difference; we may, therefore, leave out of our consideration the margarine. Whether we take margarine as food or not, or whether it is found in our body or not, is not of much consequence. It is, however, a very curious circumstance, that the wild horses of America contain larger quantities of margarine than the horses of this country, and that seems to indicate that the one may be converted into the other, or, at any rate, substituted for the other. Oleine is liquid at all temperatures. Castor-oil never throws down any deposit of stearine, for it is composed entirely of oleine. On the contrary, the butter-tree gives an oil which is always solid, and is nearly all stearine. So with palm-oil from Africa, the produce of the *Elais guineensis,* and the palm-oil obtained from the cocoa-nut palm in the island of Ceylon. This palm is cultivated in large quantities by Price's Patent Candle Company, of London, for the purpose of obtaining stearine for the making of candles. Thus, you see, stearine and oleine have different relations to heat. If you expose stearine to a high temperature, it becomes liquid like oleine.

Now there is another property which oils possess, and that is, that they are insoluble in water, and this insolubility in water is one of their most remarkable characteristics. Those of which I speak are also called fixed oils; and this arises from the property which they possess of not being easily evaporated. If you place a drop of oil on a piece of paper it will not be easily dissipated by heat. There are, however, oils which are easily evaporated, and these are called volatile oils; such as the oil of lavender, the oil of nutmeg, and oil of cinnamon. If you drop a little of any of these upon a piece of paper and hold it over a candle, it will evaporate quickly. They are formed of hydrogen and carbon with oxygen, but have a different constitution to the fixed oils.

Now let us pass from the physical to the chemical properties of oils and fats. They are principally composed of carbon and hydrogen, and on that account are highly inflammable. They burn with a flame; where we have a flame we must have hydrogen. The result of their combustion in the air is the production of carbonic acid gas and water. You may easily detect these compounds with a burning candle. If you hold a cold glass over it, taking care not to blacken it by condensing the carbon in the form of smoke, you will find water will condense in the inside. If you now take a wide-mouthed bottle and put it carefully over the candle, you will collect a gas in the inside. This gas you can prove to be carbonic acid, by pouring in some lime-water, which will immediately become turbid from the formation of carbonate of lime. The carbon was in the candle, and so we find in all these burning, oily matters, that we have carbon, which can be proved by the production of carbonic-acid gas when we burn them in the atmosphere. Any kind of oil would do just as the candle does, and yield the proof that it contains carbon as well as the proof that it contains hydrogen.

Thus much for the ultimate composition of the fatty matter. We cannot burn sugar or starch in this way, because the quantity of oxygen combined in the sugar and the starch takes away the hydrogen and leaves only the carbon to burn, and we have to add a considerable quantity of heat in order to get rid of the water before the starch and sugar will burn.

Now a very curious chemical point is, that these things, oleine and stearine, are not chemical compounds of carbon, hydrogen, and oxygen, in that form, but that they are actually put together in the form of an acid united to the base. Let me illustrate what I mean, by the composition of chalk. Chalk is a compound of an acid with a base; the acid is carbonic acid, and the base is lime: and if you pour some water on the chalk, and afterwards a little sulphuric acid, you will expel the carbonic acid.

Now stearine and oleine are just as much compounds of an acid and a base as chalk or carbonate of lime; and what we have in stearine is a quantity of stearic acid combined with a base called oxide of lipyle, but which is popularly known by the name of glycerine. Glycerine then is an oxide. Carbonate of lime is carbonic acid gas combined with oxide of calcium, and stearine is stearic acid combined with glycerine or oxide of lipyle, and this oxide of lipyle acts upon the stearic acid just as the oxide of calcium acts upon the carbonic acid.

When we take these things as food, they are not taken up as globules of oil or fat, for they would not pass through the absorbents. Nothing that will not dissolve in water will pass through the lacteals into the blood, and it is very interesting to find the same chemistry going on in our stomachs that goes on outside them. The history then of the digestion of these substances appear to be this, that in the stomach the fatty acid combines with a base so as to form a soluble compound, which is carried into the blood, where it is again formed into an insoluble compound when it is deposited as fat. This change is the foundation of the art of soap-making, and, I may say, we are indebted to the art of soap-making for a knowledge of this curious property in the oil. When we make soap we take a quantity of alkali and put it to the oil. The consequence is, that the alkali takes the place of the glycerine and combines with the stearic or oleic acid as the case may be, and a soluble stearate or oleate of the alkali is formed. In this process the glycerine is set free, and this glycerine used to be the refuse of the soap-boiler; he threw this away; he now knows better what to do with it, as glycerine is turning out to be a most useful substance in the arts.

These soaps, which are formed with potash, or with soda, are both soluble in water; but there are certain compounds of stearic acid and oleic acid, which are not soluble. Thus, we have insoluble soaps and soluble soaps. The soluble soaps are also of two kinds: there is the hard soap, which is formed by soda and the fatty acid; and there is the soft soap of the shops, which is formed by potash and a fatty acid. They dissolve in water, and form a lather. I am not going to enter here into an account of the processes of soap-making, but I would point out that one of the qualities which these soaps possess, is the property of dissolving oil. They not only are soluble themselves, but when they get on to the dirty hand—the hand having held the dirt by the fatty matter on the skin—these soaps dissolve the fatty matter; and thus it is with linen, and all substances which we wash.

Now, this property may throw some light on the way in which the oil is disposed of in the stomach. But I have said that there are some insoluble soaps. If this stearic acid were to combine with lead, or with lime, the oxide of calcium, instead of potash, then you would get an insoluble soap, which would not dissolve in water or act as a detergent. You know when you go to a chalk district, where the water contains large quantities of carbonate of lime, that, when you wash your hands, a substance rises and sticks to the skin, so that you might think it better to have no soap at all. The fact is, all this time you are forming an insoluble soap—a lime soap—the lime having taken the place of the soda. The best way, in this case, is to go boldly to work and rub away at the soap till the lime is all exhausted, and then you may wash with the soda soap. It is the same in the stomach; unless the oils meet with potash or soda, they cannot be made soluble: if they meet with lime they are insoluble. It is only by the agency of the former that they can be made soluble and digestible, and can pass into the blood. Now, this is very important; for, if we insist on cooking out of the food these soda and potash salts, there is nothing left for the saponification of the fat.

There is, however, a provision made for giving alkalies to the stomach by the agency of the liver. The liver, as I have before mentioned, secretes, or separates from the blood sent to it, a substance called bile. The bile, when mixed with oily matters, has the power of saponifying them, and rendering them easy of absorption. With the bile there is also poured into the stomach a fluid, secreted by the pancreas, which is called the pancreatic fluid. It contains a principle called pancreatin which has the power of saponifying or emulsifying the fatty matter of the food. Besides these fluids, the mucous membrane of the alimentary canal contains alkaline substances which may also exert the same action, and thus we see how ample the preparation is for the carrying readily into the system these important constituents of our diet. We must at the same time recollect that if the alkalies of these fluids are the agents of the saponification, they must be supplied in the food before they can be thrown out in the secretions.

Before leaving this subject, I would call your attention to the glycerine which is separated during the decomposition of fatty matters. It was formerly thrown away by the soap-maker: it is now, however, purified and used for many purposes. It will not burn like the acid from which it is separated, and it is that part of the fat or tallow which, when burning, gives out a disagreeable smell, so that it is now separated from the oil with which the best candles are made. The best candles are now made from stearic acid.

Glycerine is called so from its sweetish flavour. It is not, however, used at present as an article of diet, but it has been employed in the same cases where cod-liver-oil has been recommended, and I understand with considerable success. If it should turn out to be as useful as codliver-oil, it would be a great advantage, as it is much less disagreeable to take. Glycerine is also used by medical men as an external application; and where the object is the protection of the skin, it seems to act very favourably. It appears to answer the same purpose as oil in anointing, and with this advantage, that not being readily decomposed, it does not emit the unpleasant smell that oil frequently does. Glycerine has many properties that recommend it for use in the arts.*

But let us now pass on to the action of the oily and fatty matters on the system. I have classified them with the starch and sugar, because, as I said before, they are maintainers of animal heat and force. There can be no doubt that they perform these functions, and that it is no mere theory; for it is a well-known fact, that where men are exposed to cold, they consume a large quantity of fatty matters. Sir John

* See Lecture on Soap and Candles in course on Uses of Animals.

Franklin, and all Arctic travellers, have recorded their expressions of surprise at the quantity of coarse fat that the people who live in the Arctic regions will take. In his first voyage, Sir John Franklin tells us that he gave to an Esquimaux boy a quantity of tallow candles to see how many he would eat, and it was not until he had eaten 14 lbs. that Sir John became frightened for his store, and gave the boy a large lump of fat pork to get out of the bargain. Even the sailors who go out in these Arctic expeditions use a large quantity of fat, and the food which they principally used, called pemmican, contains as much as 80 per cent. of fat. Our uncooked meat, including pork, does not contain more than from 16 to 50, and our cooked meat not more than 15 per cent. of fat. Generally, the inhabitants of northern climates eat a larger quantity of fatty food than the inhabitants of southern climes. In the northern parts of Russia they get so into the habit of taking coarse fat, that when they come south they cannot do without it. An instance of the desire for this food is recorded in the case of some Russian troops, lying at one of our seaports at the beginning of the present century. The people of the town were surprised to find the oil lamps of the town went out very soon, and this could not be explained, until it was found that the Russian soldiers were in the habit of stealing out in the evening, of climbing up the lampposts and drinking up the oil. In the streets of St. Petersburg they sell meat pies, and a bottle of train-oil is always kept to supply those who may wish with this additional luxury.

Throughout the body there is a tissue, which is called adipose tissue, or fat when it is separated. This adipose tissue is present in all healthy animals. It is this tissue which disappears when people are suffering under disease, and they become thin and lean; and it is the absence of this which makes people grow thin and ugly when they are old. I use this word ugly here in contrast with the beauty produced by the rounded lines of the flesh well stuffed with adipose tissue. Now this tissue lies in little cells, and by a microscope you can easily see these cells, in which the oily matter is deposited (Fig. 2).

The uses of this adipose tissue in the system are very manifest. In the first place, it acts as a kind of supply of fuel in times of scarcity; just as we take care in the summer time to fill our coal-cellars with coal for winter use, so it would seem that nature takes care in the summer time that animals should have large quantities of this fat as a store of fuel for the cold, and we find it deposited on the backs of animals in temperate climates during the summer time. All the ruminantia become fat in summer, and the starch and sugar of the grasses which they take are converted into fat and put upon their backs. Thus the dormouse and the hedgehog, and various animals which hybernate in the winter, become fat in the summer. In their winter sleep, when they get no food, the fat is consumed during their sleep, and they wake up from their long nap thin and lean. A man is fatter in the summer than in the winter. Some persons think they get no fatter in the summer than in winter. Some persons think that they get thinner in

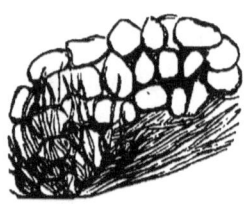

Fig. 2.—*Adipose Tissue.*

summer. But the real consumer of heat is the cold of winter, and just in proportion to the intensity of cold in the winter will be the quantity of fat which is lost; and the inhabitants of cold climates seldom get fat, for they cannot take enough fat to deposit it in their tissues and keep them warm. This has been proved in this country very conclusively. In prisons they give the same diet in winter and summer, and from careful weighing of the prisoners it has been found that they always weigh most at the latter end of summer and are thinnest at the beginning of March, and so they go on alternating. These facts show that one of the functions of fat is to supply the blood, when destitute of combustible materials, with a quantity of fuel for combustion. Then there are other purposes which it subserves, such as lightening the body. The fat man, in proportion to his size, weighs lighter than the thin one; and so it is with animals. Whales, dolphins, porpoises, and creatures of that sort, are supplied with enormous quantities of fat to enable them to move in the water; and if it were not for that, they would not be able to pursue their prey or move so rapidly through the water as they do. Fat is also a bad conductor of heat, and enables these cetaceous creatures, which are warm-blooded, although living in the cold waters of arctic oceans, to maintain their high temperature. Was it not for the large mass of fat in their tissues they would die. This is probably the cause of the large quantities of fat deposited in animals which live in cold climates. Their fat acts as a kind of packing for the body. Our muscles would not be so perfect in their action if there was not a due quantity of adipose matter deposited between them;

and we find in the system wherever there is any want of matter to make up the rotundity of form, that fat is put in, just as the potter, in sending out his ware, puts in a quantity of straw or wool to keep it from breaking.

Fat is also deposited round the joints in considerable quantities, and seems to act there by diminishing friction, just as man adds oil to the moving joints of his machinery. But there is one important action of fat which differs entirely from those which I have spoken of, and that is that we find the fat existing in the young of the higher animals, and in all cases where tissues are about to be formed. The muscular and nervous tissues, when they are beginning to grow, are accompanied by fatty matter; oil globules will constantly be seen forming a kind of scaffolding for those cells which contain albumen and fibrine. So that these oily matters are of more importance in relation to the health and maintenance of the tissues of the body than sugar or starch. This fact seems to explain what has recently been made known as a fact, that in certain forms of disease, one of the most effectual remedies which can be given is the oil of animals, more especially codliver-oil. Now, it has been known a long time that the oil of fish would act beneficially in certain forms of disease; and recent experience has shown that it is more particularly in the disease that is known as consumption that this substance acts beneficially.

By giving these oils, we supply to the system a larger quautity of fatty matter than is required for combustion, which is deposited in the tissues, and just as persons increase in weight, is their strength and general health improved. It seems to give a power of development to the nervous and muscular system upon which our lives depend. At one time it was thought that fish oils were the only oils of service, but you may give any oil with advantage, provided they can be digested and taken up into the blood. Persons who are getting thin, and especially where this depends on a tendency to consumption, may take fat meat, butter, cream, and salad oil with advantage.

Some persons are disgusted with the smell and flavour of codliver-oil, and then it may become of importance to have recourse to olive-oil, almond-oil, butter, cream, or fats. Lately, there has been brought into this country, from Australia, the oil of the dugong, which it is said acts quite as efficiently as codliver-oil. The more favourable action of the fish and animal oils probably depends on their property of being more readily saponified or emulsified in the stomach, so that they are more easily digested.

Sometimes fat has a tendency to accumulate in the system. It is one of the objects of the grazier to make his animals fat. He does this not only for the sake of the fat of the animal, but also because the flesh of fat animals is more tender than that of those which are lean. In order to effect this object, he feeds his cattle with food containing fatty matters, and, *cæteris paribus*, that food which contains most fat will have a tendency to produce most adipose tissue. There are two things which greatly contribute to the fattening of animals, and these are quietude and warmth. The history of the prize pigs and fat oxen annually exhibited at the Smithfield Cattle Show proves this.

The quantity of fat contained in the human body

varies according to circumstances. I have calculated that a man weighing 11 stones, or 154 lbs., should have in his body 12 lbs. of fat. Men, however, weigh very differently according to their height. A man who weighs 154 lbs. and is only 5 feet high, would probably be very fat; whilst a man standing 6 feet high at that weight would be regarded as thin. Dr. Hutchinson weighed upwards of two thousand men, and found their weight as follows:—Men at 5 feet 1 inch weighed 8 stones 8 lbs.; at 5 feet 4 inches, 9 stones 13 lbs.; at 5 feet 8 inches, 11 stones 1 lb.; and at 6 feet, 12 stones 10 lbs. When a man exceeds this weight, it is probably owing to the increase of fat.

This increase of size often produces great inconvenience, and leads to serious results. The heart is over-taxed, and it becomes diseased, and fatal consequences result. The causes of this fatness are both natural and acquired. Some persons, like some breeds of animals, get fat on a diet which produces no such effect in others. But many circumstances, over which people have entire control, tend to produce obesity. Indulgence in alcoholic liquors, the free use of saccharine and oily foods, sedentary habits, and living in warm rooms, all assist in producing it. Over such habits and practices all persons have more or less control. When people are not unhealthy, avoiding butter at breakfast and bread at dinner is a good rule, with only one glass of wine in the day, and no sugar in tea, coffee, or chocolate. Hard biscuits may be also substituted for hot rolls at breakfast with advantage. Regular exercise, not excessive, in the open air, should

ON OIL, BUTTER, AND FAT. 107

also be taken daily. But, alas! the obese are generally infirm of will, and perhaps their bodily state is in some measure connected with this mental condition; they will not practice the necessary denial till it is too late. Could we but insist on the discipline implied in the sentence, "six months at the treadmill," how many of our fat friends would avoid the sad penalties of their self-indulgence.

Let me now direct your attention to the source of these oils and fats which we take in our food. Now, one of the sources of oils and fats in the system is undoubtedly the starch and sugar which we take. I told you in the last lecture that starch and sugar contained a considerable quantity of water. There are 72 parts of carbon, 10 of hydrogen, and 80 of oxygen in 162 parts of starch and sugar. In oils and fats, we have 66 parts of carbon, 10 of hydrogen, and 8 of oxygen in 84 parts of fat; or we will put them thus—

	Starch.	Fat.
Carbon	72	66
Hydrogen	10	10
Oxygen	80	8
	162	84

So that you see, if we take away some of the oxygen from the first, we shall have the hydrogen left pure for combustion. Now, this change seems to be easily accomplished. When starch and sugar are taken into the system, they are usually decomposed by the action of the oxygen in the blood. The hydrogen is oxidized, and water is formed, whilst the oxygen remains with the carbon, and forms carbonic acid, which is given off; so that, as Liebig remarks, "no true combustion of carbon occurs in the living body, but the carbonic acid is formed by a process of substitution in this case—one of decay or slow oxidation from a body rich in hydrogen, the hydrogen of which is oxidized and removed, and replaced by one or more equivalents of oxygen." Now, if the supply of oxygen is equal to that of the starch and sugar, there would be no formation of fat; but, under a variety of natural circumstances, either the oxygen is deficient, or the supply of sugar and starch is redundant. Under these circumstances, other changes go on. We know, for instance, that sugar, when fermented, gives off carbonic acid, and yields a substance called alcohol, which is much richer in carbon and hydrogen than sugar. Now, it would appear that a similar process goes on in the animal body; not, however, a true alcoholic fermentation, but the sugar in the blood loses carbonic acid in such proportions that it becomes converted into fat. It appears that this process may even take place in the stomach, and that in some persons a kind of fatty fermentation, as we may call it, takes place in the food in the alimentary canal, and leads to an unnatural kind of obesity. There is some evidence to show that this change may go on in the liver, and that the sugar in that organ is converted into fatty matter. At any rate, however far we may be from comprehending the exact seat and nature of these changes, there can be little doubt that our starchy and saccharine food is capable of being converted into fat.

On this subject there was formerly a dispute between the French and German chemists, the former maintaining that all the fat of the body was derived from fat contained originally in the vegetable food of animals, and they were very diligent in their analysis of all kinds of vegetable food, to show that it contained fat. Here is a table which gives you the quantities of fat contained in one hundred parts of various kinds of vegetable food—

Potatoes	0·2	Rice	0·7
Wheat-flour	1·2	Beans	2·0
Barley-meal	0·3	Cocoa	50·0
Oatmeal	5·7	Lentils	2·0
Indian-meal	7·7	Buckwheat	1·0
Rye	1·0	Tea	4·0
Peas	2·0	Coffee	12·0

Now, if animals, such as calves or sheep, are placed in circumstances to get fat, that is, kept in warm houses, and not allowed to run about and feed with any of their ordinary food, they will have much more fat in their bodies than could be accounted for by the quantity of fat in their food.

In this controversy Liebig brought forward the case of the celebrated Strasburg goose, which is an animal that has to submit, for the sake of the luxuries of mankind, to a very peculiar operation. It is tied down to a board and put in front of a fire, which appears very cruel; but it does not hinder the animal from getting fat. It is fed with barley-meal, and it thus takes in much more starch than is necessary to maintain its heat, and the consequence is, the starch is converted into fat, and deposited in greatest abundance in the liver. The goose is then killed, the liver is taken out, and these distended livers are the precious *morceaux* contained in the *pâté de foie gras*. But there are other cases which seem to establish this great fact. Wax is a sort of fat; and Professor Milne Edwards took a number of bees, weighed them, and then put them under a glass jar with sugar. The bees were taken at that season of the year when they were making their cells and forming large quantities of wax. Next day he took the comb, and the sugar, and the bees, and weighed them. The bees had neither lost nor gained; but the sugar had lost exactly as much as the wax produced. This shows that the bees had the power of converting the sugar into wax; and in this experiment we have almost a crucial instance of the fact. Then we may conclude from this, that where fatty matter is not taken in food, there the sugar will be converted into adipose tissue. But then this process is a laborious process to the system, and there seems to be no doubt that it is more easy to supply it directly from the vegetable or animal kingdom, by taking those substances which contain oil or fat.

The sources of oil or fat in the vegetable kingdom are very numerous. Besides the articles of food I have before mentioned, a large number of seeds of plants contain oil in large quantities. Let me shortly describe some of these. A source of oil which is extensively employed in this country is the almond (*Amygdalus communis*). The seeds of this plant are known in the shops under the name of sweet and bitter almonds. The sweet almonds are eaten alone at dessert, and enter into the composition of cakes, custards, &c.; but the bitter almonds are employed only for the sake of the peculiar volatile oil they contain. They both, however, contain the bland oil which is sold as almond-oil. It is obtained by expression from the bruised seeds, which are first blanched. This process consists in removing the skins from the outside of the almond-seed. Almond-oil contains margarine, but in less quantity than olive-oil, so that it stands the cold better. The dry remains of the almonds, after the oil is expressed, is sold for detergent purposes under the name of almond paste.

The almond belongs to the same natural order of plants (*Amygdalaceæ*) as the apricot, peach, nectarine, plum, and cherry. The almonds correspond to the seeds or kernels of these fruits, and the shell of the almond is the same organ as the stone of the other fruits. The almond is covered with a dry green shell, which has none of the pleasant flavour of the same part of the fruit in the peach and other similar fruits.

The chestnut (*Castanea vesca*) is another seed containing a considerable quantity of oil, which is used by man as food. This seed does not come to perfection in this country, although we have some glorious examples of the tree, especially in Greenwich Park, of which it is the great ornament. The nuts consumed in this country are principally brought from France and Spain. They are usually eaten in this country at dessert or as a pleasant morsel; but in the south of Europe the peasantry eat them as a substantial article of diet.

Various species of plants belonging to the walnut family yield seeds which are eaten in this country, as well as on the continent of Europe and the United States of America. Besides the common walnuts, which are the produce of the *Juglans regia*, which is commonly cultivated in Europe, there is the Peccan or

Pekan nut, the produce of the *Juglans olivæformis*, and the hickory-nuts from the *Carya alba*. The Souari, Swarrow, or butter-nuts, are highly esteemed on account of their pleasant flavour. They are also obtained from a tree belonging to the walnut family called *Caryocar butyrosum*. These are all the produce of the New World.

The Brazil-nuts, which are also brought from the New World, contain a great deal of oil. They are the produce of a plant called *Bertholletia excelsa*. The seeds are contained in a hard wooden fruit, which is so large and hard in some species of the same family as to give them the name of cannon-ball trees. The Sapucaya-nuts are the produce of a tree belonging to the same family. The fruit is hard and large, and bursts by the removal of a kind of lid, which leaves the rest of the fruit in the form of a cup. These are called monkey-cups. It is said that several monkeys will thrust their hands into these cups, and when each has filled its hand, they cannot get them out again, and as they are too greedy to let go, they are often caught in this way.

The hazel-nut is another instance of a seed containing oil. It is the produce of the *Corylus avellana*. Nut-oil is expressed and used by watchmakers. The hazel is found wild in England, and is also extensively cultivated; the nuts are then called cob-nuts or filberts. Filbert is a corruption of full beard, a name given to the nut from its bracts extending over the fruit. Large quantities are also imported into this country from Spain. In addition to those grown in this country,

140,000 bushels are imported, the value of which is about £90,000.

The seeds of many of the palms yield fixed oils, especially the palm tree (*Elais guineensis*) of Africa. The seed of the cocoa-nut palm (*Cocos nucifera*) is used as a substantive article of diet in Ceylon, and many parts of the East Indies (Fig. 3). It is imported into this country for the sake of the oil it contains. The milk in the interior of the seed is a bland fluid, and, when the nut is fresh-gathered, is a cool and pleasant drink. In the young state the seeds of most palms are filled with a cool fluid consisting mostly of water. This fluid is drunk by the inhabitants of the countries in which they grow. The double cocoa-nut of the Seychelles Islands (*Lodoicea Seychellarum*) contains sometimes as much as fourteen pints of water, and is drunk by sailors touching on these islands with great relish. Even the hard ivory-nut (*Phytelephas macrocarpa*) contains, when young, a fluid which is drunk by the natives of the countries in which it grows.

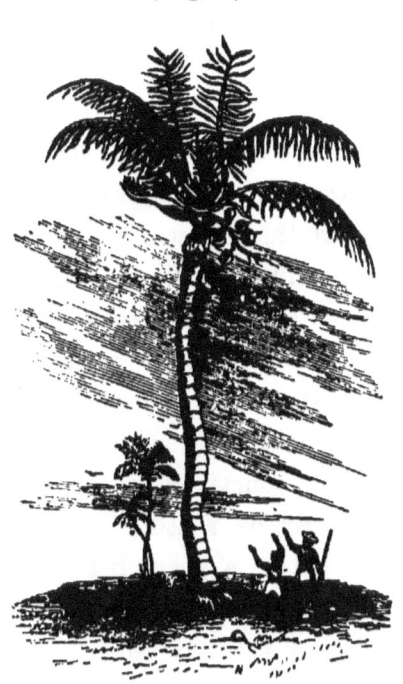

Fig. 3.—Cocos nucifera.

Another seed containing oil is the earth-nut. This is the fruit of a trailing leguminous plant (*Arachis hypogæa*, Fig. 4). It is cultivated in Africa and the tropical parts of Asia and America. The seeds yield a bland oil, which is expressed and eaten as salad-oil. The pods containing the seeds are roasted, and are thus imported into this country, and frequently eaten at dessert.

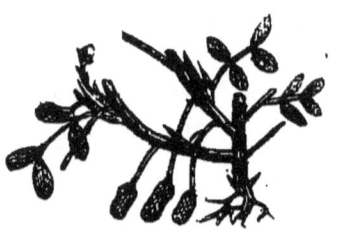

Fig. 4.—*Arachis hypogæa.*

Other seeds less known, and eaten in this country, are the Pistacio nut, the produce of the *Pistacia vera*, a tree much cultivated in the Greek Islands. It is extensively consumed by the Turks and the Greeks. Then there is the Cashew-nut (*Anacardium occidentale*), from the West Indies. The shells contain a remarkably acrid oil, which, from a recent case in the criminal courts, seems to be capable of destroying life. It should be roasted before it is eaten, and then it is regarded as a great luxury. Chicha-nuts, pine-seeds, and beech-nuts are also occasionally eaten, on account of the oil they contain.

Amongst vegetable foods yielding oil, the cocoa or chocolate plant (*Theobroma Cacao*) is one of the most remarkable. The seeds of this plant contain 50 per cent. of a hard oil or butter. Of the other dietetical properties of this seed I must speak in a future lecture.

A bread is made at Gaboon, in Africa, from the seeds of the *Mangifera gabonensis*, called Dica or Odika bread, an article of diet originally described in the *Journal of the Society of Arts*, by Mr. P. L. Simonds.

By simple boiling in water, from 70 to 80 per cent. of fat can be extracted from this bread. In this respect these seeds resemble chocolate, and it is not impossible that they might be used in Europe in the same way. They are exceedingly abundant in Gaboon.

The last plant yielding an edible oil, to which I shall allude, is the Olive (*Olea europæa*, Fig. 5). This plant is cultivated extensively in France, Italy, and Spain. When the fruit is young it is pickled in salt, and eaten to give a relish to wine. When ripe, the fruit contains oil in great abundance, and it is the only instance I know of any other part than the seed yielding a fixed edible oil. The *Madia sativa* yields oil in all parts of its structure, but this oil is not eaten. Although the olive will grow in this country in the open air, it will not perfect its fruit. Between 11,000 and 12,000 gallons of this oil are annually imported into this country. It is called salad-oil, and is principally consumed as a dressing in salads. It is much more largely consumed on the Continent, where it takes the place of butter. It is a very wholesome food, and it would be well if people in this country would cultivate a taste for its use, especially in making salads. In this country these very valuable adjuncts to our food are rendered exceedingly disagreeable; first, by the want of drying the plant used, and in the next, by its

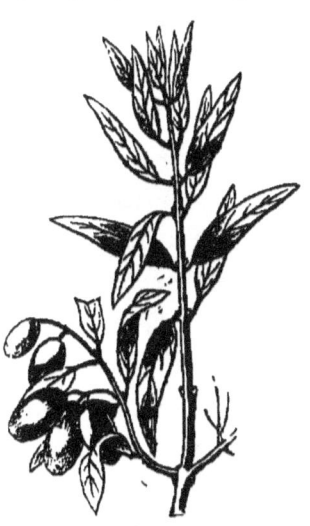

Fig. 5.—*Olea europæa*.

being deluged with vinegar. A salad properly prepared should have the leaves of the plants used dried to such an extent that they will readily absorb the dressing poured over them, which should consist of two-thirds or three-fourths olive-oil. I need not also add that the oil should not be rancid; but such is the thorough carelessness with which these articles are put on our tables, that in nine cases out of ten, the oil is rancid and unfit for use. This, perhaps, accounts for the flood of vinegar to drown its flavour.

Then the animal kingdom supplies us with a certain quantity of fatty matter, and the most important source is the milk of the higher animals, which contains 8 per cent. of carbonaceous matter, and 4 per cent. of that is butter. This rises to the top of the milk, and we take it off under the name of cream. The cream is beaten, and a certain quantity of the caseine and water which was in the cream is churned out, under the name of buttermilk. I am not able to distinguish between the action of butter and these oils. It, however, contains a substance known by the name of butyric acid, which forms compounds which, in the earlier stages of butter-making, are agreeable to our notions of what is pleasant; but it is the continued evolution of this butyric acid which makes butter so objectionable when it becomes rancid. In fact, all animal oils have the power of forming butyric acid, and those who have not smelt it may get a vivid idea of it by sniffing train-oil in an advanced state of decomposition. It does not appear to act as a poison, for sometimes persons have been recommended to take codliver-oil when it is rancid. I am not, however, aware that there is any benefit to be got out of rancid oils. In Kamschatka, and many parts of the world where they are in the habit of keeping their animal oil a long time before it is consumed, a taste for this rancidity is acquired, and rancid oil is relished more than the fresh oils.

The quantity of fat contained in different kinds of animal food differs very much. The table to which I now draw your attention will enable you to select your food according to the quantity of fat it contains. The proportion of fat is given for one hundred parts of each kind of food.

Milk (cow's)	3·5		Mutton	40·0
„ (human)	3·0		Cheese	25·0
„ (ass's)	1·5		Salmon	5·0
„ (goat's)	5·0		Herring	6·0
Pork	50·0		Mackerel	7·0
Veal	16·0		Soles	0·25
Beef	30·0		Cod	2·0

In studying this table we must recollect that the fat in the milk is what we call butter. I would call your attention to the fact that goat's milk is richer in butter than any other milk. Of course, all these substances vary in the quantity of flesh-forming matters they contain. Amongst the meats, pork has the most fat, and veal the least. Amongst the fish, mackerel and herring are those which contain most oil, and soles the least.

After saying thus much in favour of oil, I think I ought to say that in some cases it seems to act very injuriously on the sytem. The stomach gets into a state in which the oil of the food is rapidly decomposed, and butyric acid is formed. The stomach rebels at this compound, and tries to get rid of it, and that unpleasant taste in the throat is produced, which is called "biliousness." This is the very common fate of those who indulge in hot bread steeped in melting butter, or in food prepared with unctuous sauces. The cure for it is very simple, when the cause is known; but as long as people think it is bile, they will have recourse to "antibilious pills," and the results are an injured stomach, impure blood, serious disease, and not unfrequently an untimely grave.

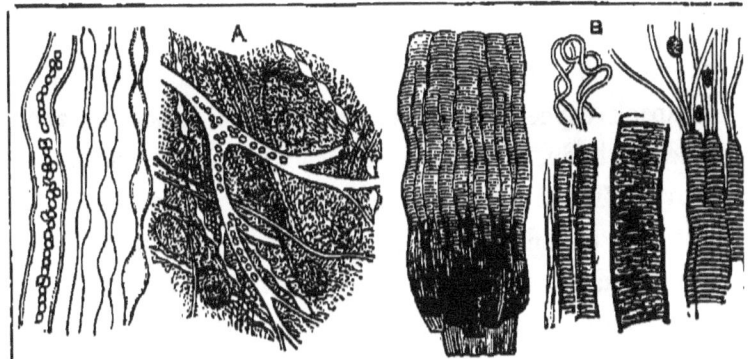

Fig. 1.
A. *Nervous tissue under microscope.*   B. *Muscular ditto.*

ON FLESH-FORMING FOODS.

IN this Lecture I shall draw your attention to the flesh-forming groups of food, and you must allow me to point once more to our table of the constituents of food. You will see we first went over the water and the saline substances of food, and then we came to the force-giving foods, and we took up, first, sugar and starch, and then oleaginous matters—the animal and vegetable oils.

Now we come to the fourth group, which are those foods that give flesh to the body. We found that the starch and the sugar and the oil were taken into the body for the purpose of maintaining animal heat. We found that some of the oil remained in the system, and formed what we call adipose tissue, but that is not a tissue that performs any distinguishing vital functions. We do not think by the aid of fat, nor form the muscles by its assistance. Then to-day I have to speak especially of those substances which, entering into the body, form those tissues by which we think and move. These foods are called nutritious; and they are not only called nutritious, but also nitrogenous. They are called nitrogenous from the fact of their containing, in addition to carbon, hydrogen, and oxygen,—nitrogen in combination. The nitrogen, then, is a distinct element of their composition—hence the term nitrogenous is applied to them.

Now, if you will consider for a moment the nature of the processes of nutrition that go on in the body—the nature of the laws of growth and decay—you will see that there must be materials supplied from day to day to enable the body to grow, to be renewed, and, in fact, to live. These processes, then, may be studied quite independent of those which I have mentioned before, which produce animal heat; and they are carried on by the agency of a set of organs which are called the nervous and the muscular systems. When we examine the muscles and the nerves under the microscope, we find them presenting the forms which you see in the accompanying diagrams. (Fig. 1, A and B.)

If we take a portion of brain (for brain is nervous matter), or a portion of muscle, and examine them chemically, we shall find that they not only contain carbon, hydrogen, and oxygen, but that they contain in addition nitrogen. Thus it is that we find these four elements in those tissues which we believe are essential to what we call vital processes. You see the fatty matter may be introduced into any part of the body quite independently of any necessity for its existence.

Persons may get very fat or very thin, and yet their nerves and muscles act in the same manner. But if the food which supplies nervous matter or muscle is diminished, then they become unable to perform the functions of life. Now these four elements, carbon, hydrogen, oxygen, and nitrogen, are called organic elements because of their universal presence in the living and growing parts of both plants and animals. We have no part of an animal and no part of a plant growing and living, and performing its functions, unless these four elements are present. Hence, when the German poet sang his punch song, he seemed to have had a prescient view of modern chemical research—

"Vier Elemente innig gesellt
Bilden das Natur bauen die Welt."

"Four elements, intimately mixed, form all nature and build up the world." And certainly that is true of the world of organic beings.

Now just in the same manner as a fire goes out unless we put on fuel—unless we put on additional material as fuel—so in the case of the action of this muscular and nervous matter we find that the material is exhausted by use. We think by the aid of our brain—of the nervous matter of which it is composed—and in this way every time we think we exhaust or destroy a certain portion of nervous matter; and if we went on thinking, if we went on feeling and perceiving,—exerting this nervous system,—the nervous system would at last become entirely exhausted, unless new materials replaced the old ones that were used. During these thinking and perceiving processes the little cells of which it is composed appear to be actually destroyed: so that every time we think we sacrifice a quantity of nervous matter. So it is with the muscles. The muscular matter is composed of little cells, which are united together in the form of fibres, which have the power of contraction, and every time a muscle is used it contracts, and there is a destruction of muscular matter. Just as we have no flame from the candle, nor heat from the fire, without fuel, so we have no nervous action, no thought, no muscular movement, no power, unless there exists the materials of change. Just as in the one case the heating process chemically changes the material on the fire, so the vital processes, incessantly acting in the system, change and consume the materials of our food. But the materials of which we now speak do not pass off directly, as they do in the case of the materials which constitute the food which gives us animal heat.

The nervous tissue and the muscular tissue, after they have performed their functions, throw back their tissue into the blood, and it is from the blood that the material is got rid of which has been consumed in the action of the muscular and nervous systems. Now that both muscular and nervous action depend upon the materials of our food, can be easily ascertained by the performance of a very simple experiment. Let a person begin his daily work without his breakfast, and when dinner-time comes go on with his work; then, whether his work be mental or physical, the missing his food will begin to tell. But let him go on, and what is the consequence? Why, we see at last a time comes when the nerves refuse to do their duty, when sensation is not present, when the brain cannot think, and persons sink into a state of unconsciousness. Not only the nervous system, but the muscular system is affected in this way, until at last the starved man is unable to move hand or foot, and dies. Here, then, lies the necessity for the taking of food; the materials of which we are composed are constantly passing away. We are in a state of perennial moult,—I use the word moult intentionally. You know that animals throw off certain parts of their body at certain seasons of the year, and we call that moulting. We apply the term to the periodical casting off of their feathers, hairs, and other epidermal appendages. Crabs and lobsters throw off their shell altogether, birds their feathers, and horses their hair; but in the human being we find this process of moulting is going on constantly—our skin rubs off, our mucous membrane wears away, and our internal organs, all of them, disappear by a similar process, so that I calculate a human being loses about the fortieth part of his weight every day, and in this way you will find that the vital organs of the human body are renewed every forty days. Physiologists formerly supposed that this was a longer process. Taking, for instance, the growth of the hair and nails in certain parts of the body, they supposed that their moulting was the measure of the duration of every part of the body; but if you examine this subject, and calculate the quantity of food we take every day, you will see the period cannot be longer than forty days, in which we take in a bulk of food equivalent to the mass of our bodies, and that this must have passed away in order to make room for the new matters. Thus there is not only a necessity for taking in food which maintains the heat of the body, but there is a necessity for taking the food which maintains the functions of the nervous and muscular systems.

Then this waste of which I have been speaking is the result of the activity of our nervous and muscular systems, and the material for its production is supplied, not by the starch, nor by the sugar, nor by the water, nor by the fat which we take as food, but by the substances of which I am now more particularly to speak.

There are two sources of this kind of food: the first is the vegetable world, and the second is the animal world. But I shall have to show you here that the vegetable—the plant—is the original source of these substances; for, although we take them from animals, they have first obtained them from plants. Thus the ox and the sheep, which we consume in the form of beef and mutton, have not fed on flesh; they have fed on the grass of the field, on hay, on oats, on peas and beans, on vegetable products, and it is from plants they have derived the flesh which we consume as food.

Let us now see what these substances are composed of. I say they are identical in plants and animals,—animals deriving them from plants,—and they undergo little or no change when taken into the animal system. We take certain substances from plants and animals, and find that they are identical in composition, and that whether we take them from the plant or the animal is a matter of indifference, provided we digest them and make them into blood.

Now the substances which we thus use as food possess considerable chemical interest, and present considerable variations in animals and plants, but I must refer you to chemical manuals for a fuller account of them than I can give here. The three most important forms which they assume in our food are called albumen, fibrine, and caseine. These substances are found in both the animal and vegetable kingdoms. Let us speak first of albumen. Albumen is a substance which is known to exist in the animal kingdom, and we are familiarly acquainted with it as contained in the white of the egg; that is one source of it which is very commonly known, and therefore I speak of it first. And also on this account: that a property which this albumen possesses is well exemplified in the very common process of boiling an egg. You know after you have broken the shell of a boiled egg you get the outside hard and white; now that outside consists of albumen, the inside yellow part called the yolk, also consists principally of albumen, and exhibits the property of coagulating by heat. There are some other places in which albumen is found in the animal system. It is this form of nitrogenous matter which is taken up into the system to form the nervous substance, and with it are formed all those delicate organisms which are called nerves. Nervous matter consists of about 7 per cent. of albumen, not a very large quantity, but still this matter must be regarded by us as an intensely interesting product, because it is the material by which we are put in relation with the external world. It is this which enables us to see, to hear, to taste, to smell, and to feel. It is this which enables us to think, to feel, and to be conscious of our existence. All this depends upon the condition of the albumen in our system. Although we may sit at our breakfast partaking of the daily egg, thinking of other things, yet the laws by which the egg becomes the source of our thought is worth a little consideration.

Another source of albumen in the animal kingdom is the blood which circulates through the system of animals. It is composed of water, of albumen, and of fibrine—of water principally. If we say fibrine about one quarter per cent., albumen 7 per cent., globules and salts 13 per cent., and water 80 per cent., you have an approximation to its real composition. From this you will see the importance of albumen. It is the material out of which all our organs are formed.

Albumen is not, however, confined to the animal kingdom. I have said all animals must obtain this substance from the vegetable kingdom, and we accordingly find it in plants. Although it is not so often present among plants as fibrine and caseine, yet we find it sufficiently frequent to be able to identify it. It is not, however, necessary to supply this substance in its pure form in order to have it deposited in the body. In the stomach there is a power of converting caseine and fibrine into albumen. The albumen that is introduced into the stomach is cooked, deprived, as it were, of the vital property, and therefore it has to be revitalised, made again into albumen and a living substance, and it is then that it is taken up into the blood. It is the same with fibrine and caseine.

Then, I say, there are some plants which contain albumen. Here I have a series of analyses containing the quantities of the flesh-forming matters, the produce of various kinds of food, and you will find that some of them contain albumen.

ON FLESH-FORMING FOODS.

Comparative Chemical Composition of one pound of various Kinds of Vegetable Food.

	Water.	Ashes.	HEAT-GIVERS.			FLESH-FORMERS.			ACCESSORIES.	
			Starch.	Fat.	Sugar.	Gluten.	Caseine.	Albumen.	Cellulose.	Gum.
	oz. gr.	oz. gr.	oz. gr.	oz. gr.	oz. gr.	oz. gr.	oz. gr.	oz. gr.	oz. gr.	oz. gr.
1 lb. of Wheat	2 106	— 112	9 242	— 84	— 385	2 21	— —	— 126	— 119	— 119
,, Barley	2 106	— 293	7 297	— 20	— 265	2 22	— —	— —	2 50	— 258
,, Oats	2 78	— 210	6 153	— 397	— 378	2 316	— —	— —	2 6	— 210
,, Rice	2 70	— 34	11 380	— 48	— 27	1 17	— —	— —	— —	— 68
,, Rye	2 35	— 122	8 79	1 —	— 262	1 318	— —	— 213	1 230	— 371
,, Maize	2 105	— 70	9 262	— 66	— 21	1 402	— —	— —	— 284	— 21
,, Beans	2 161	— 245	5 333	— 101	— 140	— —	3 368	— —	1 350	1 156
,, Peas	2 112	— 175	5 403	— 140	— 140	— —	3 324	— —	1 206	1 193
,, Lentils	2 105	— 105	5 262	— 140	— 140	— —	4 70	— —	2 263	1 153
,, Buckwheat...	2 118	— 126	8 —	— 70	— 140	1 165	— —	— —	3 114	— 140
,, Potatoes.....	12 —	— 64	2 219	— 15	— 223	— 100	— —	— —	— 224	— 30

Let us take rye: 1 lb. of rye contains 318 grains of gluten and 213 grains of albumen. Rye is a very nutritious article of diet on that account. 1 lb. of wheaten flour contains 2 ounces of gluten, and a quarter of an ounce of albumen—much less than in the rye, but still a sufficient quantity of albumen to be recognized. Potatoes also contain a small quantity of albumen, and there are other plants, carrots, turnips, cabbages, and asparagus, all of which contain albumen.

Now, by taking any of these plants, and crushing and squeezing them, you may get the albumen suspended in the water, in the same way that you get it in the white of egg, or in blood. You may easily ascertain the presence of albumen by a simple experiment, and that consists in exposing it to heat, when it coagulates. Albumen will not only coagulate by heat, but by a variety of substances. It may be thrown down from its solutions by mineral acids, especially nitric acid. In this way we may test for albumen independently of fibrine and caseine. I may just add, that alcohol throws down albumen in this way; and you may see in this fact how alcohol may prevent the proper digestion of food, especially when taken in the form of ardent spirits, as gin, brandy, whiskey, rum, &c. It throws down the albumen and wastes it, and unless the stomach has the power of taking it up again, you see, such food is lost. That is one of the great mischiefs of drinking distilled spirits: it has the power of coagulating the albumen which ought to go into the blood. To be sure, there are persons who are able to bear this, but it frequently commences that series of morbid changes which terminate the spirit-drinker's life, by depriving the nervous tissue of nourishment. This is one of the causes of *delirium tremens*, the drunkard's mania. If you withdraw the alcohol, and take every pains to introduce food which will digest, and the system has sufficient strength left, you may cure a man even of this dreadful malady.

Passing on from albumen, I come to speak of fibrine. Now, fibrine is much more abundant in the vegetable kingdom than albumen: we do not know the reason, for there is very little difference in the chemical composition of these things, very little indeed. But there is a difference in their properties—fibrine is not soluble in water, and when suspended in any liquid, easily separates. We find it in the blood at the rate of about a quarter per cent. If we draw blood, and set it aside for a few minutes, a clot is produced, and the fibrine entangles the red blood globules which circulate in the blood, and they form the clot. It is the fibrine separating from the blood which does this; this property of spontaneous coagulation is one of the characteristics of fibrine.

Then, fibrine is not only found in the blood of animals, but it constitutes the whole of their muscular tissue. Just as we find that the nervous cell is composed of albumen, we find the muscular cell is principally composed of fibrine. Fibrine may be procured from muscles, but it is more easily procured from blood. We can also obtain fibrine from wheat flour, which has the same property. Fibrine, as it occurs in plants, is called gluten. At the latter end of the last century, an Italian, of the name of Beccaria, washed flour, and got away all the starch, and found he had left this substance—a substance which he called gluten, from its adhesive, sticky nature. A curious thing about this discovery was that he described it very accurately, stated that it produced compounds precisely similar to the flesh of animals, and that in decomposition it gave out precisely the same smell; and yet no one, until lately, even suspected there was the slightest identity between this substance and the tissues of the animal. In fact, until 1838, it was generally believed that there was no nitrogenous substance in the vegetable kingdom, and you will find in the text books on physiology of that period, that whilst it was stated that animals contained nitrogen, the vegetable kingdom had none.

Fibrine is contained in a variety of plants:—wheat, oats, rye, rice, and so on. Now, it is this fibrine which supplies us with the principal materials of our nutrition, for we feed on these things in larger quantities than on the flesh of animals, or any form of food which contains albumen.

There is a third form of these substances, which is called caseine. This is the substance which we separate from milk under the name of cheese. It differs from albumen and fibrine from its being held in solution by a free alkali in the milk, and when you add the slightest quantity of acid to the milk it separates in the form of curds—you know what curds and whey are? I shall not dwell on the properties of this caseine in the animal kingdom to-day, because in the next lecture I shall allude to animal food. But I will just add, that it is found in the milk of the higher orders of animals, and also in certain plants; beans, peas, and lentils contain it, and, in fact, all plants belonging to the order or family *Leguminosæ*. It is sometimes called legumin when obtained from the seed, but in all its properties it resembles caseine, so that Liebig and other chemists have had no hesitation in pronouncing that legumin and caseine are identical.

Now, these three substances, which I have told you were present in plants and animals, were at one time supposed to be the peculiar products of the animal system, and it was supposed that the animal system had the power of forming them out of vegetable food. Thus chemists and physiologists, not suspecting that they were in the peas, beans, or anything that man ate, supposed that the system had the power of inducing the nitrogen of the air to unite with starch, sugar, and other materials, and thus to constitute the materials of our muscles and nerves. That was the theory before 1838, when Mulder, a Dutch chemist, struck with the fact that these substances were much more frequent in the vegetable kingdom than they had been supposed to be, made special analyses of all kinds of vegetable food; and found that in every case he could obtain substances closely resembling the albumen, fibrine, and caseine of the animal kingdom. But, further than this, he performed experiments which have led to the adoption of a theory of the nature of these substances which has had considerable influence on our physiological views. He submitted albumen, fibrine, and caseine to the action of potash; and, having obtained solutions of these substances, he added an acid, and he always got a precipitate thrown down which he believed to be a substance common to the whole of them. Now this substance he called protein, from a Greek word, πρωτευω, signifying "I stand first."

Mulder's protein is a substance which has produced perhaps more discussion than any other substance in the whole range of chemical inquiry; for, no sooner had Mulder announced this discovery than it was adopted by Liebig, and Liebig was the first to make known the nature and properties of protein to a British public. When Mulder accused Liebig of having announced this discovery without giving him the credit of making it, Liebig had advanced sufficiently in his knowledge of the subject to doubt the very existence of protein, and, accordingly, asked Mulder what protein was? Mulder very properly replied that as Liebig had understood it so well as to point out where it existed in a variety of substances in which he did not know of it before, and had given it a composition of his own, he probably knew as much about it as he did, and therefore declined answering the question. At the present moment the chemical world is divided. Some chemists deny its existence as a separate substance, while others say that the only consistent view of the nature of albumen, fibrine, and caseine is, that they have protein for their common base. Be this as it may, you can go and ask for an ounce of protein, and get it, in a chemist's shop. It is of no use, therefore, saying there is no such a thing. The cause of the dispute has arisen from the great difficulty in investigating the true composition of a substance composed of so large a number of atoms of the elements of which it is formed. Thus, if we write down Mulder's formula—one atom of this substance is composed of 36 atoms of carbon, 27 of hydrogen, 5 of nitrogen, and 12 of oxygen—you see what an immense number of atoms a single atom of this substance is composed of; and a chemist, in endeavouring to ascertain what the composition really is, is unable to come to a conclusion as to how protein differs from caseine, or albumen, or fibrine, more than they do from each other. That seems to me the main point of the whole discussion; the difficulty of estimating the difference is so great, that a chemist may say that he cannot make it out. But then the theory comes to help us out of a difficulty. If protein is the base of all these, it is easy to see that they can be converted one into the other. Protein serves us immensely as a general term, for frequently it is difficult to say whether you are dealing with fibrine, albumen, or caseine, so that you can speak of them as protein, or as a proteinaceous substance.

Now we find that this protein is always present, under certain circumstances in both plants and animals. If you take a vegetable cell, and examine it under the microscope, you will frequently find in it a little spot, which Robert Brown called a nucleus, and Schleiden a cytoblast. The cell appears to grow upon the nucleus. (Fig. 2.) In both the vegetable and animal kingdom we find these nucleated cells. In the interior of the cells of the nerves (Fig. 1, A), and wherever we find cells in the human body, in the animal or the vegetable kingdom, there we find nuclei, and there is good reason to believe that the cells have been

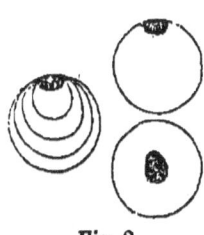

Fig. 2.

built upon this foundation. (Fig. 3.) This nucleus or cytoblast is composed of protein, so that protein is uni-

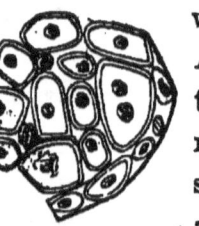

Fig. 3.

versally present in plants and animals. As I have said before, it is composed of the four elements, carbon, hydrogen, nitrogen, and oxygen, and now you see how it is that there can be no animal and no plant without these four elements, because there can be no cell without being built upon this nucleus or cytoblast, which is always composed of albumen, fibrine, or caseine. This substance lies at the foundation of all life, and is also called protoplasm. There can be no vegetable or animal life, and no cell life, unless there is this protoplasm.

Then we find no indication in the animal system that an animal has the power of forming this substance of itself. None of those minute animals that live in water,—the infusorial animalcules, or animals that live on land,—have the power of going to the mineral kingdom, and taking up in a mineral form the elements which enter into the composition of protein, but the plant has this power.

The plant has the power of converting the dead inanimate mineral substances into the necessary vital products of the whole organic kingdom. Thus we find the animal feeding upon the plant, and everywhere the vegetable kingdom is spread before us in the world as a feast for the animal creation; wherever you see minute fungi or confervæ growing in water or on land, you find animals ready to consume them, and man himself is not an exception to the law. We must ultimately obtain the fibrine, the caseine, and the albumen, from the vegetable kingdom. We take it directly from the vegetable, from peas, from beans, from wheat, oats, and maize; we take it from these directly, but we take it only indirectly when we take it from beef, mutton, game, or fish, the products of the animal world. These animals have, however, gone first to the vegetable kingdom, and appropriated the protein in their nerves and muscles, and we, for the sake of digesting such food more easily, slay these animals and eat them, and in doing this we do that which a whole group of animals are doing from day to day, and which have no power, like ourselves, of appropriating vegetable food at all.

Now let me call your attention to the vegetable food which contains these substances, reserving the forms of animal food which contain them for consideration till the next Lecture. In speaking of the albumen, I may say we have little vegetable food which contains albumen alone. All the plants, or parts of plants, we eat, contain gluten or fibrine in larger quantities than albumen. At the same time, at certain seasons of the year, we all appreciate asparagus, cabbages, broccoli, and cauliflowers, and this group of plants contains albumen; but fibrine is the form of the proteinaceous substances from which we derive the largest quantity of our flesh-forming food, and this fibrine is contained in wheat, barley, oats, rye, maize, rice, potatoes, and a great number of other vegetable foods.

You will see, in the table of the constituents of food, the proportions in which these are found; they are there presented to the eye: and we will now proceed to speak of some of the plants which produce them. Now, looking at our table, you will see that suet fat and butter contain no flesh-forming substances. Beer contains but 1 per cent. of nutritive matter, and is, therefore, not a thing to be taken for nutrition, at all. Benjamin Franklin discovered that, long before modern chemistry discovered the reason. Carrots only yield 1 per cent. of flesh-forming food, turnips only 1 per cent., and potatoes only 2; while even sago, tapioca, and arrowroot, composed principally of starch, yet contain as large a quantity of nutritive matter. You will recollect, as a practical result of our investigation, that such kinds of food should not be taken as substantive articles of diet. Those who live on turnips, potatoes, parsnips, or carrots, must, sooner or later, find out their mistake. A neighbouring nation tried to live upon potatoes, until Providence seemed to interfere to prevent the waste attendant on living on such food. It seems as if the necessity of consuming this food in such enormous quantities led to that excessive culture by the poor Irish, which at last invited, if it did not engender, that disease which destroyed the potato crop. There seemed to be a delusion about the potato crop among the Irish. They supposed that, because they got a larger quantity of potatoes than wheat by weight on a given quantity of land, that they obtained more nutriment; but a bag of 100 lbs. of potatoes contains no more nutriment than 13 lbs. of wheat.

Then there is rice, containing 6 per cent. of nutritive matter; cocoa-nibs, 10 per cent.; Indian maize, 11 per cent.; wheaten flour, 13 per cent.; barley-meal, 14 per cent.; oatmeal, 18 per cent.; dry peas, 23 per cent.; and cheese, with its caseine, 31 per cent.

Now, you see, by the table, the value of the articles of food, in relation to the nutrition of the system,—to the supply of the stuff out of which nerves and muscles are made; but what you do not see there, and which is a subject to which I would draw your attention at once,—you do not see how much of that matter would be digested if you were to take it. Now, if you will take a piece of Suffolk cheese,—and, although it is all nutritive matter, you would find, if you were to take this into your stomach, that you would not digest it. If you did not digest it, it would be of no value, as it could not pass into the blood. Now, it is one drawback upon the use of caseine as food, that, when it is once separated from the fluids from which it is obtained, it is indigestible; and it is only when it contains large quantities of oil, that it becomes more digestible. Thus, you see, peas and beans, with their great quantity of nutritive matter, not being so digestible as other substances, are not so valuable as articles of diet. It is, therefore, those substances which contain fibrine and albumen which are the most important articles of vegetable food to man. These we mostly obtain from the order *Graminaceæ*, or grasses,—wheat, barley, oats, rye, rice, maize, and the millets, which are the representatives of the others in the parts of the world where they grow. In many parts of Africa, and other parts of the world, millet is consumed in large quantities.

The cereal used in largest quantity is wheat; and I would, therefore, draw your attention to wheat first. With regard to its composition, there would appear to be quite as much, if not more, nutritive matter in oats,—a larger quantity of saline matter, and, in fact, of all those constituents of food which are necessary to the production of the tissues, the maintenance of the animal heat, and the supply of mineral materials to the body. With regard, also, to barley, we find that barley has the same capabilities as oats; it contains all the constituents of wheat and of oats. We may also say, with regard to maize, that it contains the same constituents,—starch, nutritive matter, and saline matters,—even in larger quantities than the oats and wheat; and, in addition to them, it contains a very large quantity of fatty matter— of oily matter, which is not found in wheat, in barley, or in oats. Why, then, has wheat been consumed so largely by the most polished nations on the surface of the earth? Why do barley, oats, rice, maize, and millet constantly succumb to wheat? Where wheat will grow, there it has been grown — in India and China—and where people can get wheat, they will have it. I have no other explanation to offer except that wheaten flour alone, of all these farinaceous foods, will make fermented bread. I do not know, however, that the time may not come when we shall find that the fermented bread of wheat flour is not so good as the unfermented bread from the flour of other grains, and that we may not have occasion to change our habits in this respect. But at the present time wheat is consumed. Its produce is more abundant in districts of a higher temperature than our own, and it is always cultivated in this country with difficulty. Our really natural grains are barley and oats. Barley is cultivated as high as 70° of latitude, and also in the tropical parts of the western world; so that barley has a greater range than oats or wheat. The oat has a much more northern range than wheat; and, of the three, the wheat is cultivated in our northern climate at the greatest uncertainty and expense; but still we cultivate it. Wheat does not appear to have a larger quantity of nutritive matter: it contains less protein than oats, and very little more than Indian meal; a considerable quantity, however, more than rice, but not a much larger quantity than barley-meal. It seems, then, not so much its composition, as the power it possesses of making a light loaf by fermentation, which causes it to be the favourite form of food.

Now bread is of two kinds. It is either vesiculated or unvesiculated; that is to say, it is thrown into vesicles in the form of bread, or it is not thrown into vesicles, and assumes the form of what we call biscuit, passover cakes, oaten cakes, and food of that kind. However, wheaten flour is cooked in other ways; and then it does not differ from the flour of barley, oats, or maize. It is made into puddings and pie-crusts, which may both be regarded as unvesiculated bread. At a certain temperature, from having been a thick tenacious mass, it may be cooked to any point of thickness, from the thin batter pudding to the hard Suffolk dumpling, or harder crust of biscuit. Unvesiculated bread is the unleavened bread of Scripture. The vesiculated bread may be divided into two groups; fermented and aërated bread.

In making fermented bread, you take the flour, consisting of the starch, the gluten, &c., and then some water. The starch and water are then mixed together, or rather there is placed in the flour before the water is mixed with it a quantity of yeast. This substance consists of gluten, or fibrine, or one of the proteinaceous matters in a state of change. When the brewer makes beer, he takes the barley in the form of malt, which contains a large quantity of albuminous matter, or rather gluten, which he does not require for his beer. During fermentation, this rises to the top of the beer or the wort, and then it is skimmed off in a fermenting condition. It is this yeast, then, which is mixed with the water before the flour is put to it; and when the dough thus made is exposed to heat, the effect is to cause the yeast to communicate its state of change to the gluten of the wheat, which is again communicated to the starch.

Now this starch (as I told you in the Lecture before last), under the influence of a fermenting agent, becomes converted into glucose; such an agent is contained in our saliva, and is called salivin or ptyalin. In this way we convert starch into glucose in our mouth, and in this way the same change comes over the loaf. A certain quantity of the starch is converted into glucose—only a small portion, but that glucose suffers a further change; the glucose ferments, and is decomposed, and alcohol is formed, and carbonic acid gas is given out. In the ordinary fermentation of sugar, in order to make beer or wine, you take glucose, which contains 12 atoms of carbon, 12 atoms of hydrogen, and 12 atoms of oxygen, and you get from that alcohol and carbonic acid gas. You get out 4 atoms of the carbon and 8 atoms of the oxygen, in the form of carbonic acid gas, and leave 4 atoms of oxygen, 12 atoms of hydrogen, and 8 atoms of carbon. Now, that constitutes two atoms of alcohol. Alcohol is a hydrated oxide of ethyle, and the chemists write it down thus: $HO + O + (H\,5\,C\,4)$. I will not dwell on that process now any further than just to say that the change which goes on in the conversion of starch into glucose, and glucose into carbonic acid gas in vesiculated bread, is precisely the fermentation that goes on in the fermentation of sugar, in order to make alcohol. Now, that is a fact; and at one time it was supposed that it would be an economical thing to take the bread and bake it in an oven, which was so constructed as to catch the alcohol. Five and thirty years ago, a company called the Metropolitan Bread Making Company, was established for carrying out this plan. The bread, however, was very hard, as the baking was very imperfect, in order to secure the alcohol. The company did not succeed. Those bakers who did not sell the company's bread tried to persuade people that in collecting the alcohol formed, the company kept back something the public ought to have had, and it was not an uncommon thing to see in a baker's shop window the announcement of "Bread sold here, with the gin in it."

From my own experiments I concluded that the alcohol which is formed is exceedingly small. I have taken dough and fermented it, and put it into a vessel, and tried to ascertain the quantity of carbonic acid gas that was given off. But as the bread rose, no carbonic acid gas escaped, and all that was formed was contained in the bread. Now, the quantity contained in a loaf of bread is really very small. I dwell on this because there has been a statement made that unfermented bread was a great saving of the starch,—that fermentation was a wicked process, on account of the waste of the starch. It is also stated that gluten is destroyed. This is not the case. It is also stated as a proof of the destruction of the gluten, that ammonia was formed in the baking of the bread. I have not been able to detect ammonia during the rising of bread, and I believe this also to be an error.

Then there is this matter of interest to us in the fermenting process. In certain seasons wheat begins to grow before the miller gets hold of it to make flour. During that process of growth the starch is naturally converted into sugar, just as the maltster converts his barley into malt. When germination goes on in wheat, such wheat had better go to the maltster than the miller. When the baker uses flour from this kind of wheat he puts the yeast to the flour, but the starch has already started in its progress towards sugar, and the consequence is, that the bread becomes sticky and dirty-looking. What is the baker to do? Why, there is one thing that will stop all this; and that is alum.

This is the history of the introduction of alum into bread, especially in large cities, where people are particular, and where people can afford to be particular, and where even the least opulent classes of society will have white bread. The baker has this temptation, then, to put alum into the bread; but when once the baker knows the magical effect of alum he has seldom the courage to leave it off. His bread looks so white, and people are so fond of white bread,—and can only a little alum do people any harm? Nevertheless, alum is a bad thing. We know that alum does not exist in our system among the compounds that are universally necessary for its existence, and it produces injurious effects on the system.

In making bread bakers add potatoes to the flour,

and this is sometimes regarded as an adulteration, but this is not the case; the potatoes assist the fermentation, and frequently potatoes cost more than flour.

Another addition to baker's bread is salt, which is sometimes added rather unsparingly.

By the aërated process bread is made without the introduction of yeast as a ferment, and carbonic acid gas is introduced in some other way. Now, there are two processes by which this is effected: first, by the decomposition of a carbonate; and, secondly, by the addition of carbonic acid. The first is the process by which the patent unfermented bread, recommended by Dr. Whiting, is produced; and the other is a process patented by Dr. Dauglish, and called aërated bread. Now, with regard to Dr. Whiting's process, it is very easy to understand. A little carbonate of soda is taken and put into the flour, then a quantity of hydrochloric acid is added to the water, and directly the hydrochloric acid comes in contact with the carbonate of soda, the carbonic acid is set free, and during the time the bread is being baked the carbonic acid gas is evolved, and common salt is formed. As hydrochloric acid is not always to be got pure, some persons recommend tartaric acid in its place. This forms tartrate of soda, which perhaps is not so desirable a compound as the hydrochlorate of soda or common salt. Bread thus made certainly keeps better than bread made with yeast. It is sold under the name of Dodson's unfermented bread.

The aërated bread is made by making the flour into dough with water containing carbonic acid gas in solution. This is done by using an apparatus like a soda-water machine, or gazogene, and injecting a quantity of water charged with carbonic acid into a cylinder containing the flour, and then the water is thoroughly mixed with the flour. This is done, by the aid of steam, in the course of a few minutes, and a valve in the cylinder is opened below and the dough is allowed to run out into little tin-cases, in which it is carried to the oven and baked. The carbonic acid is expelled during the baking, and thus the bread becomes vesiculated. The great advantage of this process is that, from the beginning to the end, you have no handling, no kneading, nor have you any of the waiting processes which beset the making of bread by fermentation. If you use German yeast and milk and warm water the bread will rise in three hours; if you use German yeast and no milk it will not rise under four hours; but frequently baker's bread stands nine, twelve, and even fourteen hours before it is put in the oven. This involves a great amount of human labour, and requires men to be sitting up all night. Thus it is that the baker's occupation is one exceedingly injurious to health; but by the aërated process the making of the dough is effected in the course of twenty or five-and-twenty minutes.

But the question as to whether the bread thus made is as good for health is one of great interest. It has been stated that man has eaten fermented bread from the beginning of the world, and that it is necessary he should do so, and that he instinctively prefers it, and therefore it must be best for health. Now this statement is not correct, for the great mass of mankind do not ferment bread, for they cannot ferment rice or maize. But we need not refer to Chinamen or Indians.

but to our Scotch neighbours, who, many of them, never eat wheat bread, but unfermented oatmeal, and there can be no doubt that they flourish on this diet. I think, therefore, this argument in favour of fermented bread must fall to the ground.

Then we may argue the matter as a question of taste. Well, if you like fermented bread best, there is an end of the question, and fermented bread has probably a sweeter flavour. During the fermenting process the starch has had a tendency given to it to change into glucose. In the aërated process there is no fermentation or change of the starch further than in the baking, and consequently fermented bread tastes sweeter in the mouth. The question is, is that an advantage? In some cases it is a disadvantage; as the fermented bread passes into a change further than glucose. There are many persons who cannot eat sugar, apples, pears, grapes, or anything containing glucose. They can eat a little cane-sugar, and that is all. Why? Because the stomach produces compounds which hasten the breaking up of the glucose and its conversion into acids. Thus it is that on some persons fermented bread acts as a poison. Many people can take dry toast who cannot take new or soft bread, and persons under these circumstances prefer biscuits that have not been fermented at all, and it is in these cases that unfermented aërated bread acts favourably.

I must, however, leave the question now with you to determine for yourselves. I will merely say that there is not that attention paid to the process of baking among bakers, and certainly not among people who bake at home, that there might be. The consequence

146 ON FLESH-FORMING FOODS.

is, that no two batches of bread are alike. Above all things, there is a necessity for attending to temperature during baking, and yet a thermometer, the only means by which temperature can be measured, is almost unknown among bakers. In Vienna, and many parts of Paris, they make much better bread, and a much more enjoyable bread, than any we have in London. This arises from the scientific attention given to the process. Here we carry on most of our occupations as if an entire ignorance of their nature were a means of

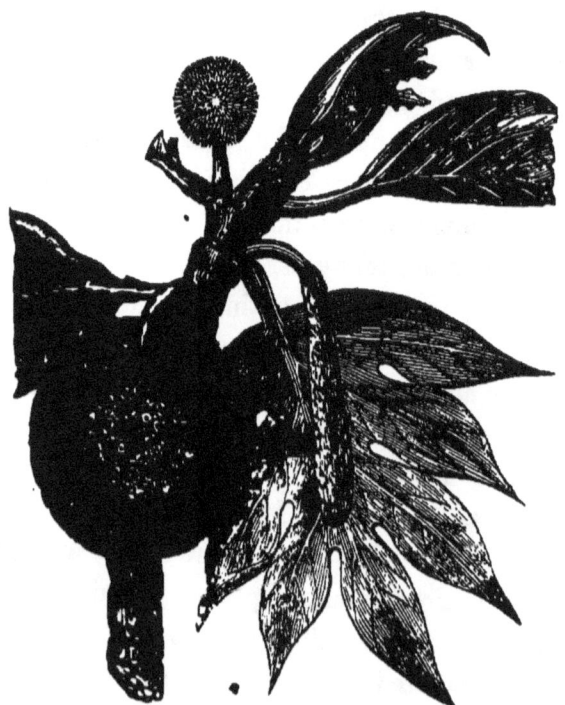

Fig. 4.—Bread-fruit Tree.

certain success. Is it then to be wondered at, that even in the manufacture of "our daily bread" we go to work in an expensive way, and produce an inferior and often injurious article?

Time will not permit me to speak of the other cereal grains, of barley, oats, maize, rye, and millet, containing gluten and albumen, nor of the leguminous seeds, peas, beans, and lentils, which all contain caseine; but I wish to mention the fact that other foods contain all the principles necessary to human subsistence. Thus there is the bread-fruit tree (*Artocarpus incisa*, Fig. 4), whose large fruits form a very delicious and substantial article of diet to the natives of the South Sea Islands. You may remember that the attempts in the last century to bring this fruit to England formed an interesting episode in the history of the voyages made to that part of the world. Most persons will have heard something of the voyage of Bligh to the Society Islands, and the mutiny on board his ship, and the escape of the mutineers to Pitcairn's Island, where their descendants are still located.

Another plant, belonging to a very different order, is the buckwheat. (*Fagopyrum esculentum*, Fig. 5.) It is cultivated in this country for the sake of its green fodder. But on the continent of Europe its ripe seeds are ground and mixed with wheat flour, and eaten as human food. The seeds contain nearly 9 per cent. of gluten, and 1 per cent. of fatty matter, 50 per cent. of starch, and 2 per cent. of sugar.

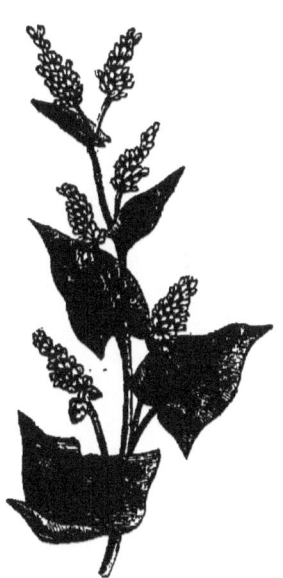

Fig. 5.—*Buck-wheat*.

In other parts of

the world chestnuts, figs, dates, and the Quinoa goosefoot, are eaten as substantive articles of food. But you will remark that no food is used as a principal support of man unless it contains from 6 to 8 per cent. of flesh-forming matters.

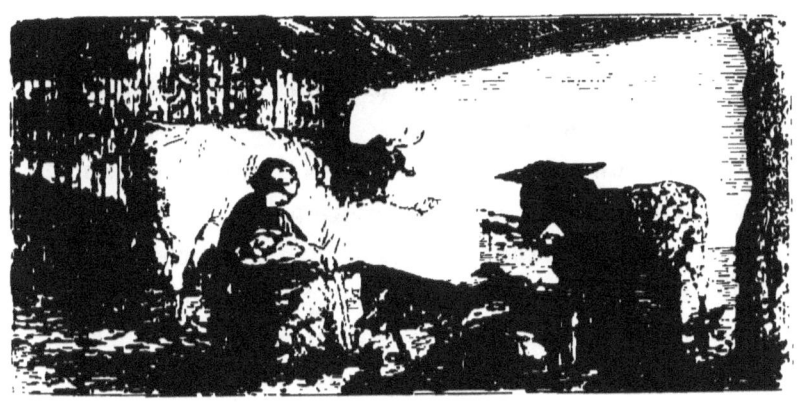

Fig. 1.

ON ANIMAL FOOD.

IN this Lecture I purpose speaking of those flesh-forming substances which we obtain from the animal kingdom. I told you in my last Lecture, that all that which constitutes the flesh of animals—that which forms the muscles and the nerves, and which we eat as food, is derived from the vegetable kingdom—from plants. There would be no flesh unless animals first fed on the vegetable kingdom—on plants. If some animals are carnivorous, we find that they feed on those animals which are granivorous or herbivorous. Thus the ox and the sheep, and various kinds of birds, all feed on grass or grain, and the flesh which we obtain from them they have derived from the plant. The plant, you will recollect, produces this flesh-forming matter in the interior of its cells, where it is known by the names of the nucleus, the cytoblast, the protoplasm, the primordia utricle, and the endoplast.

I have now to speak of the things that have thus been obtained from the plant, appropriated by animals, and made to subserve the purposes of man as articles of diet.

In casting around for something like a form of food that we could regard as a type of all others, there is none better than milk; and as milk is an animal product, I shall speak of it in detail to day. Milk really represents all the food of which we partake which is not medicinal. That milk is a type of all food, is found in the fact that the young of all the higher mammalia are fed on this food for several months many of them for above a year, and get no other, article of diet. During this period they grow very rapidly, and increase in size; consequently, they must have obtained all that which constitutes their muscle, their nerve, their bone, and other tissues, the heat they give out and the force they exert from the milk they have taken : so that, you see, milk must contain the essentials of all food; and is worthy our attentive investigation.

Let us, then first study the composition of milk. A pound of cow's milk contains about $13\frac{3}{4}$ oz. of water, which is the first substance we spoke of in these Lectures; then it contains about $\frac{1}{4}$ oz. of mineral matter, of which we spoke in our second Lecture; $\frac{3}{4}$ oz. of sugar, of which we spoke in the third Lecture; $\frac{1}{2}$ oz. of butter, one of the oily substances of which we spoke in the fourth Lecture; and then it also contains $\frac{3}{4}$ oz. of caseine, of which we spoke in the last Lecture; so that, you see, milk contains representatives of all the groups of human food. Nor do I wish you to think that such a view has in any manner originated with myself. I would here refer to a classification of food according to the late Dr. Prout, and we are probably more indebted to Dr. Prout than any other investigator in advancing our knowledge of the action of food; for before Mulder had made his great discovery, and Liebig had written and made this subject so popular, Dr. Prout had produced his celebrated work on the Stomach, in which he pointed out that milk may be taken as the type of human food. He divided food into four groups: first, the aqueous, embracing water, tea, coffee, and other watery beverages; then the second group he called saccharine, embracing such substances as sago, arrowroot, sugar, and sweet fruits, and containing from 40 to 50 per cent. of carbon; then came the albuminous group, represented by cheese and the flesh of mammals, birds, and fish; and, lastly, the oleaginous group, containing 70 to 80 per cent. of carbon, and represented by butter. Now, the deficiency of this classification is, that it does not allow for the value of the salts or mineral substances as food, which were spoken of in the second Lecture.

Different animals yield milk of a different composition, and we find a variety of these milks employed by man as food. The milk of the cow is more constantly employed in this country than any other; but in some countries the milk of the goat stands in the same relation to the popular diet as the milk of the cow does here. Again, in disease, recourse is had to asses' milk; and thus it becomes of importance that we should know something of the composition of milks.

We are not at all likely in this country to get goats' milk, but the milks we use are cows' milk and asses' milk. I have here the analyses of these milks and of human milk, and you may easily compare these milks one with the other.

1 lb. of Cows' milk contains—

	oz.	gr.
1. Water	13	333
2. Caseine	0	350
3. Butter	0	245
4. Sugar	0	315
5. Mineral matter	0	70

1 lb. of Human milk contains—

	oz.	gr.
1. Water	14	41
2. Caseine	0	210
3. Butter	0	210
4. Sugar	0	280
5. Mineral matter	0	35

1 lb. of Ass's milk contains—

	oz.	gr.
1. Water	14	76
2. Caseine	0	140
3. Butter	0	105
4. Sugar	0	420
5. Mineral matter	0	35

The milk of the mother frequently fails, and it becomes a question of importance to know what is the best substitute. Now, cows' milk is the readiest and cheapest expedient, but frequently asses' milk is preferred; because, if you take the quantity of caseine, sugar, and butter, they are nearly alike in human and asses milk; but cows' milk contains more caseine, more flesh-giving matter. Hence the practice, when cows' milk is given to children, of adding half the quantity of water; and then, in order to supply the deficiency of sugar which is thus occasioned,—for the sugar very nearly corresponds with that of human milk,—to add a small quantity of sugar. There is no doubt that this is very good theory, and that cows' milk reduced in that way nearly approaches human milk. At the same time, asses' milk has been supposed to be a better substitute than cows' milk, and it is better still if a little cream is added to it. There is no objection on the score of composition at all; and the only objection is that we do not in this country keep these animals for the supply of milk, so that it becomes an expensive article of diet. Cows' milk differs from human in its containing an excess of the cheesy, or flesh-forming matter. But a question of great importance arises here, and that is as to whether the milk we administer to infants in the condition we get it from the cow, or as sold in the shops of London, is that upon which they are likely to prosper. Now, it has always appeared to me to be of consequence that it should be given to children as soon as possible after it is drawn, for this reason, that milk is very liable to decomposition, which renders it very much less digestible than when it is fresh drawn; and not only this, but the milk gets into a state of change, in which, instead of yielding a proper amount of nutriment, it becomes a source of irritation, and, occasionally, of dangerous disease, and even death. I was so much struck at the amount of mortality among infants during the hot summer of 1859, that I made inquiries as to how children had been fed who had died of diarrhœa, and I found, in almost all cases which I inquired into, that they had been fed upon cows' milk. It was also generally admitted that the milk had a great tendency to get sour. Now, sour milk may produce dangerous disease in the stomach of a child, and it is very frequently the case, that in the height of summer children are feeble and debilitated, and ascescent cows' milk, administered in that state, is likely to produce disease, and even death. There is one thing to be remembered: a little lime-water, or a little carbonate of potash, will correct this acidity. We may also add some form of vegetable food to the milk, which will correct this tendency to decomposition, which milk possesses, and which seems to be the great recommendation of some forms of flours, which contain both nutritive and heat-giving ingredients. I speak more particularly of the flours of wheat, barley, oats, and maize. Now, I think the flour of any of these substances, especially if they are properly prepared by heating, may be added with great advantage to the cows' milk that is given to children, thus preventing that tendency to excessive change which we find in milk alone. I therefore perfectly agree with a lady who has written on this subject, when she says that one of the great sources of death in children arises from improper feeding, and that she believes where children cannot obtain mother's milk, the best substitute is cows' milk, mixed with a certain quantity of farinaceous food. It should, however, be always recollected that the mother's milk is the best food for a child till it is 8 or 9 months old, and not till that age is it natural for it to partake of vegetable food at all.

Now, I do not say that if you get cows' milk fresh, that you want a better substitute; but in London we are not in this condition. I believe, in London especially, we are liable to partake of milk produced by cows kept in confinement, which has a greater tendency to this acid condition than milk produced by cows kept in open meadows in the country. There has been recently introduced a preparation of milk called Condensed Milk. This is an excellent preparation as it prevents altogether the adulteration of milk by water.

There is another question about milk on which I would say a word or two; and that is a question raised by Mrs. Baines, the lady I have before referred to. She suggests that there may be something in the milk which we have not yet discovered,—that there may be in all milks a peculiar essence, which belongs to that milk and to no other, and which may prevent the milk of one animal agreeing with the stomach of another. It may be that there are such essences; but what I would say on this subject is, that at present we are perfectly ignorant of any such thing, and that we are not justified in acting upon such a suggestion. We have no evidence that shows that pure and well-developed cows' milk is not a perfectly healthful food; and we have the evidence of its composition that it is sufficiently like human milk to render it an efficient substitute.

Let us now proceed to examine the special components of milk

The first we shall speak of is caseine, which is one of the flesh-forming substances; and with these we have more particularly to deal. Now, this caseine is contained in milk in solution. If you recollect, I told you, in the last Lecture, that there were three of these flesh-forming substances—albumen, which you find in the white of egg, having the property of coagulating with heat, as you all know; and then there is fibrine, which constitutes the flesh, the muscle of animals, and which we also find in the larger proportion of vegetable matters used as food. Then I told you there was caseine, which we find in peas and beans, and which, in those substances, is also called legumin. Caseine, like albumen, is held in solution in animal fluids. If you take some caseine and add potash to it, you will dissolve it; and if you take away the potash, by the addition of some acid the caseine will appear directly. We know that the slightest amount of acid curdles milk; and you will see how it is that in the dairy the slightest amount of acidity, or any tendency to change in the sugar, so as to convert it into an acid, will curdle the milk. Hence, the dairy-maid must have an eye as sharp as a needle to detect the least drop of milk on the furniture of the dairy, for it soon decomposes, and she must wipe it away with a cloth; for if she touches it with her hand, and then afterwards the milk, the whole is turned into curds and whey. So, when we make syllabub, we put the milk to acid wine, and the wine separates the milk, and the curds come up. But if we allow milk to stand for a certain time, we shall find that, naturally, this caseine has a tendency to separate from the milk with the butter which is contained in it and not dissolved in it.

If you put a drop of milk under the microscope, you will see little globules of butter floating in it. Here is a drawing (Fig. 2) of the microscopic appearance of milk. The large cells are what is called colostrum, a substance found in the milk of the mammalia for a few days after the birth of their young. The smaller globules are those of butter. The butter has a tendency to separate, and this is taken off in the form of what we call cream; it is then churned, and the water and sugar and curds are pressed out of it; and thus the butter of the shops is produced.

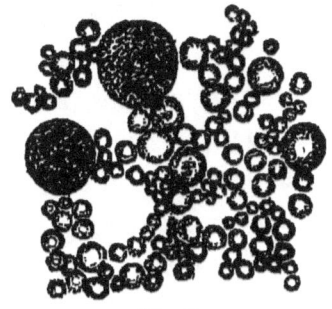

Fig. 2.

Now, when we have got the cream, we have left a quantity of milk holding the caseine in solution with sugar and water and the saline matter. If we put an acid to it, the caseine separates, and the pure whey is left. If we now evaporate the whey, the sugar of the milk is left, and this is sold in shops for dietetical purposes.

Milk sugar, or lactose, as it is called, nearly resembles grape sugar, or glucose. Grape sugar has 12 atoms of carbon, 12 atoms of hydrogen, and 12 atoms of oxygen; whilst milk sugar has 11 atoms of carbon, 12 of hydrogen, and 12 of oxygen. So you see how closely these substances are allied.

Caseine, then, is the base of the substance which we know as cheese. It is not all caseine; at least, not all cheese is all caseine, for cheeses differ rather in the butter they contain than in the quantity of their caseine.

If you take the table of the constituents of food drawn up by Dr. Playfair, and examine the proportion of caseine in cheese, you will find that it has 31 lbs. in every 100 lbs., and 25 lbs. of heat-givers. So we must not regard cheese as a flesh-former only, as it in fact contains both caseine and butter. Cheese is made by submitting the curds of new milk to a degree of pressure, which reduces them to the various degrees of solidity which we see in cheese. Our common Cheshire cheeses, Gloucester cheeses, and so on, are made of the cream and curds of one milking; but we do not value cheese so much on account of the caseine as on account of the butter, and just in proportion to the quantity of butter yielded by the cows in the various districts of this country will be the value of cheese. In the meadows of Cheshire there are large quantities of butter-forming food, which give the Cheshire cheese its value. But you may have cheese made with an extra quantity of butter, like a double Gloucester, or a Stilton. Cream taken from the milking one day is added to the milking of another day, and thus a double quantity of butter is secured, and these are the most valuable cheeses. It is not the caseine, therefore, but the butter, which makes the cheese valuable.

Now there are cases in which they skim the cream before they begin to make cheese. These cheeses are remarkable for their hardness, because caseine, independently of the butter, is an exceedingly hard substance; and these cheeses are sometimes brought into the market, and they are so hard that they are the subject of many a joke. Of such are the Suffolk-bang cheeses made by frugal housewives of that county, who first take the butter and send it to market, and then make their cheese. It is said of it in derision that "dogs bark at it, pigs grunt at it, but neither of them can bite it."

Blomfield, in his "Farmer's Boy," thus sings the virtues of his native cheese:—

> "Unrivall'd stands thy county *cheese*, O Giles!
> Whose very name alone engenders smiles;
> Whose fame abroad by every tongue is spoke,
> The well-known butt of many a flinty joke,
> That pass like current coin the nation through.
> And, ah! experience proves the satire true.
> Provision's grave, thou ever-craving mart,
> Dependent, huge metropolis! where Art
> Her poring thousands stows in breathless rooms,
> Midst pois'nous smokes, and steams, and rattling looms;
> Where grandeur revels in unbounded stores;
> Restraint a slighted stranger at their doors!
> Thou like a whirlpool drainst the countries round,
> Till London market, London price resound
> Through every town, round every passing load,
> And dairy produce throngs the eastern road;
> Delicious veal and butter every hour,
> From Essex lowlands and the banks of Stour;
> And further far, where numerous herds repose,
> From Orwell's brink, from Waveny, or Ouse.
> Hence Suffolk dairy wives run mad for cream,
> And leave their milk with nothing but its name;
> Its name derision and reproach pursue,
> And strangers tell of 'three times skimm'd skyblue'
> To cheese converted, what can be its boast?
> What, but the common virtues of a post;
> If drought o'ertake it faster than the knife,
> Most fair it bids for stubborn length of life,
> And like the oaken shelf whereon 'tis laid,
> Mocks the weak effort of the bending blade;
> Or in the hog-trough rests in perfect spite,
> Too big to swallow, and too hard to bite.
> Inglorious victory! Ye Cheshire meads,
> Or Severn's flow'ry dales, where plenty treads,
> Was your rich milk to suffer wrongs like these,
> Farewell your pride! farewell renowned cheese!
> The skimmer dread, whose ravages alone
> Thus turns the mead's sweet nectar into stone."

This kind of cheese is very indigestible, and is sold at a low price, but still it contains a large quantity of flesh-forming food. But caseine is more easily digested when combined with butter. Hence we find most other cheeses easily digestible as compared with the hard Suffolk cheese. Nor do cheeses alone differ in the relation of the caseine to the butter. It differs according to the method of preparing it. In some cases the curds are allowed to decompose a little before they are pressed. Then they are pressed with various degrees of firmness. Cream cheeses are only gently pressed, and eaten new. The colour of the milk affects the cheese, and some are high coloured, whilst others are white. In Cheshire, they colour them with annatto. We find also in Germany the cheeses have a variety of substances in them. There is the Schabzeiger, which is flavoured by the addition of the plant known in this country as melilot. This cheese finds admirers in England. The Parmesan is a cheese with much caseine and little butter. Gruyere and Dutch cheeses are alike, but the former have more butter and a richer flavour.

Taking cheese at a price of from 7d. to 10d. per lb., the question arises as to whether it is an economical article of food. It contains that form of flesh-forming matter which is furnished by Providence to young children, and the young of all the higher animals; and in the form in which it is thus supplied, there is no doubt that it is very nutritious. But when it is separated, the question of its digestibility must be considered. Where cheese is digested, there is nothing which contains so large a quantity of flesh-forming matter; but then you must not go away and think we can live on cheese. There are persons who like it, and have taken it for a time, but they have been arrested in their course by its indigestibility. But the hard-working man, who labours with his muscles from hour to hour in the open air, with his stomach in the best possible condition to digest his food, rather invests his little money in cheese than in meat, for cheese contains nearly twice the quantity of nutritive matter that you get in cooked meat. In fact, I shall have to show you that the quantity mentioned in the meat is diminished by a substance that is not nutritive at all. But then with regard to persons who do not require it as a nutritive or flesh-forming agent in their food, why is it eaten at all? It seems to possess an action which renders it desirable, and particularly after taking other foods. Caseine is easily decomposed, or easily put in a condition in which it causes other things to change. I told you in my last Lecture that we add yeast to flour for the purpose of causing fermentation. Now, I said that the yeast communicated change to the gluten, and the gluten communicated that condition of change to the starch, and the yeast is the beginning of this series of changes. Now, this caseine is like gluten. It will start a series of changes. Hence, when we put it into the stomach, it starts a change in the food, and this change seems desirable; for unless the food is placed in a state of change, it cannot be converted into chyle. So that a small quantity of cheese taken with the other food seems to facilitate the digestion, and the taking up of food into the system. Hence perhaps we may see how mankind has got into the practice of partaking of a small quantity of cheese after other kinds of food.

Then there are some persons who prefer mouldy cheese to fresh cheese; and if you take it for facilitating a change of food in the stomach, you had better take the decomposing cheese, which is more likely to effect the change

We must now leave cheese, to speak of those other flesh-forming substances which are derived from the animal kingdom, and which we know by the name of the flesh of animals. Now, the flesh of animals is composed of both fibrine and albumen. I told you that the fibrine of vegetable food was represented by the gluten of wheat-flour, and we get it in bread. Then, the albumen we obtain from asparagus, and such-like vegetables. Now, in animal food we generally find both albumen and fibrine. There are some cases, however, in which we get the albumen separated from the fibrine: this is the case with eggs. Hence the egg is an article of diet. It contains albumen both in the white and the yolk: this yolk, however, in addition to the albumen, contains a quantity of oil; so that in eating an egg, we are really eating both a heat-giver and flesh-former. But there is also much water: the white of egg contains 85 per cent. and the yolk about 53 per cent. of water. Taking 1 lb. of eggs, both yolk and white, we shall have about 12 ozs. of water, 2 ozs. of albumen, and $1\frac{1}{2}$ oz. of oil or fat; the egg also contains saline matters.

Then, again, we find the albumen exists in nerves: I speak of the fact that albumen exists in the nerves of all the higher animals; and, of course, when we eat nervous matter we partake of albumen. Albumen exists in the brains of animals; and we occasionally eat brain sauce, and it is a very palatable addition to the head of a calf when cooked. There is a considerable quantity of albumen in the blood of animals; and you should give attention to that fact because it is the source of albumen in the tissues. All the fleshy parts of animals contain blood; and the blood contains as much as 7 parts in 100 of albumen; so that, although we bleed animals generally before we kill them, we still leave a quantity of albumen in the flesh.

This leads to a question on which I wish to say a few words; and that is, as to whether we are wise economically, and are justified in bleeding animals to death and throwing away all the blood, which is, after all, good food. When you recollect that we take from 5 lbs. to 20 lbs. from a sheep or an ox, and multiply that by the number of sheep and oxen killed in the course of a year, you will find that it amounts to something which is quite frightful to contemplate. Now, I have no hesitation in saying that the blood you take away is just as good food as the blood you leave in, and that you would do much better to leave the blood in the animal. There are other ways of killing animals than bleeding them to death. These are unpleasant things to think of; but, after all, we have no hesitation in eating the mutton and beef after it is slain, and we ought to be able to give a reason for our extravagance. We do not take the blood away from hares and rabbits: they are brought to the table and eaten by the most fastidious. So also with birds: pheasants and partridges—we do not bleed them; and I tell you more—if you did, they would not be so pleasant to eat; they would lose some of their gamey flavour. Dr. Carson, of Liverpool, many years ago pointed out the great loss incurred in the present mode of killing animals, and suggested a method of killing them by which the blood was saved; and Dr. Carson induced a certain number of people of Liverpool to try meat killed in his way, and they declared it so much better, that a butcher was induced to kill his animals in that way, and the result has been that he has surrounded himself with customers. Mr. Carson, son of the late Doctor, was kind enough to send me up a quarter of a sheep which had been killed in this way; I invited a few friends to partake of it, and they one and all pronounced it delicious. Economically, this is an important question, and it ought to be a consideration whether we are justified in throwing away so large a quantity of this nutritious albumen.

The quantities of fibrine and albumen in butcher's meat are about the same; but I have now to draw your attention to another constituent, which has always figured in all our chemical analyses as flesh-forming matter. If we take a quantity of beef or mutton, or even of pork, and boil it for a certain length of time, we obtain from it a substance which thickens the water as it cools, and makes it into what we call a jelly. Now, that substance has been supposed to be the nutritive matter of the meat. It has been extracted and sold separately from the other constituents of the meat, as nutritive matter; the impression is that this matter is more nutritive than other kinds of food, and it is given to persons who are weak and dying for want of strength to keep them up; and yet I have an extraordinary statement to make to persons who believe in this, that this is not nutritive matter at all; and, although not to be objected to when mixed with other substances, alone it certainly is not capable of supporting life. This substance is called gelatine. It exists in the nerves and muscles and all kinds of flesh of animals. It forms, in fact, the cell-walls of animals. The cell-walls of plants are composed of cellulose. Both cellulose and gelatine are insoluble in cold water, and the difference between them is, that gelatine is soluble in hot water. Gelatine is obtained from all kinds of animals, and all parts, and from bone, and skin, and membrane. This gelatine is used in the arts for making size and glue, and for fining beer and wine, and various other purposes.

The sound of the sturgeon and of various other fish is composed almost entirely of this substance, and when prepared and cut into strips it is called isinglass. It is obtained commercially, for dietetical purposes, from a variety of things, from the skins of animals not sent to the curriers, and from bones, and so on; and very good gelatine is procured from the refuse of the tanner's yard. So that the substance which we know in the arts as glue and size, and as food under the name of gelatine or isinglass, is this gelatine which you can get from all parts of animals by boiling. Then, I say, it is not a nutritive substance; it is not a digestible substance, and, therefore, cannot be nutritive. Many years ago, the French, being fond of soups, and the poor living principally on soups, discovered that those persons who lived on soups suffered in their health. This became a question, of so much importance that a commission was appointed to inquire into the properties of gelatine, and the result was that it was reported that gelatine had no nutritive property. The impression on the public mind was, however, so favourable, that it was still used in France; and a second commission was appointed, and the result of its labours confirmed the conclusions of the first commission. In Belgium also a public inquiry was instituted, the result was the same conclusion as the two French commissions. You do not find this gelatine in the blood. If it were a nutritive agent, you would find it there. You do not find it in eggs, nor do you find it in milk. Seeing, then, there is no gelatine in these nutritive things, which are naturally prepared to form the parts of the body, we are warranted in concluding that it is not a flesh-forming substance at all. Then it appears that this substance is merely an accessory in our usual food, just what cellulose and gum are in our vegetable food. Hence I have called these substances accessory foods. They are not to be rejected; they do not injure; on the contrary, I believe there is evidence that they do good.

It is found in feeding horses, that if you give them beans or oats alone they will not do so well as if you mix with these more nutritive foods a quantity of chaff, chopped straw, which is little more than cellulose. It appears to me that man has the same relation to these things, and that he requires some indigestible food. In all our food there is a certain quantity of indigestible matter, and if it does not disagree it acts beneficially. This is one recommendation of brown bread, it contains more cellulose than flour. Those who can eat brown bread habitually have better health than those who cannot, or who persist in eating white bread.

If we look once more at the table of the constituents of food, you will find that the quantity of nutritive or flesh-forming matter in cooked meat is put down at 22 per cent.; that is to say, in 100 lbs. of butcher's meat there would be 22 lbs. of nitrogenous matter, but you must recollect that this includes a quantity of gelatine. The quantities of these flesh-forming matters are calculated on the quantity of nitrogen yielded by the meat. Now the gelatine contains nitrogen, and I have endeavoured to ascertain the quantities of gelatine in meat, and the question comes, whether we ought to regard all nitrogenous matter as nutritive when gelatine is present? Deducting, then, the gelatine, I find meat contains less flesh-forming matter than wheat, oats, maize, peas, and beans. But then comes the question of digestibility. There is no doubt in my mind that the fibrine and albumen contained in meat is rapidly taken up and made use of, while there is a doubt as to whether the nutritive matter in wheat, barley, oats, and maize, is all taken up. The gluten of bread, of barley, oats, and maize, is less digestible than the albumen and fibrine of mutton and beef; in the same way as the gluten of bread is more digestible than the caseine of peas and beans. You recollect the large quantity of nutritive matter in peas and beans. The quantity of caseine in peas is 23 in 100, so that they contain really more nitrogenous matter than butcher's meat; but then it is not so digestible, and this question of digestion must always be considered in the administration and consumption of food. The instincts of man seem to have guided him on this question, for when he works hard, or when he thinks hard, he has recourse to animal food, and he has discovered that it is more easily made into flesh than the same substances in vegetable food.

It is then, I think, a safe conclusion that where nutritive matters are required, beef and mutton should be given. In cooking these, however, we may endanger their nutritive qualities; and as it is sometimes a matter of importance, in cases of disease, to give the most nutritious diet, I will say a word or two on the manufacture of beef tea. You will recollect, then, that as the gelatine is of little value, and the albumen is coagulated and rendered less digestible by heat, it is not necessary to boil beef in order to make nutritive beef-tea. The beef should be cut up into small pieces, and a little soft, or distilled water, with a few drops of hydrochloric acid, and a little salt added to it; after it has stood for a few hours, the liquid should be strained off, and when taken should be heated to a temperature of about 100°. This liquid contains not only fibrine and albumen, but other compounds found in the juice of flesh. Amongst other things, it contains two substances, found in the flesh of animals, called creatine and creatinine. They resemble, in their chemical nature, quinine, and they are found in human flesh. It may be that it is those substances which give so much value to animal food. It may be that to have these things ready-made in our food may facilitate the nutrition of the muscles and the other vital parts of our bodies. Beef-tea made in this way contains also the mineral compounds of potash and phosphoric acid.

We may learn a lesson from this method of making beef-tea in the preparation of our animal food. It so happens that the creatine and creatinine, with all the salts of which I have spoken, can be boiled out of meat; and when the meat is served upon the table, and the water is thrown away, you have really got rid of some of the most important constituents of your food. If the meat is put into the water before it boils, and the albumen has time to exude, the saline matters with the creatine and creatinine will also escape, and in this way you get rid of the most important matters of the food. On the Continent they are more alive to the economy of cooking, and in consequence they use the water in which the meat is boiled for the purpose of making soup. Not only does this apply to meat but also to fish. The liquid in which fish is boiled is just as valuable as that in which any other articles of diet are boiled.

Then, with regard to the best method of boiling meat, a hint or two may be given here. Where persons have predetermined to throw away the water they boil meat in, they should recollect that albumen is contained in all meat; and if you put the meat in cold water, it gradually exudes; but if you put it directly into boiling water, you produce a covering of coagulated albumen around the meat, which keeps in, to a considerable extent, the creatine, and all the other precious products of the juice of flesh. The water should boil; that is, it should have a temperature of 212°, and be kept at that heat for ten or twelve minutes, then the heat may be reduced to 150°, and kept at this heat till the whole is cooked. We were told the other day in the papers that for the last twenty years our soldiers at home had had meat served out to them which had never been properly cooked; that it was always boiled, and boiled in such a way as to ensure the loss of all the nutritive matter; and that they were fed on merely the rags of meat. If this be true, it only shows you how practical this subject of cooking food is; which not only involves our individual comfort, but our national welfare. In order to have strong and brave soldiers, you must feed them well. It is not sufficient that you pay the highest price for the best food, you must see that it is not spoiled in the cooking. There are scientific principles lying at the foundation of the art of cookery as of every other human art; and if you neglect to apply them, if you neglect to educate your cooks in them, you must expect to suffer.

Let me add now a few words on the subject of living only on vegetable food. You know from what I have said that I am an advocate of a mixed diet for man, but I would more particularly draw your attention to a statement that is often made, that it is not necessary to partake of animal food at all. Persons who argue thus, put forth, as a first ground, the immorality of the act, and the impropriety and wickedness of taking away life at all. This is surely an absurd assumption; for the Creator has made a certain number of creatures that could not live upon vegetable food, and they naturally prey upon the lower animals which feed on the grass and the herbs of the field. The lion and tiger exist by prey; and it appears to me that man has a perfect right, without being charged with immorality or impropriety, to take the lives of the lower animals for his food.

Then anatomical arguments are adduced against

ON ANIMAL FOOD. 171

animal food. It is said that man, in his structure, is better adapted for vegetable than animal food. I must here again join issue, for I believe I can show you from his structure that man is more adapted for a mixed diet than either vegetable or animal alone. Here is a view of the jaws and teeth of a carnivorous creature. (Fig. 3). The jaws are so constructed that they will only move up and down like a pair of scissors. This is the head of a tiger. Look also at his sharp-pointed carnivorous teeth, especially the great canine teeth. They are intended for holding and cutting up living food. Now look at the horse (Fig. 4). His lower jaw is quite movable from side to side. Instead of pointed teeth, they are flat, and every arrangement is made for grinding, not cutting, the food; and this is the character of the mouth of a herbivorous animal.

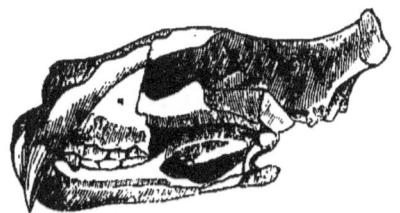

Fig. 3.—Tiger skull.

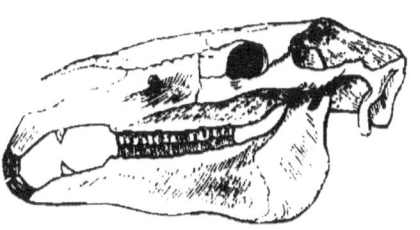

Fig. 4.—Horse skull.

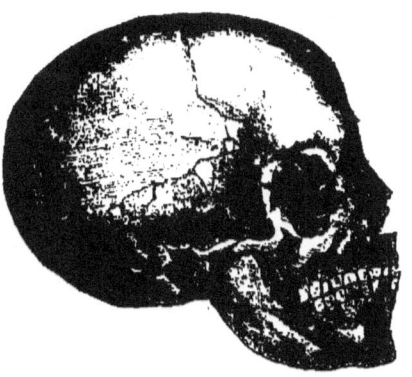

Fig. 5.—Human skull.

Now if we take the skull of a man (Fig. 5), we find he has certain teeth—canine teeth—which, like those of lions and tigers, have the power of cutting; but he has also flat teeth, and the power of moving his lower jaw laterally, and can bring these flat teeth across each other for the purpose of grinding his food; so that you see he is evidently provided with instruments to enable him to prepare for his digestion both vegetable and animal food. I might prolong this argument by showing you the complicated structure of the stomach of the sheep and the ox, and comparing this with the stomach of the lion, point to the fact that the human stomach has neither the complicated structure of the one nor the simplicity of the other. There are many other points of structure in which man seems to stand between these two groups of animals—the herbivorous on the one side and the carnivorous on the other—which would seem to indicate his adaptation for taking both kinds of food.

But whatever may be the arguments of the vegetarians, they do not practically carry out their doctrines, for they partake of considerable quantities of animal food. They take milk and butter and cheese and eggs. Dr. Carpenter states, in a recent review, that he had taken a vegetarian cookery-book, and calculated the quantity of milk, butter, and eggs employed in their food, and found that, if a vegetarian family lived in accordance with the rules of this book, each member would consume half an ounce more animal food a day than he did in his own family,—and he was no vegetarian. So that you see people are deceiving themselves who enforce such a doctrine as this.

On the other hand, there are some persons who advocate a diet of purely animal food. I had a book sent me the other day, written by a gentleman at Liverpool, who states that he has discovered that the panacea for all human evils is the taking of animal food alone; and he takes the opportunity of stating that he is looking for some young lady of similar principles and practice who will link her fortunes with his own and establish a family of carnivorians.

There is no question that man may live on a purely vegetable diet; but the question is as to whether that kind of diet is best for the community. We find in the history of man that those races who have partaken of animal food are the most vigorous, the most moral, and the most intellectual races of mankind. You find that the ancient Jews, although they had certain sanitary regulations with regard to killing and eating animals, partook largely of meat, and were amongst the most vigorous people of their day. We find in modern Europe that those nations who take the most animal food are the strongest; and amongst ourselves, it is just in proportion as we give our labourers animal food, or wages to procure it, that they are stronger and better able to do their work. It is vain for a man to expect to get through intellectual or physical labour without an abundant supply of the material of thought and of physical power, and I have shown you that animal food is one of the readiest means of affording this supply.

Before concluding this lecture I would refer to the fact that by pressing the lean of meat we get a liquid which is called the "juice of flesh." It is free from the fibrine, albumen, or gelatine of the meat, and contains principally the mineral matters of the flesh with creatine, creatinine, moric acid and osmazone. By evaporating this juice, the compound known by the name of "Extract of Meat," or "Liebig's Extract of Flesh" is made. This substance itself contains little or no nutritive or flesh-forming matter, but it renders all food more digestible. It acts in fact as a stimulant to a weak stomach and enables it to digest what otherwise would become a source of irritation and disturbance.

I might now proceed to discuss more fully the qualities of this compound and the various kinds of animal food which we eat, but my time is exhausted, and I must leave what I have said as hints for your future guidance. I hope I have succeeded in showing you that the subject of food is one deserving your attention. The question of food lies at the foundation of all other questions. There is no mind, no work, no health, no life, without food; and just as we are fed defectively or improperly, are our frames developed in a way unfitted to secure that greatest of earthly blessings—a sound mind in a sound body.

SECOND COURSE.

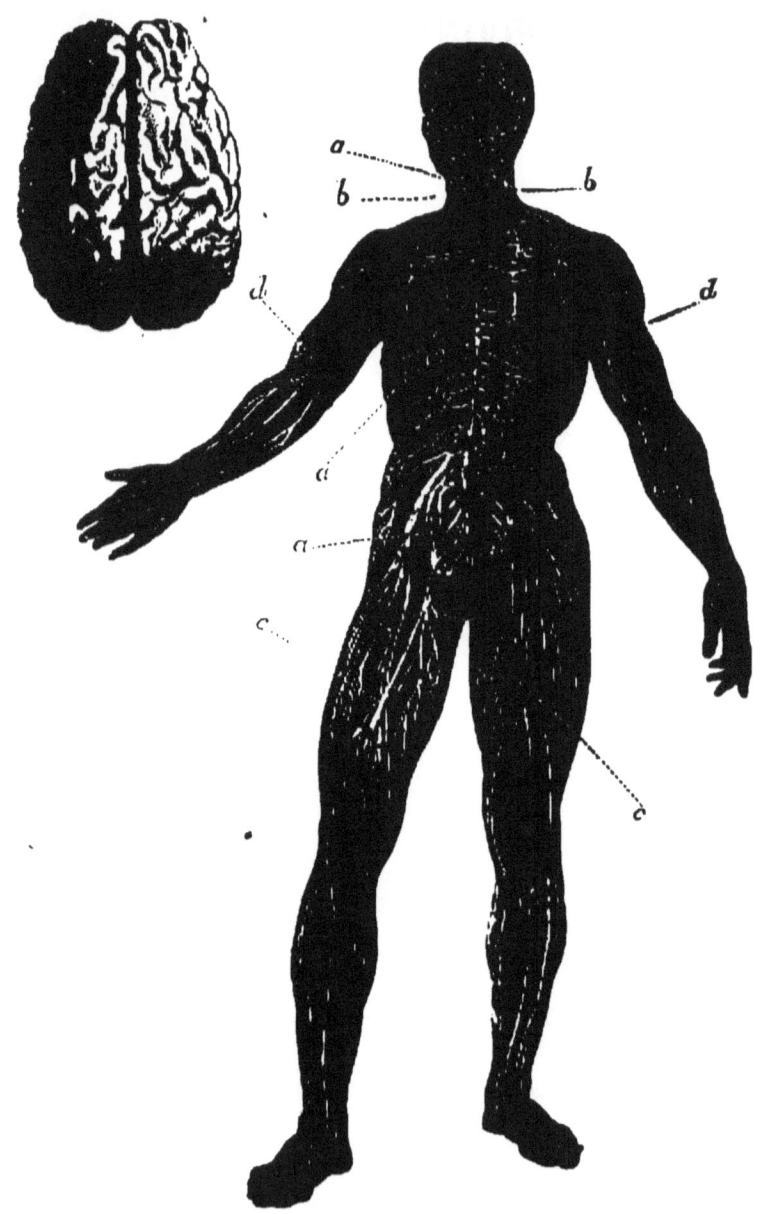

DIAGRAM OF NERVOUS SYSTEM.

a a a Spinal Cord.
b b Sympathetic Nerves.
c c Nerves of Leg.
d d Nerves of Arm.
e Nerves of Head.
f Brain.

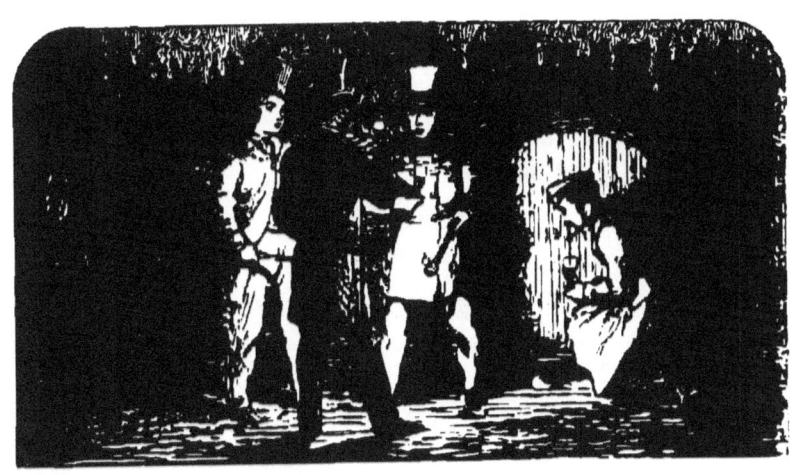

ON ALCOHOL.

IN this lecture I shall take up the second great class of foods. You will recollect that I divided food into two principal classes: the first consisting of those substances which are *necessary* to our daily life, and of which I have spoken at length; and the second, of substances which, although playing an important part in food, are yet of such a nature that they may be regarded rather as *auxiliaries* in the great work of maintaining life, than as necessary to life. I also stated that they acted as many medicines do, and met rather those wants of the system which resulted from a tendency to a diseased condition; and hence I called them *medicinal*.

When you recollect that this class of substances includes alcohol in its various forms, condiments and spices, tea, coffee, chocolate, and tobacco and opium, you will at once perceive how different they are from the last class of which I have spoken. Some persons even deny the right of these things to be called food at all. They say that they enter the system and pass from it without forming part of the tissues of the body, and without being changed, and ought not to be called food. This seems to me a hardly justifiable attempt at appropriating the word food in an unpopular sense, and we shall scarcely be able, I think, to persuade people to regard beer and wine and tea and coffee as things not coming within the meaning of the word food.

The substances of which I have now to speak all agree in one common action, and that is, they all act on the nervous system. On this account it will perhaps be better that I should give you a slight sketch of the nature of the nervous system. In the lecture on flesh-forming foods, I told you that nervous and muscular tissues were ultimately composed of cells, and that the nervous tissue consisted principally of albumen. In the human body this nervous matter is arranged into a system, of which there are three principal parts—the brain, the spinal cord, and the nerves. The nerves perform two functions,—those of sensation and volition. They receive impressions from without, and carry them up to the great centres, the spinal cord and the brain. The impression thus produced is registered, as it were, on these centres; and the result is a corresponding action, and a nerve of motion distributed to a muscle is brought into play. Thus all motion is brought into action by sensation. The spinal cord is the centre of a series of actions of which the mind is not cognizant: hence the movements performed under its influence are said to be involuntary, and it is regarded as the centre of a system, which, independently of the brain, is called excito-motor. In the lower animals, which have no brain, the nervous system is entirely of this character.

But in the higher animals and man there is a brain. The brain is the seat of the intellectual functions, the emotions, consciousness, and volition. It is connected on the one hand with a number of nerves, which are called the nerves of special sense, which go from the eye, the ear, the nose, and the tongue; and on the other hand, with the spinal cord and the nerves of motion. In animals possessed of a brain it gives a controlling power over the action of the nerves of motion. Hence movements effected under its controlling agency are called voluntary. The nerves distributed to the muscles by which we move are more or less under its influence, and they are called *nerves of volition*, and the muscles are called *voluntary muscles*. (See diagram of nervous system.)

Now, without going further into the anatomy or physiology of this highly-interesting system, I would call your attention to the fact that it is on this system which the alimentary substances of which I shall now speak more particularly act. They strengthen, weaken, or derange the nerves of sensation and motion; exalt, depress, or change the action of the spinal cord; and in the same manner act on the intellectual, emotional, volitionary, and conscious functions of the brain. Medicines which thus act upon the nervous system are called narcotics; and did not this term convey the impression that the production of sleep is the result of the use of substances to which it is applied, it would be unobjectionable. I do not like the multiplying terms, but I think the word *neurotic* would be preferable, as applied to these substances, as simply indicative of their action on the nervous system.

Let us, then, without further inquiring into their action here, speak of these nerve-influencing foods. I speak first of alcohol, as by far the most important, and as in some measure, in its action, typical of the rest. Alcohol is a substance which is formed by the decomposition of sugar in fermentation, and is the basis of the fermented beverages known as wines, spirits, beer, &c. If we take any of the forms of fermentable sugar which were brought before you in a previous lecture, and place them in circumstances to undergo change, you will find that the elements of the sugar will arrange themselves in a different manner, and that you will have as the result carbonic acid and alcohol. Let us see how this is. Grape sugar (glucose) contains 12 atoms of carbon, 12 of hydrogen, and 12 of oxygen; or, if we put it into weights, 180 pounds of grape sugar contain 72 pounds of carbon, 12 pounds of hydrogen, and 96 pounds of oxygen. Now during fermentation a certain portion of this carbon unites with the oxygen, and forms carbonic acid, which passing off, leaves the remaining carbon and oxygen with the hydrogen, in the form of alcohol. Or perhaps you will understand the change better by the aid of this diagram:—

ON ALCOHOL.

One atom of grape-sugar contains—

Carbon.	Hydrogen.	Oxygen.
12 atoms.	12 atoms.	12 atoms.

These are converted into two atoms of alcohol, containing—

Carbon.	Hydrogen.	Oxygen.
8 atoms.	12 atoms.	4 atoms.

And four atoms of carbonic acid gas, containing—

Carbon.	Hydrogen.	Oxygen.
4 atoms.	0	8 atoms.

	Carbon.	Hydrogen.	Oxygen.
Thus—	12 atoms,	12 atoms,	12 atoms (grape-sugar).
	8 atoms,	12 atoms,	4 atoms (alcohol).
	4 atoms,	—	8 atoms (carbonic acid).
	12	12	12

Alcohol, then, is composed of 6 proportions of hydrogen, 42 of carbon, and 2 of oxygen; or put into weight, 94 parts will contain—

	PARTS.
Hydrogen	6
Carbon	72
Oxygen	16
	94

But it is not in reality so simple a body as here represented. A part of the oxygen and hydrogen exists as water, whilst the carbon and the hydrogen form a compound called ethyle; and just as in carbonate of potash, the carbonic acid is united to the oxide of potassium, so the water in the alcohol is united to the ethyle, forming a hydrated oxide of ethyle. By adding sulphuric acid to alcohol we take away the water, and the oxide of ethyle can be distilled; we then know it under the name of ether—sulphuric ether. This change is interesting to us, for it is in this way we can explain the *bouquet* of wines and the flavour of spirits. They are in many cases due to ethers formed out of the alcohol they contain.

Alcohol is very volatile, and can be distilled from the water of the liquids in which it is formed. It has, however, so great an affinity for water, that pure alcohol cannot be obtained. It is a powerful solvent, dissolving oils, resins, and other substances, and is, on that account, used in the arts.

Alcohol is very combustible, and gives out an intense heat, and is used on this account by the chemist for lamps. Whilst burning in the air its hydrogen and carbon unite with oxygen, forming water and carbonic acid gas. It coagulates solutions of albumen; and when mixed with water and placed in an animal membrane, it is found to pass through the membrane with less facility than the water. These are two important physical characters of alcohol in its relation to the animal system as an article of diet; and perhaps we cannot do better than commence our consideration of the action of alcohol on the system, by considering the effect of these physical properties of alcohol on the food and the stomach.

By coagulating the albumen of the chyle, it is probable that alcohol may seriously interfere with its due and easy absorption. The curious fact, too, of the more rapid absorption of water than alcohol by an animal membrane may explain one of the injurious effects of alcohol upon the membranes of the stomach. If the membranes of the stomach have the same power of separating water from alcohol out of the living body, then the stomach is constantly exposed to the action of a highly-concentrated solution of alcohol, which may serve to increase its injurious effects on the system. In estimating, however, the effects of alcohol on the system, it should always be recollected, that the form and quantity must have a great effect. Thus, taking the two immediate effects to which I have just now alluded, it will be evident, that the stronger the alcoholic solution, and the larger the quantity, the more decided must be its effect. So important is the comprehension of this fact, that I would point out to you that many things which are poisonous and destructive of life in large quantities, and in a pure form, may be taken with impunity in small quantities and diluted. Thus salt, when taken in large quantities and undiluted, has a most injurious and poisoning effect, but in small quantities it is necessary to life. I mention this, because one of the most distinguished writers on the use of alcohol has not hesitated to commit himself to the fallacy of attempting to conclude what must be the effects of small doses of alcohol daily, by the effects of large and poisonous doses on the system.

We may then, I think, conclude, from the physical facts I have just stated, that the stronger forms of alcohol, as distilled spirits and strong wines, are likely to interfere with the digestion and absorption of our food by their physical action on its constituents. But this action is not, I believe, confined to the food. The inner walls of the stomach are lined with a delicate mucous membrane and glands, whose functions are carried on by the aid of delicate cells, the structure of which is entirely destroyed by the action of alcohol.

There is no better ascertained fact in the whole range of pathological research than that the mucous structure suffers material and dangerous degradation in the habitual spirit-drinker. I would also draw your attention to the fact, that this effect is much more likely to occur when alcohol is taken on an empty stomach, than when taken with food. I have observed, that persons who drink mixed liquors directly after a meal suffer less than those who take them on an empty stomach, the disturbing effect of the alcohol on the food being less serious than that on the mucous membrane of the stomach. This is true of all forms of alcoholic drinks. They are more likely to exert an injurious effect on an empty than on a full stomach, and they are more injurious in both cases the less diluted they are. With regard to the action of alcohol by the more rapid absorption of the water, I would just say, that I believe it is more injurious in the form of spirits and water than of wine and beer; the water apparently separates more rapidly in the former than in the latter case.

As far, then, as its physical action is concerned, I do not know that we can say anything good of alcohol at all; it may seriously interfere with the functions of absorption, and injure the coats of the stomach, and when taken injudiciously, a very long way short of producing any effect on the nervous system, it may yet prevent the proper nutrition of the system, and insidiously lay the foundations of incurable disease. The practical admonition which this part of our subject conveys is this: Avoid taking wines, spirits, and beers, on an empty stomach. In cases where they must be taken, let them be as dilute as is compatible with the object sought to be obtained by taking them. This leads to a very practical question, and that is, how much pure alcohol, in proportion to a given quantity of water, may be taken with impunity? Of course, this is a difficult question to solve, as the quantity which might be taken with impunity by one man might be injurious to another. At the same time, as a matter of experience, I may say, that I have seen little or no inconvenience following the taking, in moderate quantities, the weak table beers of this country. The quantity of alcohol in them is about half an ounce to the pint. I present you here with a table of the quantities of alcohol contained in various fermented beverages, by which you will see that they all contain a larger quantity of alcohol than I think can be taken without running the hazard of injury.

——	Water.	Alcohol.	Sugar.
	oz.	oz.	oz. grs.
London Stout	18½	1½	0 281
London Porter........	19¼	0¾	0 267
Pale Ale	17½	2½	0 240
Mild Ale	18¾	1¼	0 280
Strong Ale	18	2	2 166
Table Beer	19½	0½	0 100
Port	16	4	1 2
Brown Sherry	15½	4½	0 360
Pale Sherry	16	4	0 80
Claret	18	2	—
Burgundy.............	17½	2½	—
Hock.................	17¾	2¼	—
Mosolle..............	18¼	1¾	—
Champagne	17	3	1 133
Madeira	16	4	0 400
Cider................	19	1	0 400
Braudy	9½	10½	0 80
Gin, best	12	8	—
Gin, retail..........	16	4	0½ 0
Rum	5	15	—

But let us now turn to the question of what becomes of the alcohol after it is absorbed into the system. That it is absorbed, there is no doubt. It gets into the head, and, in order to get there, it must be first carried into the blood. We will first confine ourselves to its action on the blood. In the first place, then, the alcohol, on entering the blood, seems to exert the effect of setting free certain fatty matters, which had been previously dissolved in the blood. How it effects this it is difficult to say; but recent experiments have shown this, and some persons have not hesitated in attributing the fattening effects of small doses of alcohol to this action. The fat in the blood is apparently prevented from being carried off in some other form, and is arrested by the adipose tissue. If this should really turn out to be the case, it might be well to pursue the question as to how far such an effect may not assist in that fatty degeneration of the tissues which is one of the most frequent causes of the predisposition to fatal diseases. The probability of such a result should awaken all who indulge in alcoholic drinks, however far short of any immediate unpleasant effect, to the almost irremediable condition of disease into which they are getting, and which may be only made evident when too late to be removed.

As to whether alcohol has any further direct effect on the blood I do not know. I would, however, mention a curious fact related to me by Dr. Addison, and that is, that sherry wine, on being applied to the blood, alters the form of the red corpuscles, and gives them a stellate, instead of a round appearance.

I now come to consider the question, whether alcohol undergoes any chemical change whilst in the blood, or in the tissues to which the blood comes. The ready way in which alcohol becomes oxidized and burned in the air has led to the supposition that it undergoes this change in the blood. This doctrine has received the support of the great German chemist, Liebig, and on this ground he places alcohol amongst the heat-giving foods. The following passage from his "Animal Chemistry" gives this view :—

"Besides fat, and those substances which contain carbon and the elements of water, man consumes, in the shape of the alcohol of fermented liquors, another substance which, in his body, plays exactly the same part as the non-nitrogenized constituents of food. The alcohol taken in the form of wine, or any other similar beverage, disappears in the body of man.

"Although the elements of alcohol do not possess by themselves the property of combining with oxygen, at the temperature of the body, and forming carbonic acid and water, yet alcohol acquires—by contact with bodies in the condition of eremacausis, or absorption of oxygen, such as are invariably present in the body—this property in a far higher degree than is known to occur in the case of fat and other non-nitrogenized substances.

"Decisive experiments have proved that the secretion from the kidneys after moderate use of wine, contains no appreciable trace of alcohol ; it has even been found that the condensible fluid obtained by passing the expired air through a cooling apparatus—that is, the perspiration of the lungs—is, in the same circumstances, entirely free from alcohol. From these facts we can draw no other conclusion but this, that the elements of the alcohol consumed have been given out as oxidized products, the carbon as carbonic acid, the hydrogen as water. If, moreover, we reflect, that after the use of wine, the proportion of carbonic acid diminishes in a certain proportion, obviously corresponding to the hydrogen of the alcohol, no doubt can remain that the elements of alcohol are available for the respiratory process, and are actually employed in respiration.

"It is plain that the quantity of alcohol which can be given out in the form of an oxidized compound in a given time depends on the quantity of oxygen taken up or capable of being absorbed in the same time. If the amount of carbon taken up in the form of alcohol be greater than the amount of oxygen contained in the body, and necessary for its conversion into carbonic acid and water, then the excess of alcohol must pass off as such, or in the form of a lower stage of oxidation, such as acetic or butyric acid; or else it must be discoverable in the body."

The opinion here expressed by Baron Liebig has gained extensive credence, and alcohol has been everywhere regarded as a heat-giving food. The main arguments on which the theory rests are: 1. The easy way in which alcohol is oxidized out of the body. 2. The fact that persons taking much alcohol in their food require less sugar, starch, or fat, and *vice versâ*. 3. That alcohol when taken into the body is not detected in the breath and in the secretions.

Now, taking these arguments in their order, it appears that although alcohol is easily oxidized out of the body, there is no proof that this change goes on in the body. In a series of experiments recently performed by Messrs. Lallemande, Perrin, and Duroy, in France, for the purpose of ascertaining the nature of the action excited by ether, chloroform, and alcohol in the system, no indication of the union of oxygen with alcohol was found in the body. The fact also of the quantity of carbonic acid not being increased after the taking of alcohol would also seem to render it improbable that this gas is formed as the result of the oxidation or combustion of the alcohol.

With regard to the second argument, it may be quite true that persons who drink alcohol do not require heat-giving food, and the contrary; and yet the alcohol be not consumed by a process analogous to that accompanying the destruction of starch, sugar, and fat.

With regard to the third argument, that alcohol is not found in the secretions, this seems not to be the fact. It is well known that for some time after persons have taken alcoholic beverages the odour of alcohol can be detected in their breath. Messrs. Lallemande and others found in their experiments that, not only were ether and chloroform returned from the system in the secretions unaltered, but also alcohol. Dr. Edward Smith, of London, also was able to detect alcohol in the human breath, and in the perspiration from the human skin after the taking small quantities of alcohol. It seems to me, therefore, that we have no right to assume that alcohol is oxidized in the blood until we have further confirmatory evidence. At the same time it must be admitted that no one has at present demonstrated that all the alcohol taken into the system passes off from it unchanged.

There are, indeed, some further changes which take place in the body from the action of alcohol on the blood and tissues that would lead us to suppose that its elements must undergo some change. Thus I drew your attention to the very curious and well-established fact that beer-drinkers and wine-drinkers, and especially port wine-drinkers, are liable to attacks of gout. It does not occur in spirit-drinkers, nor does it happen to water-drinkers. The sugar and the acid of the wine seem to have little or no influence in the production of these effects; we must therefore attribute them to the alcohol. Now my friend Dr. Garrod has shown most clearly that gout depends on the presence of lithic acid in the blood; and the question comes up for answer, as to the manner in which alcohol produces this effect, whether by a chemical change in its own constitution, or by some physical effect which it produces on the tissues. I bring this fact before you both as an illustration of the action of alcohol and as a phenomenon requiring explanation.

It is mainly through the blood that alcohol acts on the nervous system. Before, however, we speak of these special effects, we may refer to some of the other organs to which the blood conveys this substance, and whose functions are affected thereby. The liver receives all the blood from the abdominal viscera, and we should expect it would be affected by the presence of the alcohol. The tissues of the liver seem to have a peculiar affinity for alcohol, and all observers agree that in animals to which alcohol has been administered, the liver has given the most abundant evidence of its presence. It has also been observed that the administration of alcohol increases at first the secretions of that organ. It produces more bile; and if you recollect, I told you in a former lecture that the liver secretes sugar, or a sugar-forming substance (hepatine); and it has been found that alcohol develops the quantity of this substance. The consequence of taking habitual over-doses of alcohol are, first, congestion and enlargement of the liver, and subsequently an inflammatory stage sets in which tends to diminish its size. A small, contracted, inefficient liver is the result. This condition of the liver is so commonly known amongst gin-drinkers, that medical men know it by the name of "gin-liver."

I pass on now to speak of the effect of alcohol on other organs. The blood goes to all organs, and some part or other of the nervous system supplies all organs, so that it is difficult to separate the effect of the alcohol, as exerted physically in the blood, from the effect produced upon the nervous system and through it upon the various organs of the body. Thus alcohol speedily acts upon the heart, but this is probably through its action upon the nervous system. Nevertheless, we may consider its effect on this organ as independent of those especial effects upon the nervous system to which I shall have presently to allude. It is either by its direct or indirect effect upon this organ that alcohol exercises its most obvious action on the system. Unless the nervous system is affected by very large doses of alcohol, or the heart is beating rapidly from nervous exhaustion, the effect of alcohol upon this organ is to quicken its action. If the heart is beating slowly, a dose of alcohol will make it beat less slow; if it is beating quickly it will make it beat more quickly. When beating feebly in disease so as to threaten fainting, it restores its action and prevents the fainting. It thus acts as a stimulant. It is on account of this action that it becomes a most valuable medicine. It restores the flagging powers of the heart in exhausting and depressing disease, and medical testimony is almost universal as to its beneficial action under these circumstances. By thus increasing the action of the heart, effects are produced on the most distant organs. The arteries carry more blood in a given time, and the minute capillary vessels, which connect the arteries with the veins, are the recipients of a larger quantity of blood. As long as the interchange between the two sets of blood-vessels is kept up, the organs thus supplied with blood are only healthfully excited; but the time comes, sooner or later, if the stimulus is supplied, when the capillaries refuse to do their duty, and congestion or stagnation of the blood is the consequence. This will account for the fact that, when only small quantities of alcohol are taken from day to day, a beneficial action of the organs is the result, whilst an excess from day to day may produce the most disastrous consequences.

The organs whose functions are more or less affected by the increased action of the heart are the skin, the lungs, and the kidneys. The great function of the skin is to regulate the heat of the body. This is effected by the conversion of a certain quantity of water into vapour; the water, in passing into vapour, making latent or rendering inactive a certain quantity of heat. For this purpose the skin is supplied with a set of glands (Fig. 1), called sudoriferous, or perspiratory, which are brought into action by anything that increases the heat of the body. Now, any increased action of the heart increases the oxygenation of the blood; and the heat of the body, which is thus developed, is brought down by the action of the perspiriferous glands of the skin. It is in this way that alcohol acts as a diaphoretic and increases the action of the skin.

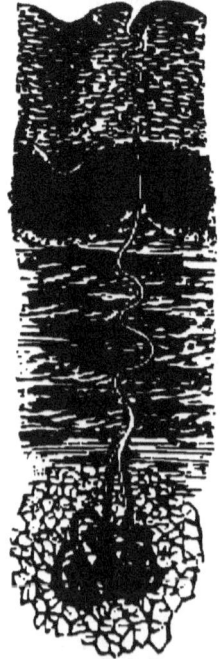

Fig. 1.—*Sudoriferous Gland of Skin.*

An attempt has been made to show that this action

of alcohol does not take place; that so far, indeed, from its increasing the functional activity of the skin, it diminishes it. I am not aware of any direct experiments on this point, but such is the inference drawn by a recent experiment on the action of alcohol on the system. Now I think this is contradicted by the experience of every one who is in the habit of drinking alcoholic beverages. Who has not taken a draught of beer on a hot summer's day, and has not felt almost immediately its effect on the skin, an effect much greater than if the same quantity of water had been taken? The same effect follows the taking of wine, brandy, and whisky. Under these circumstances, I think, we are justified in regarding alcohol as a diaphoretic. I do not know that this would modify in any manner our view of its action as a food, but it is of some importance with regard to its action as a medicine.

Passing on from the skin, we now come to speak of the action of alcohol on the lungs. All the blood of the body is sent through the lungs, and during its passage through the capillaries of these organs it gives off water and carbonic acid, and takes up oxygen. I have told you that as far as the experiments of Vierordt, Becker, and others, go, it would appear that the quantity of carbonic acid expired, after the taking of alcohol, is below that of the quantity expired when only water is taken. So that, from these experiments we cannot conclude that the excretory function of the lungs, as far as carbonic acid gas is concerned, is increased.

I ought to mention here, however, that, according to Dr. Edward Smith's experiments, some fermented beverages have the power of increasing the quantity of carbonic acid expired, whilst others diminish the quantity below that which is thrown off when only water is taken. Dr. Smith attributes these results to the fact that, in the case of wine, spirits, and beer, as ordinarily drunk, other substances are taken into the system besides alcohol. There is no doubt in my mind that not only the composition of the beverages drunk, but also of the state of health and other circumstances connected with the individuals experimented on by Dr. Smith, have led to some of these anomalous results. They do not, however, generally affect our views of the action of alcohol on the system. The expiration of carbonic acid is only one of the results of the changes produced by the action of food on the system, and there can be no doubt that its redundancy or deficiency may be compensated for by other actions going on in the system.

The other constituent thrown out from the lungs is water; and we might anticipate, on two grounds, that the water thrown out from the lungs during the action of alcohol would be increased. If, according to the theory of Liebig, the alcohol is burned by contact with oxygen, not only would carbonic acid be produced, but water. We might also anticipate that as a larger quantity of blood was passing through the lungs, if their function of excretion depended on this blood, the excreted water would be increased. Now, according to the experiments of Dr. Becker, the quantity of water thrown off from the lungs is not only not increased, but actually diminished. We can, however, account for this fact by the increased function of the skin. There is, indeed, no better established physiological fact than that, where two organs get rid of the same product from the body, when it is augmented in one it is decreased in the other, and *vice versâ*.

I now come to speak of one other important action of alcohol. During the time that it is circulating in the blood it is brought in contact with all the tissues of the body: it is carried to the nerves, to the muscles, in fact, to every tissue of the body. Now, the living functions of these tissues are carried on by the agency of changes that go on in their structure. The albumen of the nerve, the fibrine of the muscle, and the gelatin of all the tissues, are changed in their composition, and they are conveyed back into the blood in the form of a compound no longer fitted for the purposes of life. This compound, which is known by the name of cyanate of ammonia, or urea, is composed of the same elements as albumen, fibrine, and gelatin, but they are arranged in a different manner. Instead of being a plastic and permanent compound, it is utterly unorganizable, and readily decomposed: dissolved in the water of the blood, it is carried away by the agency of the kidneys. Just in proportion to the quantity of change which the organs of the body undergo is the quantity of this cyanate of ammonia which is got rid of from the body. It is regarded, therefore, as an index to the quantity of change going on in the tissues. Now this change may be of a healthy or of an unhealthy kind: it may go on too quickly for health, or it may not go on rapidly enough.

Now the quantity of this substance which passes off from the system is diminished by the action of alcohol.

This is one of the most important facts in the history of the action of alcohol on the system: it accounts for some of its well-known effects. Thus, there is no better-established fact than that alcoholic drinks give a tendency to the production of such diseases as rheumatism and gout, which depend on the formation in the blood of certain compounds which ought not to be there. These compounds are probably due to this action of alcohol on the system.

On the other hand, it is well known that in certain states of the system, when change in the tissue is going on too rapidly, that alcohol acts most beneficially. Thus, with the aged and infirm, small doses of alcohol arrest the too rapid changes of the tissues, and give them increased vigour and strength.

Sanctorius called "wine the milk of old age," and its value in certain cases of senile exhaustion can hardly be overrated. It is also undoubtedly due, in some measure, to this conservative action of alcohol, that it has been found of so great value in the treatment of diseases attended with rapid change of the tissues and great exhaustion.

I now come to speak of the action of alcohol on the nervous system. I have already given you some account of the nerves, and the great nervous centres, and their functions. It is upon this system that this remarkable substance exerts its greatest effects. These effects are the result of its direct application to the nerves, or of its indirect effects through the agency of the blood. If we apply alcohol directly to a part, it acts immediately upon the nerves of that part, and excites their activity. In this way it is said to act as a local stimulant. If we take a little brandy and apply it to the naked arm, it stimulates the nervous action, and we feel a tingling sensation. The effect of this stimulation of the nerve is not confined to the nervous system, for we find that the nerves are so closely associated with the blood-vessels, that we cannot act on the one without producing an effect on the other. The result, then, of stimulating the nerves, is to quicken the action of the blood-vessels; and if the alcohol is applied sufficiently long to a part, the result will be congestion of the blood-vessels and inflammation. Now these effects which take place externally on the skin, undoubtedly take place when alcohol is applied to the membranes of the stomach. The effect of small or weak doses of alcohol is to excite the nerves and blood-vessels of the stomach. It is by this action that we can explain both the beneficial and injurious action of alcohol.

In cases where the nervous power of the stomach is feeble, and the glandular apparatus not performing its duty for the want of a sufficient supply of blood, alcohol, by its action on the nerve of the part, at once, as it were, brings the flagging organ up to its duty. It is in this way that it acts beneficially in many forms of indigestion arising from want of power in the stomach. It is in this way, too, that it acts beneficially in that large class of cases comprising individuals whose minds are intensely engaged, and in whom the whole nervous energy of the body seems concentrated in the brain-work that is going on. Alcohol, in the form of wine or beer, seems to make that impression on the stomach which calls the nervous energy from the remoter organ and concentrates it upon the important work that is going on in the stomach. Whatever may be the effects of alcohol on other organs or other parts of the system, the daily experience of thousands will testify to this action of alcohol in the work of digestion.

Just, however, as in other cases where we have seen alcohol acting beneficially, an excess of the same action proves injurious. The dose that improves digestion may easily be increased so as to interfere with it. The membranes of the stomach under the influence of overdoses of alcohol become congested and inflamed; the secretions become changed; the gastric acid is no longer healthful; and some of the worst forms of indigestion can be traced to the pernicious effects of over-indulgence in alcoholic beverages.

Passing on, then, from these direct effects of alcohol on the nerves of the stomach, I come to speak of its action on the nervous system after it has got into the blood. I have spoken of its effect on the heart, on the skin, and on the lungs. Now as all these organs are supplied with nerves in the same manner as the stomach, it is difficult to separate the effects of alcohol from its actions on the nervous system. If it quickens the heart's action, it is through its effect on the nervous system; and if it increases the function of the skin, it is through the same agency; and, in fact, so susceptible is the nervous system to the action of this agent, that it is impossible to administer alcohol without its being affected. It is, however, more to its action upon the great nervous

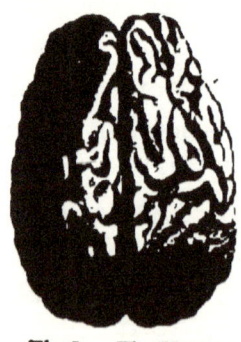

Fig. 2.—*The Human Brain.*

centres, and more particularly to the brain, that I now wish to call your attention. The brain is the seat of the intellectual functions, the emotions and feelings, the consciousness and the will, whilst the spinal cord is the great centre through which the functions of sensation and volition are performed. (See Fig. 2 and compare with diagram.)

When persons unaccustomed to use fermented beverages take only small quantities of alcohol, its effects on the brain become quickly apparent. The whole of its functions become more or less quickened or excited. The intellectual functions are more active, the observing powers are excited, the judgment becomes quickened, and it is under the influence of this agent that the most brilliant sallies of wit have been displayed. The effect is still more obvious on the feelings, and one thing is very generally observed, that the feelings excited are those of a pleasant and hilarious character. Persons habitually melancholy lose somewhat of their solemnity under its influence, whilst the social feelings are most strongly developed. It is worth, perhaps, just a moment dwelling on these effects, because, whether desirable or not, they are the effects which give to alcohol its hold upon the affections of men, and a place amongst his household gods that no other article of food or luxury that he consumes could for a moment claim. This position it has maintained in spite of all opposition, and with the known evil effects of over-indulgence constantly presented to the observation of men.

From the days of Jehonadab, the son of Rechab, down to those of Father Mathew and John Gough, there have never been wanting prophets to denounce and predict the awful consequences of indulgence in alcoholic beverages; there have never ceased apparently from the earth a large class of men who have demonstrated the possibility of living in health, comfort, and prosperity without this substance passing their lips; yet in every civilised community in the world at the present day the presence of some form of alcohol is regarded as necessary to the happiness and comfort of the social gathering. The sovereigns of the world at their feasts and the humblest denizens of huts and cabins have alike recognised its presence as an assuager of sorrow, and the active agent in the development of those feelings which render human intercourse agreeable and pleasant.

That an agent with such powers should be regarded as powerfully medicinal we cannot be surprised, and accordingly we find that medical men in all ages have prescribed it in those diseases which are attended with depression of the feelings, and diminished activity of the mental powers. It is true that it has been asserted that the excitement and exhilaration thus produced are accompanied by a corresponding depression, and that such stimulation is only obtained by an exhaustion that is injurious to the human system. This statement must, however, be met by the daily experience of a large proportion of mankind, who take small quantities of alcohol from day to day, and who, whilst they experience its exhilarating effects, are not aware of any painful depression as its result.

There is a limit, however, beyond which alcohol cannot be taken without producing not only depression after the excitement, but various serious derangements of the system which it so obviously affects. By taking large doses of alcohol, the brain becomes preternaturally excited, the intellectual functions are rapidly performed, the feelings are intensified, and the will loses its ordinary power of control over the mental and moral powers. The senses perform their functions irregularly, sight is deranged, in this state men see double, the spinal cord and its nerves are affected, the gait is unsteady, men reel, and are drunk. This state may pass into one in which the brain loses all power, in which the sensations are so dull that external objects are neither seen, heard, tasted, nor felt. The man is "dead drunk." He is in a state of anæsthesia, such as is brought on by the inhalation of the vapours of ether and chloroform, and operations have been performed on persons when in this state, without their being conscious of pain.

It is impossible that such a state of the nervous system should occur without serious effects; and it is well known that exhaustion, nervousness, depression of spirits, and a greater or less amount of inability to perform its ordinary functions come on in the nervous system after such debauchery. That alcohol can be taken to this extent frequently without producing permanent derangement of the nervous system is too well known to need any lengthened demonstration. The works of those who have written on the abuses of alcohol give copious illustrations of the terrible consequences of such indulgence.

When alcohol is taken from day to day, to an extent even short of producing drunkenness, its effects upon the nervous system are very disastrous. The functions of the nervous system are more or less imperfectly performed. The want of a proper controlling influence of the nervous centres is seen in the trembling hands and shambling gait; the brain, through over-excitement, is under-nourished, and there is a want of intellectual power and decision of will. Sleep, the great restorer of nervous power, is irregular and disturbed; the membranes of the brain become congested, and there is headache; giddiness also frequently occurs on any sudden movement. The intellectual functions are sometimes greatly disturbed, and hallucinations of various kinds are observed. The feelings also become blunted and perverted. If timely warning is not given and taken, derangement more or less complete of the cerebral functions comes on, and the person becomes insane. The records of our lunatic asylums afford abundant evidence of the fact, that undue indulgence in alcoholic beverages is a frequent cause of insanity.

There is still one other result of indulgence in intoxicating liquors which I have to mention, and that is, the production of delirium tremens, or the brain fever of drunkards. This disease may come on as the result of a long course of alcoholic stimulation, or it may appear suddenly as the result of a continued state of intoxication. In this disease the drunkard becomes delirious, and his insanity assumes a very definite form. In all cases he is the victim of painful delusions. He suspects those who are about him. He is the subject of spectral illusions, always of a painful and distressing nature. He is surrounded with imaginary horrors, and is frequently violent in his efforts to avoid them. Sleep almost entirely flees from him, and he is restless in the extreme. He is constantly striving to change his place or position. He trembles all over; his pulse beats rapidly, and the action of the heart is unusually violent. All these symptoms indicate a brain thoroughly disorganized, and, in a large number of cases, the disease proceeds till coma or convulsions terminate the existence of the unhappy victim. That this disease is entirely dependent on the action of alcohol is seen by the fact, that, in cases of recovery, the symptoms subside just in proportion as the alcohol is given time to pass out from the system. So dependent are the symptoms of this disease on the want of sleep, that it would appear that the alcohol acts on the brain by over-stimulating it and preventing that rest in sleep which is necessary for its nutrition. The delirium is generally arrested when the patient gets sleep, hence the general practice of medical men in this disease is to give opium till sleep is procured; at the same time, it has been shown, that by waiting till the alcohol gets out of the system, natural sleep comes on, and the affliction disappears without the administration of opium at all. This fact is a very important one, as there is not wanting evidence to show that the administration of opium may hasten that comatose state in which the patient is sometimes carried off.

I have thus finished the sketch of the action of alcohol on the system, and I have dwelt on this subject at greater length because of the momentous consequences to society involved in the action of this substance on the human system. So shocking and tremendous have been the evil consequences of an abuse of alcohol, that in all times there have been persons who have denounced its use, and declared their conviction that the evils of its action were so great, that no amount of good that could be claimed for it would justify the conscientious man in its use. It is on this account that I have been anxious to give you as full an account as my time would permit of its effects upon the animal frame. It will be for every one to decide for himself how far he feels justified in using it as an enjoyment or as a benefit when he becomes aware of the evils that arise from its abuse in others. With that question, however, I have nothing to do on the present occasion; and, in conclusion, I invite you to some considerations on this substance as a food, a medicine, a luxury, and a poison.

I will not enter into the question of whether we ought to call alcoholic beverages Food. It is sufficient for my purpose that, in one form or another, it enters largely into the diet of mankind, and the question is, as to whether such use is, on the whole, beneficial or deleterious. I have already shown you, that when taken to excess, its effects are very injurious to the system in a variety of ways. But a very practical question arises here as to what is excess. Unfortunately, we have no rule which we can lay down by which the dangers of excess may be avoided. The power of resisting the effects of this agent varies with age, sex, climate, natural constitution, and occupation. The young and the aged suffer more from excess than the adult and those of middle age. Women are less able to bear its action than men. More alcohol can be consumed with impunity in cold than in hot climates. Those who are engaged in sedentary pursuits need be more cautious in its use than those who live much in the open air. The more dilute alcohol is taken, the less likely is it to produce injurious effects.

Such are some of the general facts which apply to its use; but I will not undertake to say what is the precise quantity of alcohol which a man may take as a general rule without doing him any harm. There is one physiological law, however, which, if recollected, might, in some measure, control the evils that arise from taking alcohol, and it is this: that substances which have a tendency to act injuriously on the system may be taken with impunity, provided time is given for the special effects of one dose to be eradicated before the next dose is taken. Now I am not going to commit myself to an opinion as to how many hours it may take for the system to get entirely rid of the effects of half a pint of table-beer or a pint of wine; but I will express my conviction that those suffer least from the effects of alcohol who take it but once in the twenty-four hours; whilst those who are imbibing all day long keep up in their systems an action which is likely to be permanently injurious. The occasional drunkard appears to me to suffer less than the perpetual toper who never betrays the extent of his libations.

With regard to the effects upon the duration of existence of taking a moderate quantity of alcohol daily as against the entire abstinence from it, I am not aware of any decided evidence. Most of the facts that have been brought forward in favour of total abstainers have been by comparing them with classes which include both moderate drinkers and drunkards.

It is very difficult to separate the class of moderate drinkers from drunkards, as, unfortunately, most persons who drink more than is good for them are aware of the degrading character of their vice, and are careful to conceal it from observation. Limited experiments on workmen will scarcely decide the question of the beneficial or injurious tendency of small quantities of alcohol added to our daily food. There is no doubt, however, that it is the conviction of the great bulk of those who have studied this question carefully, that the daily consumption amongst adults of from half an ounce to an ounce and a half of alcohol according to circumstances, is not only not injurious, but conducive to the well-being of mankind. I know that in making this statement I shall be reminded of a certain declaration signed by a number of distinguished medical men in London; but I also know, from a very extensive acquaintance with medical men in London, that whatever interpretation may be put upon their expressed opinions, the instances in which they themselves or their families abstain from taking some form of fermented beverage is very small, and altogether exceptional.

If a few of those who might be thought competent to form a scientific judgment, led by their hearts rather than their heads, would reject alcohol as an article of diet, there are few indeed who would disclaim it as a Medicine. Individually, I hesitate to assign to it the position of importance given to it by a distinguished physician recently deceased; but that a man so capable of forming a judgment, and with such extensive opportunities of witnessing its effects, should have formed so favourable an opinion of its remedial action in disease, is sufficient reason for inquiring as to whether this agent has not a more powerful action in disease than has been usually assigned to it. Dr. Todd, at any rate, employed it in a wider range of diseases than had hitherto been considered proper. Its great action in disease seems to be to suspend the disintegrating processes engendered by morbid actions, and thus to give time for new and healthy actions to set in. Our physiology and pathology are not at present in a position to explain how a substance, in merely passing through the system without undergoing any chemical change itself, should yet exert so powerful an action on the vital processes. At the same time, it should be remembered that water itself acts in the same way; and no one doubts the beneficial action of water both in health and disease. In fact, in this case, as in the other, we must be guided by experience; and though in individual cases this may be fallible, yet that of the great bulk of the medical profession can be relied on, and would lead us to regard alcohol as a remedy equal to, if not greater than, any other which Providence has placed in the hands of man for the purpose of combating disease. I will not here detail my experience; but I hope one day to give you some further account of the action of this agent in disease.

Perhaps of all substances used by man as food, alcohol is most frequently taken as a Luxury. I mean by luxury, that it is consumed, not as an essential of life, but as the minister of sensuous pleasure and gratification. That certain things which are not necessary for our existence or comfort may be thus lawfully employed I think there can be no doubt, when we see how abundantly the kind Father of all has provided for the enjoyment of that which is pleasurable, whether it addresses the eye, the ear, the taste, or the touch. What painting is to the eye, and music to the ear, sweet and pleasant flavours are to the taste. In all nations and in all climes man has indulged in the pleasures of the palate. Wine and strong drink was the promise of the prophet of God to His people for obedience to His laws. The Psalmist thanked God for the wine that made his heart glad. Our blessed Saviour wrought His first recorded miracle on earth to contribute to the pleasure of the guests at a wedding feast; and we cannot but recognise this as one of the most important relations in which alcohol stands to man. In the terrible power which this substance possesses of drawing man from the obedience he owes to the laws of God, we may, perhaps, see one reason why man is permitted to employ it. It may be that he is thus reminded that he is expected to exercise the greatest vigilance and self-control when he is enjoying the highest pleasure. It may be that this is a part of that discipline which we have to go through whereby we may strengthen those volitions which give the highest character to man.

I have said also that alcohol is a Poison. In common with other things which we take as food, as common salt and oxalic acid, it is a poison. In common with many medicines it is a poison. Taken in an overdose it kills as quickly as strychnia or arsenic. It may act as a slow poison by oft-repeated small doses; but this is no argument against its use. Many substances, when taken in small quantities, act as invigorating medicines on the system, which, when taken in large quantities, destroy life. This shows us how careful we need be in its employment, and how necessary it is for all who take it, or are responsible for the administration of it to others, to know the nature of its action upon the system.

I have endeavoured to give you in this lecture an explanation of the action of alcohol on the system, and I trust that every one who hears me will remember how potent an agent it is for good or for evil. It would be better for those who cannot resist its seductive influence that they had never tasted it. It would be better for the world that it had never been known, unless it is employed rationally and with a sense of the responsibility it involves. It is one of the temptations that daily beset us in life, and from the evil influence of which we should daily pray to be delivered. It is one of those creatures of a kind Providence by the abuse of which we bring down upon ourselves an everlasting curse, and by the right use of which our highest and best feelings may be kindled towards the Maker and Giver of all good.

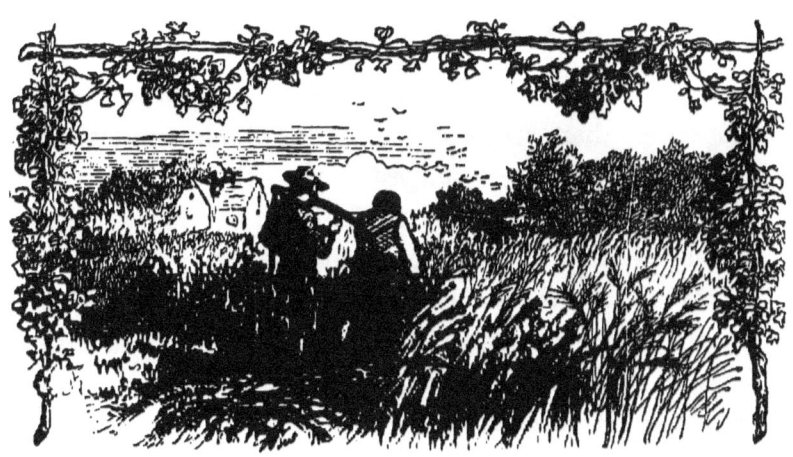

ON WINES, SPIRITS, AND BEER.

HAVING drawn your attention in the last lecture to alcohol, I will now proceed to speak of those beverages of which it is the most distinguishing ingredient. Although the various liquids which we drink under the names of beer, wine, and distilled spirits have very different flavours and properties, yet they all agree more in the possession of alcohol as a constituent than in any other property. I would caution you, however, against supposing that the quantity of alcohol these beverages possess alone determines their price or consumption. I calculate that in the form of beer the alcohol costs on an average about twopence an ounce, in the form of ardent spirits it costs from threepence to sixpence an ounce, whilst in the form of wines it costs from sixpence to two shillings an ounce. It is very clear, therefore, that these beverages possess other properties than those depending on their containing alcohol. It has been suggested that the alcohol itself may be different in character in these beverages; but, as far as its chemical composition goes, this would appear to be impossible. Alcohol, like water and a hundred other chemical compounds, has a fixed and definite character, and would not be alcohol were its properties so changed as to produce different effects on the system. I have suggested that alcohol, on being temporarily mixed with water, may be in a different physical condition as compared with its state in wines and beers, and may thus produce a different effect on the membranes of the stomach. But we have no evidence that the alcohol itself differs in the composition of the various forms of fermented beverages.

It will be, therefore, my task, in this lecture, to draw attention to those other constituents which enter into the composition of beer, wines, and spirits, and which seem to modify to a very considerable extent the action of alcohol, and which also address themselves to the palate, and constitute the basis on which the choice of these substances as articles of diet depends.

I begin with Beer, as the beverage which is most commonly drunk by the large mass of the people in this country, and also as a good example of the modifying influence which other agents exert upon alcohol in a beverage. The practice of making a fermented liquor from wheat or barley seems to have been known from an early period among mankind. Herodotus tells us that the Egyptians made a fermented drink from barley, and Tacitus states that the Germans made an intoxicating liquor from wheat and barley. In our own country beer appears to have been made, at a very early period, from wheat; but the beer manufactured in Germany, under the name of "mum," was preferred, and it was not till the reign of Queen Anne, when a duty of fifteen shillings a barrel was put on Brunswick mum, that brewing, as a trade, began to flourish in this country. We are now the greatest brewers in the world, and the extent of the production of beer at present in England is something almost fabulous.

All beers, ales, and porters are manufactured from malt, which is usually produced from the parched grain of the germinating barley. It can, however, be made from the dried germinating grain of wheat and other seeds. The fact is, any substance containing sugar may be made to yield a wort or solution, which may be fermented and converted into ale or beer. Sugar and water, with the addition of ginger, is largely used in this country, for the purpose of making what is called ginger-beer.

The seeds of all plants contain starch, either in their albumen or their cotyledons. (Fig. 1.) When a seed is cast into the ground or placed in contact with moisture the little embryo or young plant begins to grow or germinate. As the young plant grows the starch is converted into sugar. This conversion of starch into sugar takes place under the influence of a nitrogenous principle contained in the seed, which is called diastase, and the process is very similar to that which takes place when starch is converted into sugar by contact with the saliva in the mouth. The sugar in the seed is intended for the nourishment of the young plant, and it is at the period when the sugar is most abundant in the germinating seed, that the vital changes are put a stop to by heat, and malt is formed.

In this country the whole process of malting is carried on under vexatious excise regulations, which prevent to a considerable extent any improvement in the circumstances under which it is produced. Barley is the grain that is usually employed, although the law does not forbid the use of wheat should the maltster wish to employ it, but barley-malt makes a more agreeable beverage than that from wheat. The business of malting is carried on in large buildings called malthouses, in which arrangements are made for the growth of the barley and its conversion into malt. The grain of the barley is first *steeped* in cold water for a period of not less than forty hours. After the steeping it is thrown upon the floor of the malthouse to a depth of about sixteen inches, which is called the *couch*. It is allowed to remain in this situation for twenty-six hours. It is then turned by means of wooden shovels, and the depth of the couch is somewhat diminished. This process is repeated twice a day or oftener, and the depth of the barley is gradually diminished. In this state the barley absorbs oxygen from the air, and gives out carbonic acid, the temperature of the barley in the mean time being greatly increased, so that it stands at a temperature of ten degrees above the external atmosphere. This has sometimes been regarded as a genuine respiratory process going on in the young plant, but it seems rather to arise from a process of decomposition going on in the constituents of the seed, and to resemble the giving out of heat that takes place in any heap of decomposing vegetable matter. It is probable that the nutrition of the young plant is carried on by the agency of the carbonic acid thus given off, and that this decomposition of the seed is a provision for supplying it with this food before it can obtain it from external sources.

At the time this part of the process is going on, the barley gives out an agreeable odour, like that of apples, and becomes covered with moisture. The appearance of this moisture is called *sweating*. If the grains of barley are examined at this stage it will be found that the young embryo has begun to send down its rootlets or radicles—these are three in number—and shortly after the little plumule (Fig. 1) which is to become the stem appears. This is called the *acrospire*; but the process of growth is arrested before it pushes itself beyond the surface of the grain. The interior of the grain by this time has undergone considerable change, its colour has become whiter, and from being firm and dense it has become loose, and crumbles to powder between the fingers. The grain is now taken to the kiln, and exposed to a heat of 90°, which is gradually increased to 140° or even higher. It is then cleared of the rootlets, and is named *malt*. If we now examine the grain, we shall find that a great change has taken place in its

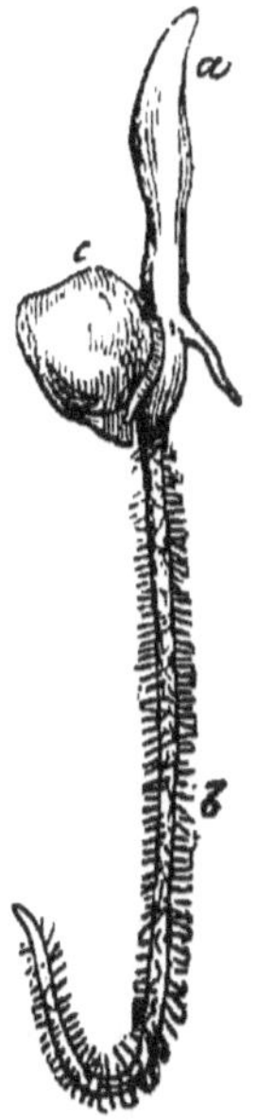

Fig. 1.
(a) *Plumule.*
(b) *Radicle.*
(c) *Albumen of seed.*

chemical composition. Dr. Thomson gives the following analysis:—

	Barley.	Malt.
Gluten	3	1
Sugar	4	16
Gum	5	14
Starch	88	69
	100	100

This is not, perhaps, a very accurate analysis, but it will give you an idea of the changes which take place during the process of germination.

Brewers use three kinds of malt, which are known as pale or amber malt, brown or plain malt, and roasted or black malt. The first only is fermentable, the second is employed to give flavour to beer, and the last is employed as a colouring matter, to give a dark colour to porters and stouts. The two last malts are made by carrying the roasting process so far as to destroy the sugar; whilst in the black malt it is charred by the heat to which it is exposed.

You see, then, that malting is an elaborate process, adopted for the preparation of the sugar which is to be converted into alcohol during the process of brewing. But before describing this process, let me call your attention to the plant which is added to the beer, and which at the present day gives to beer and ale their universal distinction. This plant is the hop—one of the most elegant and ornamental of all the plants which man cultivates for his use. The history of its first use as an addition to the fermented wort of barley is lost in obscurity. You will find a most interesting and learned account of all that is known of the history of this plant in "Beckman's History of Inventions." It grows wild in Great Britain, and is indigenous in most countries in Europe. It belongs to the same group of plants as the nettle, the hemp, the mulberry, and the fig. It is a climbing plant, with rough leaves, and has its stamens on one plant and its pistils on another. The part that is used in making beer is the head, or cone, which contains the pistils. (Fig. 2.) This is com-

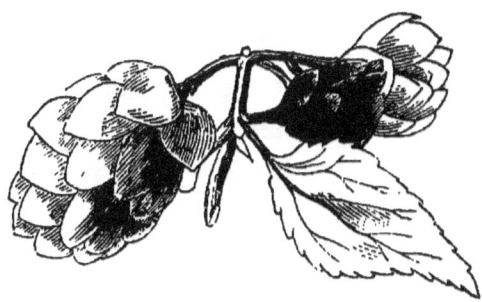

Fig. 2.—Hop Plant.

posed of a number of bracts or scales, which are green, and at the base of each is seated the pistil containing the seed. Surrounding the pistil are a number of little grains, which may be easily removed, and it is found that all the active properties of the hop are contained in these grains. They have been called lupuline, and are separated for medicinal use. Lupuline is composed of resin 55 parts, lignine 32, a bitter extract called lupulite 10 parts, and a volatile oil 2 parts. The lupulite and the oil give to the hops their bitterness and aroma.

Great medicinal virtues have been attributed to hops; and we are told they are "tonic, febrifuge, anthelimentic, antelithic, and hypnotic." But with the exception of the tonic action of the bitter extract, these virtues are altogether doubtful. In estimating, therefore, the action of the hop and the malt, it appears to me that this is the only action that need be regarded; and I may add, that I believe the same effect might be obtained by many other and less costly bitter extracts. But, then, the Government gets a revenue out of hops, and you are obliged to drink your beer with hops in it. That our beers and ales will improve, as all other departments of manufacture have done, when the Government can afford to give up the beer licence, the malt tax, and the hop duty, I have not the least doubt. The worst feature of all taxes of this kind is, that they embarrass industry, and prevent improvement, and eventually, I believe, damage the revenue in other directions.

Hops seem to have been cultivated in Germany in the 11th or 12th century; but they appear not to have been known in England till a much later period. They were at first considered a dangerous thing, as most good things have been, and the planting of them was forbidden in the reign of Henry VI. In 1530 Henry VIII. issued an order forbidding the servants of his household to add hops or sulphur to his beer. Later than this the Common Council of London petitioned Parliament against the use of hops, "in regard that they would spoyl the taste of drinks, and endanger the people."

So much for malt and hops. Now let us begin to brew. In this process the first operation is to grind the malt, which is done either by millstones or iron rollers. The grist thus produced has now to be *mashed*. For this purpose the malt is put into a mashtub, and then hot water is let in upon it and run off by taps from the bottom of the mashtub. Successive quantities of hot water are thus run through the malt, and the worts thus obtained are mixed together, and introduced into a large copper. The hops are now added and the liquor is *boiled*. After boiling, the liquor is strained from the hops and let into vessels to *cool*. When brought down to a proper point, they are passed into the fermenting tun. Here a quantity of yeast is added; and when the fermentation has brought down the quantity of sugar to a certain point, the yeast is cleared away, and this process is called *cleaning*. The beer is now run into vats or casks, which is called *racking*. It is still, however, thick and muddy, and a solution of gelatine or isinglass is added, for the purpose of clearing or *fining* it. The beer is now bunged up, and it is ready for use at various periods.

Now beer can be made to vary greatly in its quality according to the way in which this process of brewing has been carried on. Of course, the stronger the wort the more sugar, and the more alcohol as the result of fermentation. But you may carry the fermentation up to various points. You may make, at first, a sweet beer or ale by stopping the fermentation, but which eventually shall become very strong by age and fermentation. Such are our sweet ales, and ales that get strong by keeping. By carrying on the fermentation you may exhaust all the sugar, and by using malt free from gum you get a clear pale ale, and by adding a larger quantity of hops, our pale bitter ales are produced. The fermentation of these ales being over, they can be sent to a distance: hence the practice of sending such ale to India. They are, however, generally strong ales, on account of the completeness of their fermentation, and are objectionable on that account. I find that our ordinary bottled pale ale contains more alcohol than hock, claret, or Moselle wines, and as much as Burgundy.

The brewing of the pale and bitter ales for the Indian market has led to a great change in public taste for beer, and milder pale and bitter ales are extensively brewed for domestic consumption. My own conviction is, that an immense benefit has accrued from this, as the strong and sweet ales formerly drunk were objectionable on many accounts. In the first place, they caused a greater consumption of alcohol than was beneficial; and in the next place, the sugar became a source of disorder and disagreement in the stomach. The increased quantity of hop also secures in the mild bitter ales a tonic effect which is very beneficial. For habitual consumption in families the mild bitter ale, with not more than half an ounce of alcohol in the pint, is to be commended above all others.

London porter, of which prodigious quantities are consumed daily in this metropolis, is coloured with the black malt. It contains about three quarters of an ounce of alcohol in the pint, and more sugar and less hops than the pale ales. It is, however, miserably drugged in the public-houses. Its strength is reduced by water, and its qualities are brought up again by treacle, liquorice, and salt, and various narcotic agents are added to make up for the loss of alcohol. To such a condition has the porter-drinking population been brought, that they do not know genuine porter when they drink it, and having acquired a taste for its wretched substitute, they reject the unadulterated article.

Stout is only a stronger form of porter. Good draught stout contains one ounce and a half of alcohol in the pint.

All beers, ales, and porters may be bottled; and this is done before the active fermentation is over, so that this process engenders in the bottled liquid a quantity of carbonic acid gas, which converts the stouts and porters which contain a great quantity of gum into one mass of froth. It is not quite so bad in the pale ale, but here it is not uncommon to lose half the ale by its seething over the glass when poured from the bottle.

Bottled ales are generally stronger than those on draught; and with some persons the frothing state of the beer seems to agree better than the less lively condition of that from the cask. It is the same with wines and water; and carbonated waters and effervescing wines have the same recommendation.

I have not time to dwell on the varieties of beers, ales, and porters sold in this country. But they differ very much; and the impossibility of brewing the same beer in two different districts is an interesting fact. One of the most remarkable facts of this sort is the generally acknowledged excellence of the Burton beers. Now it appears there is only one condition at Burton that causes its beer to differ from all others, and that is, the presence in the water of a certain quantity of sulphate of lime. My friend, Dr. Letheby, has pointed out that this is the real cause of the success of the pale ale breweries of Burton. He says, such water will not extract the saccharine and albuminous matters of malt so fully as others, and that this is desirable in the manufacture of pale ales. I would, however, bear my testimony to the great intelligence and care with which the great pale ale breweries are conducted at Burton-on-Trent. Such prevision and intelligence brought to bear on the minutest details of a great manufactory, cannot fail to be productive of the best results.

Then you see, from what I have stated, the beers contain water, alcohol, sugar, and the bitter principle of the hop. In addition to these things, beer always contains a certain quantity of acid. This acid is acetic acid, or vinegar. It is naturally produced by the exposure of the alcohol to the action of the oxygen of the air. The change that takes place is the conversion of alcohol, which is a hydrated oxide of ethyle into acetic acid, which is a hydrate of the teroxide of acetyle. This is sometimes called the acetous fermentation; but it is not a process like fermentation, but an oxidation or slow combustion of the alcohol. This process goes on in beer after it has been put in the cask, and it is in this way that beer gets sour. In some parts of the country the beer is preferred a little tart; but in proportion as it gets acid it loses strength. The hops suspend this process; and bitter beer is much less liable to this change than sweet beers. The same changes occur in wines, especially sweet wines; and an extensive manufacture of vinegar from wine is carried on.

I now come to speak more particularly of Wine. The term wine is generally applied to fermented liquors to which no additional ingredient is added. Thus the fermented wort of malt is called malt-wine when hops are not added. The term wine is, however, specially applied to the fermented juice of the grape. Of all fruits, this one affords the best material for making wine, and there is a curious chemical reason for this which I may at once explain to you. The various fruits which can be fermented and made into wines contain organic acids. Now these acids vary in chemical composition and flavour. Thus in apples and pears we have malic acid, in oranges citric acid, and gooseberries, currants, and other fruits, also citric acid, mixed with some other acid. Grapes also contain tartaric acid. These acids do not exist in these fruits in a pure form, but in combination with the alkalies or earths forming salts. These salts are super-salts, that is, they contain a superabundance of the acid, and taste acid in the mouth. With one exception these salts are soluble in water, and that exception occurs in the grape. When the tartaric acid of the grape combines with two proportions of the acid to one of potash it forms an insoluble salt known as supertartrate of potash or cream of tartar. It is the formation of this salt in the wine made from the grape that causes the deposition of a large quantity of the tartaric acid, and the wine is thus prevented from tasting too sour. In the case of other fruits, the acid remains in the wine, and renders necessary the addition of sugar to take away the excessive acidity. This gives to other wines an objectionable character. What are called British wines, made from the fruits of the currant, gooseberry, or the orange, require the addition of sugar in order to take away the sourness of the acids they contain.

The grape vine (*Vitis vinifera*), from the fruits of which wine is made, seems to have been one of the earliest useful plants known to man. The first recorded history of the employment of wine is found in the account of Noah's drunkenness. From that time reference to this beverage is frequently made in the Bible, and we find amongst the early nations of antiquity that it was the most generally known form of fermented beverages.

Like most extensively-cultivated plants, it is very difficult to ascertain of what country the vine is originally a native. It is among the plants of which we have the earliest records in the Books of Moses, and from which it appears to have been made use of in the same manner as at the present day. Although the vine is found in many places of Judæa wild, it may still be doubted whether it is indigenous there, on account of its frequent cultivation. There seems to be little doubt of its being truly indigenous in the East, in the district between the Black and Caspian Seas. In the forest of Mingrelia and Imiretia it flourishes in all its magnificence, climbing to the tops of the highest trees, and bearing bunches of fruit of delicious flavour. In these districts no cultivation of the vine exists, and the inhabitants seldom harvest the abundance of the fruit that is produced. It is not probable that these vines are the remains of former vineyards, as plants mostly degenerate when they become wild after cultivation, which is not at all the case with these grape vines. It is probable that the wild vines found along the borders of the Caspian Sea, throughout Persia, in the north of China, and in the Deccan and Cashmere, are all indigenous, although the plant is cultivated in these districts.

In many spots in France, Germany, Portugal, and Italy, the vine is found wild, but the fruit is very generally of an inferior kind, and it is probably not indigenous in any part of Europe. We have no accounts of the introduction of the vine into Greece. It was evidently cultivated there before the time of Homer, and is supposed to have been later introduced into Italy, and the Romans probably spread it through the north of Europe, and introduced it into Great Britain. Bede, writing in 731, says there are vineyards growing in several places. These vineyards in Great Britain were generally connected with monasteries, as the inhabitants of those places paid great attention to the cultivation of fruit. When monastic institutions were abolished, vineyards very generally disappeared in this country, probably both on account of there being no monks to attend to them, and better wine being obtained from the fruit of other countries. Much has been written about the reintroduction of vineyards into Great Britain. There can be no doubt that grapes could be produced in abundance, and acquire a certain degree of ripeness in this country; but our clouded skies and high latitude must prevent the production of fruit in this country equal to that of the lower latitudes, and under the brighter skies of the continent of Europe.

The cultivation of the vine extends from near $55°$

north latitude to the equator, but in south latitudes it only extends as far south as 40°. It is cultivated at various elevations. In Middle Germany it ceases from about 1,000 to 1,500 feet above the level of the sea. On the south side of the Alps it reaches 2,000 feet; in the Apennines and Sicily 5,000 feet; and on the Himalaya as high as 10,000 feet above the level of the sea. The point of the greatest importance in the ripening of the fruit of the vine is the length of the summer. Thus, although the maximum of summer heat is as great at Moscow as in Paris, yet the vine will not ripen its fruit in the former place; and this arises from the fact that although the greatest heat of the months of June and July are as great as that of Paris, the months of August and September are several degrees below. Nor will the mean temperature serve as a rule to indicate where the vine may be cultivated. England has a mean temperature as high as many parts of the world where the vine flourishes in the greatest perfection; but it will be found that although England is warmer than these countries in the winter, it is not so warm in the months of September and October, at which time the vine is ripening its fruit. The vine will bear any degree of heat, and is cultivated in some districts close to the equator. It will not, however, bear heat combined with moisture, and the fruit in European countries is never so good in wet seasons. This, then, will account for the different points of latitude at which the vine ceases to be cultivated in Europe. In France it extends as far as 49° north latitude on the western borders of the Seine. In England, although much cultivated, the fruit seldom ripens properly in the open air. At Berlin, in 53° north latitude, the fruit is poor. Konigsberg has a north latitude of 54° 42', and is the extremest point at which the vine can ripen fruit. On the Rhine its cultivation extends down to Cologne, and even Düsseldorf. Throughout the middle and south of Europe, to the borders of the Mediterranean, between the Black and Caspian Seas, in Astrachan, in the north of China, in Hindostan, throughout Persia, along the borders of the Euphrates, in Syria, Lower Egypt, Abyssinia, and in Barbary, the vine is cultivated. In the New World, both in North and South America the vine flourishes. In South America, it is cultivated and used for making brandy and wine at Guyaquil-Pisco, in the northern provinces of Chili, at Valparaiso, and is found at Valdavia in the fortieth degree south latitude. On the other side of the continent, at Buenos Ayres, and in various parts of Brazil, it is extensively cultivated. In North America its culture is known to extend as far as 37° north latitude on the Ohio, and on the north-west coast as far as St. Francisco, in 38° north latitude. The vine is also growing now in the southern parts of New Holland and has been introduced from America into the Sandwich Islands.

The fruit of the vine is used as an article of diet in several ways. Its agreeable sweet acid flavour, when ripe, has always rendered it a very desirable food when fresh. The ancients also, there can be but little doubt, were in the habit of drinking the expressed juice of the grape before fermentation. Grapes are also dried and used under the name of raisins. The drying is generally effected by cutting half through the fruit stalk while they are suspended on the tree. Grapes thus dried are called muscatel raisins, and are principally brought from the Levant and from Spain. There is another dried grape used much in this country, called *currants* or Corinths, but which are very different things from the common currants of our gardens, and are the produce of a vine which grows in Zante and Cephalonia. Raisins and currants contain less water than fresh grapes, and when eaten alone they are liable to produce indigestion.

The most extensive use of the grape is for the purpose of making wine. In an unripe state the juice of the grape contains malic, citric, and tartaric acids, bitartrate of potash, sulphates of potash, and lime, with other inorganic salts in less proportion, a little colouring and extractive matter. As the fruit ripens, gum makes its appearance, and grape sugar is formed at the expense probably of the citric and tartaric acids. When ripe, the principal ingredients are sugar, gum, malic acid, and bitartrate of potash.

With its extensive cultivation, it is not to be wondered at that a great number of varieties should be described. The lists from the vineyards of the Continent and from the forcing-houses of England give several hundreds. In most of them the principal difference consists in the form and colour of the fruit, and the shape and clothing of the leaves. So great is the difference in some cases, that Professor Link of Berlin is of opinion that all our cultivated grapes are the products of the hybridization of several species. Independent, however, of any externally different characters, there is great variety observed in the wines they produce, which depend on causes that have hitherto escaped observation. There are instances of the same variety of vine being planted on the side of a hill or mountain, and the wine which is the produce of the grapes from the highest parts of the mountain will differ essentially from the wine which is the produce of the grapes of the lower parts of the mountain. The wines known by the names of Johannisberg and Rudescheimer, in Germany, are the produce of vines growing close together, and resembling each other in external characters. The vineyards also that produce the Leistenwein, Wurzberger, and Steinwein, are very near to each other. It has been supposed that this difference is owing to the composition of the soil, but much is undoubtedly due to the care which is taken in preserving the fruit from the influence of adverse circumstances. Thus, with regard to the vineyard of Johannisberg, which produces the most costly wine in the world, it is well known that it is surrounded by a wall that protects the grapes from the cooling and disquieting influence of winds, and all that requires attention during the culture of the grape is ensured in these magnificent vineyards.

The fruit of the grape is either purple or white, and the grapes have various sizes and are of very different flavours, but these points are but of little importance in the manufacture of wines. The purple grapes do not necessarily make red wines, nor do the white grapes make white wines. Although the flavour of some grapes is so strong as to give a taste to the wine, as in the case of the muscat grape, yet the flavours of wines are independent of the flavours of grapes.

When wine is to be made, the grapes are gathered and placed in vessels from which their juice is expressed by pressure. The juice before it is collected is called *must*. Of course it consists principally of water, which holds in suspension and solution a variety of substances. The chief of these is sugar—sugar in that form which is called glucose, grape, or fruit sugar.* Then we have gum, fat, wax, albumen, and gluten, tartaric acid free, and tartaric acid combined with potash as cream of tartar; we have also racemic acid, malic acid, and malate of lime, and then there are varying quantities of salts, as the oxides of manganese and iron, sulphate of potash, common salt, phosphate of lime, and even silicic acid. Thus you see this must is a very compound substance, but the three things of most importance in relation to wine-making are the water, the sugar, and the albumen and gluten.

The quantities of these ingredients vary in different seasons, and this will account for the difference in the wines made from them. Quantity, however, does not always indicate the difference that will be found in the wine. There may be much sugar, but it may not ferment well, or the grapes may be damaged so as to interfere with the fermentation, but generally the quantity of sugar is an indication of the goodness of the grape, and its fitness for making wine. Grapes are in best condition for making wine when the summer is hot and the season dry in which they are gathered. The heat and light of the sun principally develope the saccharine qualities of the grape. But however much

* See Lecture III.

sugar there may be, if the grapes are wet, or get mouldy or decayed before they are gathered, the fermentation is imperfect, and the wines are weak, and sour, and flavourless. This is why there are bad wine, good wine years, and middling wine years. Thus it is known that the good Port wine years have been, for this century, 1802, 1803, 1804, 1806, 1810, 1811, 1815, 1820, 1821, 1822, 1827, 1830, 1834, 1840, 1842, and 1850. In the same way lists can be made out of French and German wines, and it is curious to observe that the good years of one wine are frequently the bad years of another.

One of the great difficulties of the wine-maker is to get the must at the right time, and if the grapes have not all ripened equally, this is a great difficulty. If the grapes are gathered too soon the wine becomes sour and hard when old. If they are gathered too late, they ferment in the cask, and also become sour, but from the very opposite reason of the sourness which comes on when the grapes are gathered too soon.

The quantity of sugar in grape juice varies from 13 to 30 per cent. When the fermentation is complete, the whole of this sugar is converted into alcohol. The proportion which the alcohol forms to the sugar is about as 1 to 2, so that we may reckon that the wine will contain half as much alcohol as the must contained sugar. This is generally true of the unbrandied wines of France and Germany. In seasons when the must is deficient in sugar, cane-sugar or raisins are added to it in order to increase the quantity of alcohol, but this destroys the flavour of the wine.

After the juice of the grape has passed from the wine-press, it is placed in vats, where the process of fermentation is allowed to take place. It is not necessary to add a ferment to the juice of the grape, as the nitrogenous matters contained in it speedily enter into a state of change, which is communicated to the sugar, and the result is the production of alcohol by the series of changes which I mentioned in my last lecture. During this process the juice becomes more turbid, bubbles of carbonic acid gas appear in it, and a froth or scum is formed upon its surface. It becomes more liquid by the conversion of the sugar into alcohol, and various matters which were at first held in solution are now thrown down. The fermentation goes on more or less rapidly according to the temperature. It is more rapid in high than in low temperatures, and generally attains its height in three or four days. In this state it continues for some days longer, and when clear it is run off into another vessel, in which a diminished amount of fermentation goes on for some months. The wine is drawn off from these vessels into casks, in which it is kept till it is bottled.

Now I might detain you here to speak of the treatment of wine after it is put in bottles. It is put into bottles for the sake of keeping it, and the placing these bottles in some safe and convenient place called a cellar is technically called cellaring. Some wines are not much improved by bottling at all, and these you may drink directly from the cask. In wine countries it is not an uncommon thing to drink the wine directly from the cask as we do beer. This is more especially done with the weaker and cheaper wines, and wine is occasionally thus consumed in this country. " Wine from the wood" is sold in some of our wine shops. Inferior red wines, sherries, and Marsala, are said to improve more whilst on tap in the cask than when bottled. Weak wines cannot be kept long in the cask without a danger of the oxygen of the air converting their hydrated oxide of ethyle (alcohol) into the hydrated tri-oxide of acetyle (vinegar), which is a result very much to be avoided by those who attach importance to the flavour or strength of their wines.

Wine in casks gets altered by the evaporation of the water and the alcohol into the air, and also by the absorption of one or the other by the wood. These changes cannot happen when the wine is put into glass bottles. Wine can thus be kept longer in bottles without change than in wood. There is a notion that wine gets stronger by keeping, but this is erroneous. If fermentation goes on a little more sugar would be converted into alcohol, but this is not large even in the case of effervescing wines. It is, therefore, a false notion that wine gets stronger by keeping. Strong wines undoubtedly keep best. Wines get altered by keeping, and they get weaker by keeping. They should not be kept in hot cellars, nor cold cellars, nor cellars with a changeable temperature. It appears that a uniform temperature of between 50 and 60 is the best for all kinds of wine. Wines are said to ripen sooner in warm cellars than in cold ones, and it is very certain that new wines may be made to assume the flavour of old ones by exposing them to high temperatures, and letting them cool again. This, however, belongs to the art of " doctoring" wines, a practice that very few private individuals care to enter upon, and which, when earnestly pursued, is done with a view to deception and fraud.

Let me now direct your attention to the composition of all wines, and point to those constituents which, in larger or smaller quantities, give flavour and character to them. These constituents are *water, alcohol, sugar, acids, bouquet, colouring matter,* and *salts.*

Of course, I need say nothing about the water; that will always be in proportion to the absence of other things. I may as well, however, say that it is never less than 75 per cent., and seldom more than 90 per cent., in wines.

Alcohol is the constituent which distinguishes wine as well as other fermented beverages. It is not, however, the quantity of alcohol that determines alone the price of wine. Taking, for instance, the analysis of hock wines, as given in Dr. Bence Jones's translation of Mulder's "Chemistry of Wines," you will find that Marcobrunner, worth, perhaps, fifteen shillings a bottle, does not contain so much alcohol as Geisenheimer, which is sold at two shillings a bottle. Fiery ports, with 25 per cent. of alcohol, are worthless compared with old ports, containing not more than 20 per cent. of alcohol. Here, as in so many other articles of food, it is the flavour which gives the value.

The quantity of alcohol per cent. in different wines may be seen in the following table, given by Dr. Bence Jones, as the result of a long series of analyses:—

In Port	... ...	from 20·7 to 23·2	per cent.
Sherry	... ...	,, 15·4 ,, 24·7	,,
Madeira	... ...	,, 19·0 ,, 19·7	,,

In Marsala	... ...	from 19·9 to 21·1 per cent.
Claret	... ...	,, 9·1 ,, 11·1 ,,
Burgundy	...	,, 10·1 ,, 13·2 ,,
Rhine wine	...	,, 9·5 ,, 13·0 ,,
Moselle	... ...	,, 8·7 ,, 9·4 ,,
Champagne	...	,, 14·1 ,, 14·8 ,,

You will see, from this table, that the favourite wines of this country are the strongest. This arises, probably, from two causes: first, our natural love of strong drink; and, second, from the fact that we pay the same duties on strong as on weak wines. I am afraid, as long as the latter cause exists, it will lead to the consumption of the stronger wines. This is to be regretted, as there can be no doubt that the temptation is stronger to take more alcohol than is good with strong than with weak wines.

The quantity of alcohol in wine, when genuine, is dependent on the quantity of sugar in the grape. But there is considerable doubt as to whether the quantity of alcohol in our ports and sherries is always the result of the fermentation of the sugar naturally in the grape. It is a fact well known, that with regard to the greater proportion of Ports and Sherries drunk in this country, they have alcohol added to them, both in the countries in which they are made as well as in this country. There can be no doubt that if the taste could be generally diffused for the genuine wines of the Rhine and France, it would be better for the wine-drinking classes of the community.

Sugar is the constituent of wine, which has the nearest relation to alcohol. If the whole of the sugar in the juice of the grape is converted into alcohol, then there is none left in the wine. But it frequently happens that there is more sugar in the grape-juice than can be converted by the natural ferment of the juice—the albumen—into alcohol. Thus we have two sorts of wines—*sweet* wines and *dry* wines. Even strong wines may have sugar left, so that we have strong sweet wines and strong dry wines, and we may have weak sweet wines and weak dry wines.

The following are the quantities of sugar found in one imperial pint of several of the commoner sorts of wines:—

	oz.	grains.
Port	1*	2
Madeira		400
Brown Sherry		360
Champagne		133
Pale Sherry		80
Claret		None.
Burgundy		,,
Hock		,,
Moselle		,,

Some wines contain a great deal more sugar than any of these,—as Malmsey, Tokay, Samos, and Cyprus, which give from two to five ounces in a pint. Sugar is purposely added to some wines, to take off their acid flavour. This is the case with those wines which are called "British," and which contain acids that are not precipitated during the making: such are orange, gooseberry, currant, rhubarb wines.

The sugar in wine is in a condition in which it is easily decomposed: hence persons with weak stomachs cannot drink it without producing heartburn. It is also one of the elements of wine which appears to en-

* One ounce contains 437½ grains.

gender that condition of the system in which gout comes on. It is well known that gout comes on in port-wine drinkers; and looking at the foregoing table, you will see that it contains more sugar than any of the wines ordinarily drunk in England. Sugar alone will not produce this disease; but sugar in conjunction with alcohol, as in ports and sherries, will produce it. Sugar is found in the same state in beer. Gout is found amongst port, sherry, and beer drinkers, whilst it is almost unknown amongst spirit, claret, and hock drinkers.

If wines are bottled before the fermentation is over, the carbonic acid is retained in the wine, and what is called an "effervescing" wine is produced. There are certain kinds of wine which are favourable to this process; and in all countries effervescing wines are produced. In this country we are best acquainted with the effervescing wines of France, which are generally known under the name of Champagne. Hocks, Moselles, and even red wines, are treated thus; and when the cork is removed from the bottle, the carbonic acid begins to escape, and gives them their sparkling, effervescent character. When such wines contain much sugar, the fermentation in the bottle is arrested before all the sugar is consumed, and they are sweet effervescing wines. In other cases the sugar is all exhausted in producing the carbonic acid, and such wines are then said to be dry.

Sparkling or effervescing wines are agreeable to the palate, and, in the same way as bottled ales, they sometimes appear to assist the digestion of the food with which they are taken. In some cases, however, there can be no doubt that they produce injury. When new, they communicate the state of change in which they are to the contents of the stomach, and interfere with the healthy process of digestion. They are less liable to disagree when they are dry and contain but little sugar, than when they contain much of this substance. The quantity of sugar varies in champagne from one hundred grains in the pint to considerably above an ounce.

We now pass to the acids in wine. There are two sorts of acids, or, I may say, three. There is tannic acid, which gives the astringency to red wines, and is the principal agent in the formation of the crust; then there is the tartaric acid which gives acidity to wine; and there are the acids which, uniting with compounds in the wine, form the flavours and bouquet of wines. It is to the tartaric acid I would now draw your attention. The tartaric acid is the acid which distinguishes the fruit of the grape: it occurs in varying quantity in grapes, but it is always found in wine made from grapes. Mülder says there is from 2 to 7 parts of perfectly pure tartaric acid in 1,000 parts of wine. Then the bitartrate of potash is after all slightly soluble in water, and assists, by its solution, in acidifying wine.

Then there is always a small quantity of acetic acid, or spirit of vinegar, in wine—Mulder says from $\frac{1}{4}$ to 2 parts in the 1,000 of wine. You know that the old-fashioned way of making vinegar is to expose wine to the air, and the oxygen of the air uniting with the alcohol converts it into vinegar,—thus accounting for the old pronouncing puzzle—

"White Wine Vinegar is Very good Victuals I Vow."

Well, this oxidation of the alcohol will always take place in making wine; it takes place much more in making beer. Hence the acetic acid is always greater in beer than in wine; but then, beer contains no tartaric acid.

Sugar hides the flavour of acids; so that a sweet wine may really contain much more acid than an acid wine. You will see the quantities of tartaric acid in different wines, and acetic acid in beer, in the following table. The quantities are grains in an imperial pint.

	Grains.
Port	80
Brown Sherry	90
Claret	170
Burgundy	160
Hock	130
Moselle	140
Champagne	90
Madeira	100
London Stout	54
Porter	45
Pale Ale	40
Cider	120

The cider contains malic acid.

The action of these acids on the system has been much misunderstood. It has been supposed that acid wines are bad where there is acidity of the stomach. Now, acidity of the stomach more frequently arises from the decomposition of sugar than anything else; and wines which have sugar enough to cover their acidity have been taken to prevent this state of the stomach, whilst acid wines which contain no sugar have been avoided. Neither tartaric, acetic acid, nor any other acid, has a tendency to favour the development of more acid in the system. I think this should be generally known; for there seems to be a prejudice against the acid wines of France and Germany in this country, as though they were capable of producing the pernicious effects of our own saccharine beers, ciders, and wines.

I now come to speak of the flavour of wines, or of the bouquet, as it is sometimes called. But flavour and bouquet are two different things. The vinous flavour is common to all wines; but the bouquet is peculiar to certain wines. All persons are more or less acquainted with the vinous smell. Persons who have drunk much wine are redolent of this odour, and it is especially detected when such persons first come into a room where this odour had not before existed. This smell is very different from that given out by beer or distilled spirits. The substance which thus characterizes wine is called œnanthic ether. It is evidently formed during the fermentation of the grape-juice. This ether is formed in the same way as alcohol. Alcohol, you know, is a hydrate of the oxide of ethyle ($HO + O + C\ 4, H\ 5$). Now, if we put œnanthic acid ($C\ 14, HBO\ 2$) in the place of water, instead of the hydrate of the oxide of ethyle, we get the œnanthate of the oxide of ethyle, and this is the substance which gives the smell to wine. When separated from the wine, it is anything but pleasant; but many tastes and smells, which are unendurable in their concentrated forms, are exceedingly pleasant when diluted.

Now the special bouquets or flavours of wines are formed on the same principle as œnanthic ether. Some compound of carbon and hydrogen, like ethyle, the basis of alcohol, unites with some acid, and forms an ether which gives the surpassing excellence to favourite wines. These ethers can actually be manufactured and added to wines, so that common wines may be made to taste like those of great price; but the cultivated taste can detect the cheat. These artificial mixtures never equal the natural product. So it is with all artificially-formed essences, spirits and water. You cannot deceive the cultivated olfactory nerve by the artificial scents which are so abundantly manufactured; nor can you deceive a palate accustomed to Nature's most delicious beverages by the products of the chemical laboratory.

The compounds which are formed in wines by keeping, and which give such value to them, are combinations of the oxides of ethyle and of amyle (C 10, H 11) with acetic, propionic, pelargonic, butyric, caproic, and caprylic acids. Of course I quite despair of giving you anything like a knowledge of the combinations of those compounds which produce the various odours or flavours of wines. You can, however, understand the principle. Just as water combines with the oxide of ethyle to form alcohol, so any one of the acids mentioned can unite with oxide of ethyle or oxide of amyle to form an odorous compound. Let me give you an example or two.

Acetic ether (acetic acid, the acid of vinegar, and oxide of ethyle) is found in most wines that have been kept for a long time. You can buy it of the chemist, and ten or twelve drops will give a bottle of new wine a sort of flavour of old, quite enough to deceive people who never take wine but when they go out to a dinner party.

Then there is butyric ether. It is a compound of

butyric acid with oxide of ethyle. Butyric acid is the stuff that gives the rancid smell to butter, but when united with oxide of ethyle it gives the smell of pine-apples. This ether is found in many of the most famous wines. It can be bought of the chemist under the name of oil of pine-apples, and the fraudulent wine-dealer knows how to make use of it to get a higher price for his common Hocks.

These, then, must suffice as examples. If you want to study this subject in all its relations, you must understand the nature of compound radicals, and especially that series which form ethers with the organic acids. The history of many of these compounds you will find given in Mulder's "Chemistry of Wine."

The colouring matters of wines do not much affect their action on the system. Nevertheless one of the most obvious distinctions between the various kinds of wines drunk in this country is their colour. Thus, we have Port wines and Sherry wines, the one of which is red, and the other yellow or brown. The same distinction holds good between Clarets and Burgundies, and Moselle and Rhine wines. These differences depend on the presence in varying quantities of three substances: a brown colouring matter, a blue colouring matter, and tannic acid. The brown colouring matter is present to a greater or less extent in all the wines we call light or white wines. It scarcely exists at all in some Rhine wines and Moselles, whilst it is present in considerable quantities in Madeira, brown Sherries, and Tokay. This brown colouring matter has no very definite chemical composition, and resembles what the chemists call extractive matter. It exists in greatest quantities in those white wines in which the skins of the grapes are fermented with the juice, as the skins contain more of this kind of matter than the grape. The darker the wine is from the presence of this oolouring matter the more highly it is valued. This arises from the fact that the more alcohol the wine contains the more of this colouring matter will it take up. This is known to wine makers and wine sellers, and they frequently add burnt sugar to their light brown wines to give them the colour of strong wines.

The blue colouring matter is found in red wines. These wines are made from purple or black grapes in which the skins are allowed to ferment. This blue dye, like all blue colouring matters, becomes red by contact with acid; hence the tartaric acid of the wine gives it a red colour. Red wines have also the brown colouring matter, as is shown by the fact that they sometimes lose or throw down the whole of their blue colouring matter, and become brown or yellow. This is seen in very old Ports, and the tendency to it is observed in what is called " twenty Port."

When wines are kept they have all a tendency to throw down their colouring matters. This tendency is very much increased by the presence of tannic acid. This acid, which is present in oak-bark and many other substances used in tanning, is much more abundant in red than in white wines. It is especially present in Port wine and Claret, less in Burgundy. The presence of tannic acid gives an astringent property to red wines not possessed by white. The large quantities of tannic acid in new Port, give it also that tendency to deposit what is called a crust on the lower side of the bottle in which it is kept: this crust consists of the oxidized tannic acid, which becomes insoluble, and carries down with it the blue colouring matter and a certain quantity of the saline matters contained in the wine. The longer Port wine is kept, the larger the quantity of this crust which is thrown down. As this proceeds at the same time with the development of the flavouring substances I have before mentioned, the Port wine loses its colour and density, acquires a finer flavour, and its price is proportionately enhanced. When the Port wine was originally good, these changes give it so great a claim on public favour in this country that at the present day Port wines which have been kept for twenty, thirty, or forty years obtain almost fabulous prices in the market. Of course, this is a mere matter of taste; and such wines have no dietetical or medicinal qualities commensurate with their price.

Some writers and experimenters have, indeed, endeavoured to show that the new qualities developed in wines by keeping have much to do with their action on the system. Too little, however, is known on this subject for anything precise or positive to be laid down with regard to the action of these etherial qualities of wines.

The last substances contained in wine which I need mention here are the saline matters,—the ashes. If you evaporate a wine and then expose the residue to heat, you will get a quantity of incombustible matter, which, when examined, differs both in quantity and quality in different wines. These ashes, when analyzed, present us with the fact that there are held in solution in wines the following salts:— Bitartrate of potash (cream of tartar), tartrate of lime, tartrate of alumina, tartrate of iron, chloride of sodium, chloride of potassium, sulphate of potass, phosphate of alumina. These salts occur in the proportion of from one part to four in the thousand parts of wine. They do not make much difference in the flavour or action of wines; but Mulder says of them,—

"As distinctive marks of the genuineness of wine, they are of the greatest value. Let any one who wishes to convince himself whether a particular wine is adulterated or not, direct his attention to this point, and compare the ash with that of a genuine wine of the same kind as that under examination."

Before leaving wines there are two beverages extensively drunk in some parts of England, and which are truly wines, but which are known by the names of Cider and Perry. The first is made from apples, the second from pears. The juice of the apple and pear is procured by pressure, and it is submitted to a process of fermentation in the same way as the juice of the grape. In Worcestershire, Herefordshire, and Devonshire large quantities of these beverages are consumed, and they are drunk by the people of these counties in the same way as beer is consumed in other parts of the country. The same general principles which apply to the manufacture of wine are applicable to them. Those sorts of apples and pears which contain the most sugar will yield in fermentation the largest quantity of alcohol. Cider and perry, when carefully made and kept, undergo those changes which result in the production of bouquets, which render those beverages more highly prized, and some of the better sorts are valued as much as wines. There is more cider manufactured than perry, and that which is generally consumed amongst the population contains about the same quantity of alcohol as beer. The quantity of this substance in the pint varies from half an ounce to two ounces. The acid, however, in cider and perry is not tartaric acid, but malic acid. Consequently this acid is retained in the liquor when it is drunk.

Some persons ascribe to cider very beneficial properties, but I have not been able to make out that it acts on the system differently from ales and beers containing the same amount of alcohol.

In conclusion, I will just glance at Distilled Spirits. These alcoholic drinks differ from wines and beers in the fact that they are distilled from some form of fermented liquor. We may obtain the alcohol from beer or wine, or from any substance containing sugar which is fermented. As an illustration of the sources from which alcohol may be obtained, Loudon in his "Encyclopædia of Gardening" tells the story of an Irish gardener who was always drunk, yet no one ever knew where he got the means to indulge his propensity. It was not till he was watched with great perseverance that the source of his inebriety was discovered. It was found that he had ingeniously contrived to make a small still out of two watering-pots, attached by their spouts. Into one of these he introduced a mash of fermenting carrots, from which, by the aid of heat from an oil lamp, he was enabled to obtain a coarse imitation of his beloved potheen.

Alcohol, then, under the form of distilled spirits, may be procured from any saccharine substance in a state of fermentation. Arrack is made in the East Indies from fermenting rice or palm sago. Aqua ardiente is made in Mexico from the sweet juice of the American aloe (*Agave Americana*). Araka is made in Tartary from fermented mare's milk, arika from cow's milk. Kirschwasser in Germany is distilled from fermenting Machaleb cherries. Maraschino is made in Dalmatia from the macaiska cherry. Show-choo is a Chinese spirit distilled from rice-wine. In fact, there is hardly a race of men under the sun who have not learned the art of distilling alcohol after its formation during the fermentation of sugar.

In this country we are more particularly acquainted with brandy, gin, whisky, and rum. The word brandy is of German origin, and is a corruption of brantwein, or burnt wine, meaning wine that has been acted on by heat. The best brandy is obtained from wine, but inferior kinds of brandy are made from malt, potatoes, beet-root, carrots, pears, and other vegetable substances. The brandy of France, which is made from white wine, especially that made at Cognac, in the department of Charente, is regarded as the best. When first distilled brandy is white, but it acquires a colour from the casks in which it is kept. British brandy is distilled from fermented malt, and attempts are made to imitate the flavour of French brandy by the addition of a variety of ingredients. Brandy, like wine, contains œnanthic and acetic ethers, and is said also to owe its peculiar flavour to the addition of peach kernels, to the liquor from which it is distilled. Like wine also, it developes by keeping in bottles some of those flavouring substances which give the peculiar value to wine.

The consumption of brandy is very large. It is estimated that 15 per cent. of all the wine of France is made into brandy, and that 20,000,000 of gallons are annually made in France, of which at least one-third is exported.

Brandy, like wines and other alcoholic drinks, varies considerably in the quantity of alcohol it contains. At the same time it should be recollected that good brandy should contain from 50 to 55 per cent. of alcohol. Thus a pint of Cognac brandy will contain about ten ounces and a half of pure alcohol, the rest being water. Brandy also contains more or less sugar. Pure French brandy contains about 80 grains of sugar in the pint. It also contains acid, probably acetic acid, in the proportion of from 10 to 20 grains in the pint.

The spirit next in importance is Gin. This word is a corruption of Geneva, as that is of the French word *genièvre* or juniper. Gin is also called Hollands. Geneva, however, is not gin, but a kind of liqueur made from the berries of the juniper, which contain as much as 34 per cent. of sugar, and may be easily fermented. Gin was first made in Holland, and was brought into this country as Hollands gin. It is distilled from corn malt, and various substances are added to it to give it flavour. The most common substances of this kind are juniper berries, but a variety of substances are added to suit the taste of the consumer, so that no two gins are alike. In this country every gin distiller uses his own ingredients, whilst the retailer of gin has also his particular receipts for rendering his gin profitable or palatable, or both. Sometimes injurious substances are added to gin to make it taste strong, as sulphuric acid and sulphate of zinc; these, however, are adulterations.

The substances used for flavouring gin are numerous enough. Thus, I find enumerated bitter almonds, turpentine, creosote, lemon, cardamoms, caraways, cassia, garlic, Canada balsam, horseradish, Cayenne pepper, and grains of Paradise. None of these things are poisonous, and probably all of them assist in determining the action of the alcohol of the gin as a diuretic. Gin does not usually contain so much alcohol as brandy, not more than eight ounces to the pint being found in the best gins. Sugar is added by many distillers, but others do not add this ingredient. Gin, as it is retailed, always contains sugar, and not frequently more than four ounces of alcohol to the pint. It is consequently a weaker spirit generally than brandy, and so far is perhaps less injurious when taken raw. I have, however, before stated that the taking raw spirits is a very hazardous proceeding, and cannot be habitually indulged without danger.

Whisky is the form in which distilled spirits are most popular in Scotland and Ireland. It is distilled principally from corn, although occasionally sugar and molasses are used. It is usually sold stronger than gin or brandy. It has frequently a slight smoky flavour, supposed to be derived from the manner in which it is prepared. This is more particularly the case with what is called small-still whisky. This spirit, as it is generally sold in England at the present day, is more free from flavouring ingredients than any other form of distilled spirits.

Rum is less generally consumed in England than the other spirits, but from the fact of its being supplied by the Government to our soldiers and sailors, large quantities are entered for consumption in Great Britain. It is principally made in the West Indies, and our supplies are almost wholly drawn from Jamaica, where it is manufactured from the fermented scum of the sugar-boilers, and molasses. A flavour is often given to it by the addition of slices of pine-apple. It is usually sold considerably above proof, so that a pint of rum will contain 15 ounces of alcohol. It has a peculiar odour, which is due to butyric ether. Like brandy, it improves by keeping, and probably developes the same class of bouquets as wine. The action of the alcohol of rum is of course the same as that of other fermented liquors, but Dr. Edward Smith has pointed out a curious fact in its action on the system, and that is, that it increases the quantity of carbonic acid thrown out from the lungs. This may be due to the butyric ether. Whether this suggestion be correct or not, it is a curious fact, resulting from Dr. Smith's experiments, that whilst other alcoholic drinks decrease the expiration of carbonic acid, rum should increase it.

I must now, however, draw this long lecture to a close, and the next time we meet I propose to discuss the nature and action of those substances which we add to our food under the name of condiments, spices, and flavours.

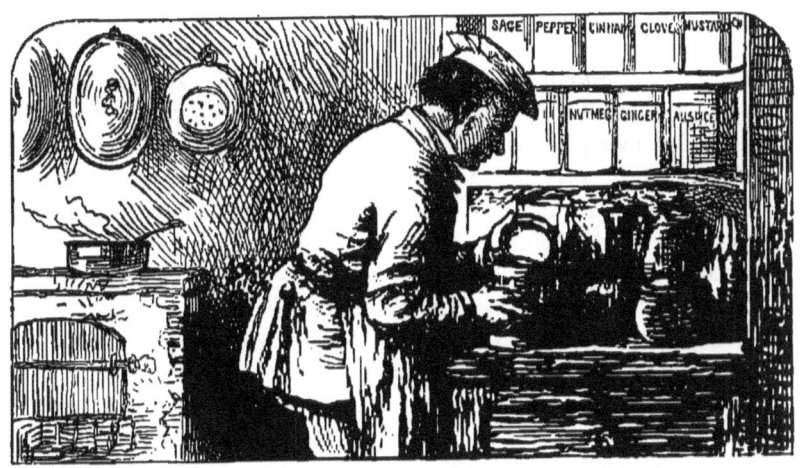

ON
CONDIMENTS, SPICES, & FLAVOURS.

A PASSAGE occurs in the life of a practical philosopher which is well known to a large number of readers in England, and which so well illustrates the subject of this lecture that I may perhaps be excused for introducing it.

"Weal pie," said Mr. Weller, soliloquising, as he arranged the eatables on the grass; "Wery good thing is a weal pie, when you know the lady as made it, and is quite sure it an't kittens; and arter all though where's the odds, when they are so like weal that the wery piemen themselves don't know the difference?"

"Don't they, Sam?" said Mr. Pickwick.

"Not they, sir," replied Mr. Weller, touching his hat. "I lodged in the same house with a pieman once, sir, and a wery nice man he was—reg'lar clever chap too—make pies out o' anything, he could. 'What a number o' cats you-keep, Mr. Brooks,' says I, when I'd got intimate with him. 'Ah,' says he, 'I do—a good many,' says he. 'You must be wery fond o' cats,' says I. 'Other people is,' says he, a winkin' at me; 'they ain't in season till the winter though,' says he. 'Not in season!' says I. 'No,' says he; 'fruits is in, cats is out.' 'Why what do you mean?' says I. 'Mean!' says he; 'that I'll never be a party to the combination of the butchers to keep up the prices o' meat,' says he. 'Mr. Weller, says he, squeezing my hand wery hard, and vispering in my ear, 'don't mention this here agin, but *it's the seasonin' as does it*. They're all made o' them noble animals,' says he, a pointin' to a wery nice little tabby kitten; 'and I seasons 'em for beefsteak, weal, or kidney, 'cordin' to the demand; and more than that,' says he, 'I can make a weal a beefsteak, or a beefsteak a kidney, or any on 'em a mutton at a minute's notice, just as the market changes, and appetites wary!'"

Well that is the text of this lecture, "*it's the seasonin' as does it*," and you know that condiments and spices are the seasoning with which we make our food pleasant; and, after all, if you consider what makes the difference between the various kinds of food, you will find that Mr. Brooks's philosophy is the correct one. It is the taste which food possesses that gives it most value in our estimation.

Now the nervous system is as much formed for the appreciation of these tastes and flavours, as the ear is for sound, and there is the same relation between the different flavours addressed to the palate, as there is between sounds addressed to the ear. The analogy is also correct in its minuter details just as some combinations of colour produce a pleasing impression on our minds, and others produce an unpleasant effect, or as one set of sounds produce discord and another set harmony, so there are some flavours that will not harmonise on the palate, and others that will produce the most pleasing and satisfactory results. Some persons may be offended by this analogy. They have so exalted a notion of the lofty tendencies of the cultivation of the arts of music and painting that to mention the art of tasting in the same category is offensive to them. Yet we should recollect that the same Creator who made the eye for vision, and the ear for hearing, made the tongue for tasting, and that no less elaborate provision is made for the one function than the other, and, in fact, we might claim for the palate, as guiding in the selection of proper food and the rejection of that which is injurious, a higher and more necessary function than could be claimed for either appreciation of colour or sound.

The tongue is the organ of taste, and it is so constructed as to allow the substances we put into our mouths to be readily applied to the nerves by which it is supplied. If we examine the structure of the tongue we shall find that its surface is covered with little projections which are called papillæ. Into these papillæ the nerves are carried which contribute to the sense of taste. The same nerves are also capable of common sensation, and are used as organs of touch. The tongue is moistened by the constant flow of saliva over it, and it is only when moistened that any sense of flavour is communicated to the consciousness.

The tongue, alone, however, is not concerned in this appreciation of tastes and flavour, for we find that the sense of smell is jointly occupied with it; for there are certain flavours that we should hardly taste at all had we no nose, and there are certain of our foods which altogether address themselves to the sense of smell. Take cinnamon, nutmegs, or cloves, for instance; if we put any of these into the mouth and close the nose, we can hardly appreciate the flavour; so it is evident that we frequently use the sense of smell in conjunction with the organ of taste. It is a curious fact that the same nerves which give the sense of taste or flavour are the nerves of common sensibility, that is to say, those by which we feel the *touch* of any object upon the external surface of our bodies by friction or otherwise. When considering the fact which I have just mentioned, that some things are not really tasted at all unless they are smelled, some persons have supposed that there is no real function of taste, but that what we say we taste, we either smell or feel, or that the sensation of taste is compounded of both. The better way to test that is to apply something to a different part of the body, such as quinine or sugar to the leg, and you will find that they produce no impression of taste or flavour in the leg; although if you put quinine upon the tongue, you will have an excessively bitter taste, and with the sugar as well as sugar of lead and other substances, a sweet taste, and a salt taste with salt, sulphate of soda, and a number of other things; so that we can thus prove that there are certain things which we really taste and which have no smell. Now we will call these substances which are tasted *sapours*, in opposition to those which are called *odours*.

Passing on from the nerve of taste I would observe with regard to the nose that it is the organ of smell, and that it has a distinct nerve of smell. This nerve is the first nerve which passes from the brain, and is called the olfactory nerve. It passes by a number of twigs through a little sieve-like bone, which covers over the upper part of the cavity of the nose. Now there are certain things which address the organ of smell which are not taken into the mouth. Thus we have a variety of gases and things which we call scents, odours, perfumes, smells, and stinks, which address themselves to the olfactory nerves alone. We find that this function is developed greatly in the lower animals, and even among the wild races of men this power of detecting the odoriferous particles of matter is very much greater than among cultivated and civilised races. The fact of man having senses to guide him in taste and smell is of importance where our intelligence fails to tell what is good for us, as sometimes happens in the case of persons in illness judging as to what is good for them better than the doctor. Doctors have sometimes yielded to a patient's wish for some particular food in consequence of this instinctive desire, and the patient has been very much the better for it. Unless the desire evinced by a sick person for some particular article of food is evidently traceable to a depraved appetite, it is frequently a part of judicious treatment to yield to the desire of the patient.

As instances of the use by the lower animals especially of the sense of smell, I may refer to the fact that they will instinctively reject food which is poisonous, however carefully you may wrap it up, even when pressed by much hunger. Monkeys, cats, dogs, and animals of the higher class will pertinaciously reject such food, this action being determined on their part by the sense of smell. It is not, however, only by the olfactory nerve that provision is made to guard against the destruction of the animal; a man may be sometimes placed under circumstances in which he will be exposed to carbonic acid, chlorine, or a variety of gases which, if taken into the system, would destroy him; he has then, besides the sense of smell, by which some of these gases may be detected, a set of nerves which produce the sensation which we call sneezing. These are titillated by various powders and gases which would act injuriously if they went into the lungs. The act of sneezing is the act of throwing away or getting rid of that which if a man got into his lungs would injure him. When a man sneezes he draws back, in cases where if he went forwards he would endanger his life. The taste has reference to food, the smell has reference to that which probably may be good or bad for food. The olfactory nerves are excited to action by substances capable of being applied through the atmosphere to the mucous membrane of the nose.

Now let us pass on to consider a little more attentively the nature of the various kinds of sapours and odours which we find in our food. To a thoughtful mind there are many ways of classifying these, but I may speak of them as agreeable and disagreeable odours and flavours, addressing both the organs of taste and smell. In the first place, we have a number of agreeable odours, and these odours may or may not accompany our various kinds of food. Such odours as those exhaled by nutmeg, cinnamon, cloves, lemon-peel, pine-apples, lavender, oil of bitter almonds, and vanilla, are employed both to flavour our food and give scent to our perfumes. Then, again, we have another set of odours which are disagreeable, arising from the mineral, the vegetable, or the animal world. Vegetable and animal substances decomposing produce sulphuretted hydrogen, which has a disagreeably offensive odour, and is injurious to health. The carburetted hydrogen of the gas which we burn gives out a disagreeable odour. Sometimes these disgusting odours, by custom and habit, become agreeable, and sometimes, in the same way, disgusting food, by custom and habit, becomes agreeable food. We have an instance of this in the preference which some persons give to food which has been kept till it is tainted by decomposition, as in the case of game and venison. There is a story told of a prince who was confined in a prison a long way from the seashore, where they never could get oysters until they were what is called a little gone; being fond of oysters, he became accustomed to the semi-putrid flavour of his dead oysters, and afterwards preferred to eat them in this condition. You will find it very difficult to make children take things which, when they grow up, they acquire a taste for—take olives or tobacco as instances.

The tendency to partake of food in a state of decomposition is natural in some classes of animals. Thus, we find some of the infusorial animalcules are brought into existence under the influence of decomposing animal and vegetable matter in infusions. Some tribes of beetles and shell-fishes prefer decomposing food. The sturgeons amongst fishes, the crocodiles amongst reptiles, and the vultures amongst birds, are instances of creatures which, for beneficent purposes, are endowed with an instinctive tendency to prefer garbage, carrion, and offal, to better kinds of food.

However well these animals are adapted to endure

and flourish on, such a diet, it is very certain that man sometimes suffers severely from such food. I have told you that water charged with decomposing animal and vegetable matter produces disease. During the prevalence of cholera, the cases were very numerous where persons were attacked shortly after eating decomposing food. During the epidemic of cholera in London, in 1849, it was found that poulterers, fishmongers, and greengrocers, suffered more than any other classes from cholera, and I think it is highly probable that this occurred from such persons eating rather of their damaged stock of goods than that which was sound. I have before referred to the mortality of infants during the hot summer of 1859, and which I attributed to the use of decomposing or acescent milk.

The way in which those substances injure the system is by imparting to the fluids of the body the same state of change in which they are themselves. It is not all persons that are susceptible of such an action. Most people in health have the power of producing a gastric juice in their stomachs which will restrain the injurious tendency of decomposing food, and thus no evil results. It is more particularly in warm climates and in warm seasons that these effects take place, and the more common forms of disease produced by this food are diarrhœa and cholera.

Let us now examine a little more closely the nature of those substances which are more commonly used for giving a relish to our food. I have before spoken of the four elements, carbon, hydrogen, oxygen, and nitrogen, and although they assume very different forms, they are still the elements whose compounds form the basis of all sapours and odours. Of these there is a series which are called essential oils, and another which we may refer to a class of bodies called ethers; but before speaking of essential oils or ethers particularly, I will call attention to the production of common ether. Ether is a very volatile body, and its odour, when exposed, is speedily diffused through the atmosphere. Now, ether is made from alcohol. Alcohol is the result of the decomposition of sugar. If we take grape sugar we find it composed of 12 parts of oxygen, 12 of hydrogen, and 12 of carbon; and alcohol, which is the substance at the foundation of all our odours, is composed of 4 of carbon, 6 hydrogen, and 2 oxygen, arranged as 4 of carbon, 5 hydrogen, 1 of oxygen, and 1 atom of water. Now, if we take away from it the water, we have ether left, which is an oxide of a substance called ethyl, composed of 4 atoms of carbon and 5 of hydrogen, the same elements that are found in coal gas. This substance ether, the oxide of ethyl, will combine with acids, so that we have sulphates of the oxide of ethyl, tartrates and citrates of the oxide of ethyl, &c. A distinguished French chemist has discovered that one compound of oxygen and hydrogen and carbon, combining with chlorine, with iodine, and with nitrogen, is capable of producing 1020 different compounds. There are probably thousands of compounds which may be similarly produced, and which give flavours, and odours, and scents, and peculiarities, in directions which we know of, and in thousands of directions which we know nothing of, and the discovery of the nature of these compounds is the direction that organic chemistry is taking at the present day.

It is one of the most curious features in the history of modern chemistry, that not only has the chemist been able to show the nature of these compounds by pulling them apart, but he has begun to find out the way to put them together again; and the chemist can now produce in his laboratory what is ordinarily produced by nature in the laboratory of the plant or fruit. One of the first things that was formed in this way was the oil of bitter almonds. You know that bitter almonds contain an oil which may be extracted from them, and has a very pleasant flavour or scent. It is used in custards, puddings, cakes, and in a variety of other ways. There are two or three substances ordinarily sold in the present day for oil of bitter almonds, which are obtained from very different sources from those from which it is manufactured in nature; there is, for instance, a substance called benzol, which is a compound of carbon 10 and hydrogen 6. Now, this benzol can be formed artificially, just in the same way as the chemist can form ether, by decomposing certain compounds, and leaving the carbon and hydrogen in the above proportion. This substance is sold in the shops under the name of benzol, benzine, and benzoline, and is probably known by some persons present on account of its being used for cleaning gloves, silk, and other things, as it possesses a greater solvent power in relation to dirt than ether or alcohol.

This benzol is obtained from coal tar, which is a most valuable substance; and although it is rejected at the gas factories, it is likely to become of most essential service to man in the manufacture of very many things.

ON CONDIMENTS, SPICES, AND FLAVOURS. 263

By adding nitric acid to benzol we obtain nitro-benzol, or artificial oil of bitter almonds.

There is another substance, hippuric acid, extracted from the drainage of our cowhouses and pigstyes, which, when submitted to the action of heat, can be made into nitro-benzol; so that, as I have said in a former lecture, there is no such thing as real dirt, for dirt is merely matter not in its proper place; the elements are pure, and only have to be again reunited. Although this acid is obtained from such objectionable sources, yet its product is introduced into the most delicate soaps and applied to our faces. And this is only one of a series of similar compounds which are found naturally in plants, but which can be imitated by the art of the chemist.

There is a substance for which we in England have long been celebrated, called pear oil—in the manufacture of which no pears are used at all. There is a compound called amyl, which is produced by the decomposition of starch, and which can be got from potatoes; it is composed of Carbon 10 and Hydrogen 11, and when united with common vinegar or acetic acid, we get a substance which cannot be distinguished from the smell of the jargonelle pear. It is with this manufactured pear oil that cheap lozenges, which are sold in the shops at a penny an ounce, are flavoured. There is another of these manufactured essences, called pine-apple oil; it is introduced into a variety of forms of confectionary, and in this case we have our old friend ether coming in again. You have all smelt rancid butter, which has been long kept; distil that rancid butter and you will obtain butyric acid, mix that with ethyle and it becomes pine-apple flavour. Now, nature has done the same thing; there has been a manufacture of butyric acid and ethyle going on within that beautiful fruit which we call the pine-apple, and the flavour is the same in the one case as the other. It is this butyric ether which gives the flavour to rum.

Then there is the oil of apples. There is an acid in the substance known by the name of valerian, which has an exceedingly unpleasant smell. There are things which for a moment are exceedingly pleasant, but by taking too much they become exceedingly unpleasant. Valerian is a substance of this kind. It contains valerianic acid, and that combined with the oxide of amyl constitutes what we know by the name of apple oil, which is used for flavouring confectionary. The pleasant taste of the apple is produced in that way. Now, this oxide of amyl can be got from potatoes, coal tar, and other substances, so that there is no difficulty in making these oils, and so many of them have been made, that we shall soon have no difficulty in procuring them, without having recourse to the vegetable kingdom. That these things are composed of carbon and hydrogen may be discovered in a variety of ways. By their inflammability, for instance. You may take them and burn them as you would spirits of wine in a spirit lamp, and the result will be carbonic acid and water, from the union of the carbon and hydrogen with the oxygen of the air.

You see what an interesting field of inquiry this branch of chemistry opens up; but I must leave this subject, and say a word with regard to the action of these substances on the system. When taken into the stomach they act upon the nervous system as well as on the organs of taste and smell, and produce an effect upon the stomach, increasing the secretion of gastric acid, and promoting digestion. We instinctively add to meat stews Cayenne pepper, and things of that kind, which act as stimulants to the stomach—they act as alcohol and stimulate the nervous system. Persons can get tipsy upon oil of cinnamon and oil of cloves, just as they can upon hydrated oxide of ethyle. For instance, there is a *liqueur* which has lately become celebrated on account of its killing so many Frenchmen—it is called absinthe, and is prepared from wormwood. The wormwood contains a volatile oil, which not only acts as a stimulant to the stomach, but also has a narcotic effect upon the nervous system; and a distinguished French chemist, the newspapers inform us, has just discovered that this wormwood contains seventeen deadly principles, any one of which would kill an individual who would venture to take it. Absinthe contains, however, as much as 20 per cent. of alcohol; and perhaps the pernicious effect of this liqueur may be traced as satisfactorily to the alcohol as to the volatile oils it contains.

Let me now speak of the classification of these Sapours and Odours. I have found considerable difficulty in this, arising from the various terms that are given to them; but I have arranged them under the heads of Condiments, Spices, Flavourers, and Bouquets, and to these I would now draw attention.

Now what is a condiment? Well, I have not been able to get a satisfactory answer; but I have thought that those substances which contain volatile oils, or ethers, or whatever you may call them, which can be taken with salt are condiments, and that those, on the other hand, that can be eaten with sugar are spices. I have classed among the condiments as being flavours agreeable with salt—garlic, leek, onions, mustard, pepper, Cayenne pepper, capers, pickles, parsley, celery, coriander, thyme, sage, mint, fennel, mushrooms, morels, truffles. Now, looking at these condiments, you will find that they all of them contain different kinds of essences, oils, or ethers, and some of them so distinct as to admit of definite classification. Thus garlick, leek, onions, and assafœtida are condiments. Persons fond of onions will get from onions to leek, from leek to garlick, and from garlic to assafœtida; and thus it is that, in the City, if you go to a chophouse, and ask for your steak with a little higher flavour, they take a warm dish, rub a little assafœdida on it, and put the steak on it. You do not perhaps know that you are eating assafœtida; but you find it agreeable. Now how is this? If we take some of these chemical bases from the sources of our pleasant scents and odours, and add to these bases, instead of oxygen, a little sulphur, then you will get things with sulphur smells, such as onions, leeks, watercresses, cabbage. When cabbage is boiled there is the sulphur smell which ascends to the drawing-room, and the exclamation occurs, "Pray shut the kitchen-door: you are boiling cabbages."

Now, in the case of onions, garlic, leek, chalots, and assafœtida, we are dealing with a substance composed of hydrogen and carbon, called allyle (C 6, H 5). Just as ethyle unites with oxygen, and forms our strong-

ON CONDIMENTS, SPICES, AND FLAVOURS. 267

smelling ether, so allyle unites with sulphur, and produces the strong-smelling sulphide of allyle.

This group of strong smelling and tasting plants belongs to the fair lily tribe (Liliaceæ), and all belong to the same genus, *Allium:* hence we call them alliaceous plants. I give you their formidable Latin names in a diagram :—

Onions .... *Allium Cepa.*
Garlic .... *Allium sativum.*
Shalots .... *Allium ascalonicum.*
Chives .... *Allium Schœnoprasum.*
Leeks .... *Allium Porrum.*
Rocambole .... *Allium Scorodoprasum.*

They have all the same substance to recommend them. In the large Spanish onions there is more starch and less oil, so that they may be eaten as a substantive article of diet.

In the case of the bitter taste which gives so pleasant a flavour to mustard, horse-radish, watercresses, radishes, and cabbages, we have the same element of sulphur as in the onions; but another powerful chemical compound is combined with sulphur. This substance is cyanogen, the same compound which, uniting with hydrogen, forms hydrocyanic acid. Now cyanogen contains nitrogen, and thus the flavouring essence of the Cruciferæ differ from that of the onion by containing this element. We have here, in fact, a sulphocyanide of allyle ($C_2 N S_2 + C_6 H_5$).

The most curious thing with regard to this compound is, that it does not appear to exist in the mustard-seed, for if we express mustard-seeds we get only a bland fixed oil, but if we moisten the powdered seed then this oil is developed. This arises from the action of the caseine of the mustard-seed, which acts as a ferment upon its other constituents and develops this powerful oil.

I have said all these oils act as stimulants; but they have other properties. The oil of mustard, for instance, is acrid, and when taken in sufficient quantities will produce vomiting. This is a fact worth knowing, that in the mustard-pot we have one of the safest and swiftest of emetics. Every one should bear this in mind, as in cases where persons swallow poison the speedy recourse to the mustard-pot may save life. A table-spoonful of ordinary mustard mixed in a wine-glassful of water, will seldom fail to produce sickness.

The acridity of this mustard oil is so great, that when applied alone to the skin it speedily produces vesication, and when the powder mixed with water is put to the skin in the form of a poultice, a wholesome irritation is produced. Mustard poultices are amongst the safest, most efficient, and most managable of counter-irritants. Every mother of a family should be acquainted with the uses of a mustard poultice.

Of course, mustard is much too common and valuable a thing not to be abused. I remember some time ago some foolish person wrote a book recommending mustard-seed to be swallowed whole as a remedy for indigestion. Of course, if he had recommended people to swallow live frogs, he would have found some stupid people to believe in him, and so people swallowed whole mustard-seeds. I very well recollect having been called, when commencing the study of medicine, to watch the sufferings of a man who had swallowed quantities of these mustard-seeds. He died; and when we came to open him, we found pints of these mustard-seeds impacted in his bowels. In some spots they were beginning to germinate, for the vital powers of the stomach had not overcome those of the grain, and the distention of the seed by this process seemed to be the cause of the death of the patient.

The acrid flavour of the horse-radish is dependent on the same oil as that of the mustard. We add it to our food under the same circumstances as we use mustard, and it acts in the same way. The oil in the horse-radish is contained in the root, and as this root is not unlike some others, it has led to mistakes occasionally fatal. The most disastrous accidents have occurred from taking by mistake the root of the common monkshood or aconite (*Aconitum Napellus*) instead of that of horse-radish. The root of the monkshood is darker and more fibrous than that of the horseradish, and the mistake can only occur through great carelessness or ignorance.

The next group of condiments to which I would refer is what we call peppers. Thus, we have black and white pepper, long pepper, and Cayenne pepper. The black and white peppers are made from the fruits of a plant known by the name of *Piper nigrum*. These fruits are sometimes used whole, but they are mostly ground in a mill, and sold powdered. The "black pepper" consists of the dried berries ground down whole. The "white" pepper is formed from the same berries, but their dark husk is first removed. The long pepper is produced by another species of plant, the *Piper longum*. This latter form is not much used in Europe; it is, however, extensively employed in the East as a masticatory. In this way it is employed in conjunction with the betel-nut, which is the fruit of a species of palm (*Areca Catechu*), and contains tannic acid. The stimulant oil of the pepper in conjunction with this powerful astringent forms an agreeable combination, which is not only consumed by the natives of Eastern countries, but by Europeans, who have contracted the habit of masticating it in the East.

The active principle of these peppers is a substance called piperine. It contains carbon, hydrogen, and oxygen, and resembles in its nature such substances as quinine, being capable of uniting with acids like an alkali. Of its action on the system we have no precise account. It has been supposed, from its use in the form of the long pepper, to be a narcotic, but of this effect we have no very definite information.

Cayenne pepper is produced by a very different family of plants, belonging to the natural order *Solanaceæ*, a family of plants that yields the potato, the deadly nightshade, henbane, and tobacco. Cayenne pepper consists of the dried fruits of two species of capsicum, the *Capsicum annuum* and the *Capsicum frutescens*. These plants are natives of America, and are cultivated in the East and West Indies. They contain an active principle like piperine, which is called capsicin. It is very stimulant, and is taken on account of its flavour, as well as its stimulant action on the stomach. It enters into the composition of curry powder, a compound of condiments and spices used extensively as an addition to food in Europe, more especially in this country, and originally imported from the East.

Another group of condiments are those which are familiarly known by the name of "mints." They belong to a family of plants called *Lamiaceæ* or *Labiatæ*. This family is remarkable for containing in their leaves and all parts of the plant minute receptacles filled with volatile oil. These oils have many of them an agreeable scent, and yield the perfumes of lavender, patcholi, and many others. Many of them are cultivated in gardens under the name of pot-herbs. The peppermint (*Mentha piperita*) is a British wild plant, and its leaves are distilled with spirits of wine, forming essence of peppermint. The oil is also distilled alone, and is called oil of peppermint. The oil is used for flavouring peppermint lozenges. The whole plant is also distilled with water, and sold in the shops under the name of peppermint water. It is a useful stimulant for the stomach, and often employed as a medicine.

To the same family also belong sage and thyme. The leaves of these plants are used fresh or dry, and form the flavouring of those ingredients which are put into the inside of ducks, geese, roast pigs, sausages, and other animal food brought to the table. "They are warm and discussive, and good against crudities of the stomach," according to an old writer on this subject.

The rosemary belongs to this order, and although not much used at the present day, sprigs of it were formerly stuck into beef whilst roasting, and are said to give it an "excellent relish." Basil, summer and winter savory, and sweet marjoram, are all used in this way, whilst ground ivy, horehound, and pennyroyal are used as medicines on account of the volatile oils they contain.

These oils are all of them compounds of carbon, hydrogen, and oxygen.

Amongst plants which yield volatile oils added to food, must be placed the umbel-bearing plants, or *Umbelliferæ*. The fruits of those plants, which are called seeds, as caraway seeds (Fig. 1), dill seeds, and the like, are remarkable for possessing elongated tubes, or receptacles called *vittæ*, which contain volatile oils. Many of these fruits are added to food to give it a flavour, as caraways, coriander, fennel, and anise. (Fig. 2.) Sometimes this oil is found in the whole, as in the celery (Fig. 3), fennel, and samphire. The wild celery (*Apium graveolens*) contains so large a quantity of an acrid oil as to be poisonous, but when cultivated, that portion of the plant which is kept under ground produces only a sufficient quantity of this oil to give it a pleasant flavour. Large quantities of this plant are consumed, and its beneficial action on the system is probably to be looked for in the mineral substances it contains, as I explained in the second lecture.

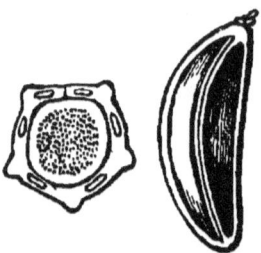

Fig. 1.—*Fruit of Caraway.*

Fig. 2.—*Fruit of Anise.*

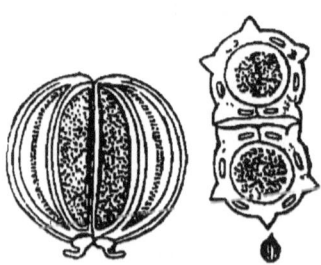

Fig. 3.—*Fruit of Celery.*

The leaves of the fennel (*Anethum fœniculum*) are

ON CONDIMENTS, SPICES, AND FLAVOURS. 273

more used than its fruits (Fig. 4), and the peculiar flavour of its oil is supposed to be more agreeable with fish than with other animal food. It is said to attract fish, and the angler puts a few leaves of fennel into his box with bait.

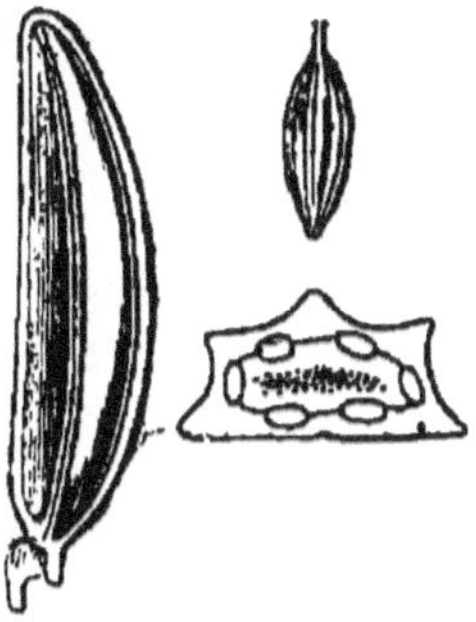

The samphire (*Crithmum maritimum*) has a poetical interest, and is one of the plants of Shakspeare. The "dangerous trade" of the samphire-gatherer arises from its growing on the sides of steep cliffs; and one of the most ornamental features of the white cliffs of Albion is the dark-green patches which this plant produces where it grows. It is gathered for the sake of the pleasant oil which is diffused throughout the whole plant, and which renders it an agreeable addition to our food, especially when used in the form of pickle.

Fig. 4.—Fruit of Fennel.

There is one other group of plants which, although I might have spoken of them under more substantial articles of diet, are, nevertheless, more frequently employed as condiments than anything else. I allude to the Fungi. The late Dr. Badham, in his beautiful book on the "Esculent Funguses of England," says of their odours and tastes, that "both one and the other are far more numerous in this class of plants than in any other with which we are acquainted."

Some of them yield powerfully-disagreeable odours as the *Phallus impudicus* and the *Clathrus cancellatus*, whilst others give out the most agreeable of perfumes. I shall not, however, pretend to give you an account here of all the fungi which the Doctor recommends to be eaten either as substantive articles of diet or pleasant additions to sauces. You will be surprised to hear that he enumerates no less than forty-eight species all good to eat. But fungi have this drawback: that some of them are very poisonous, and mistakes occur so often that only persons skilled in distinguishing the various species ought to be trusted for administering them indiscriminately as food. In the markets of the Continent persons are specially appointed for the examination of fungi, and only those which are uninjurious are allowed to be sold. Dr. Badham says that the majority of funguses are harmless; nevertheless, the frightful accounts he gives of their poisonous symptoms and the *post-mortem* appearances of the brains and bowels of those who have died of them, are enough to alarm the most stout-hearted. I shall, therefore, only refer to those which are eaten generally in England, and which may be taken with impunity.

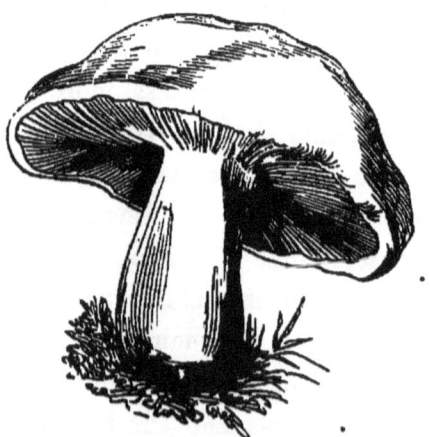

Fig. 5.—*The Common Mushroom.*

The first of these is the common mushroom (*Agaricus campestris*). (Fig. 5.) It is so well known that

I need not describe it here. When eaten it should be fresh-gathered, as after keeping it acquires properties that render it liable to disagree. They may, however, be dried quickly and kept wholesome for any length of time, or they may be powdered, and thus kept. When salted fresh and pressed they yield the sauce known by the name of "ketchup" or "catsup." The mushroom gives a fine flavour to soups and greatly improves beef-tea. When arrowroot and weak broths are distasteful to persons with delicate stomachs, a little seasoning with ketchup will frequently form an agreeable change.

The mushroom itself may be cooked in a variety of ways. Some roast them, basting with melted butter and serve with white wine sauce. They may be made into patties and added to fricassees. In France they steep them in oil, adding salt, pepper, and a little garlic; they are then tossed up in a small stew-pan over a brisk fire, with chopped parsley and a little lemon-juice.

The morell (*Morchella esculenta*) (Fig. 6) is occasionally found in Great Britain, and is considered a great luxury by fungus-eaters. It is cooked in the same way as the common mushroom, but has a more delicate flavour. Although usually obtained from our Italian warehouses, if sought out it may not unfrequently be found in our orchards and woods at the beginning of summer.

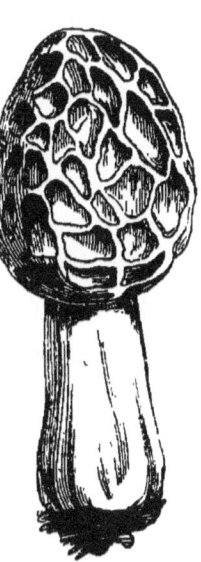

Fig. 6.
The Morell.

T

The truffle (*Lycoperdon Tuber*) (Fig. 7) is another fungus found in the markets of England. It is more rare in England than the morell, but it is brought in considerable quantities from France. They grow entirely underground, and in France dogs and even swine are trained to discover them. They give a delicate flavour to soups and gravies, and enter into the composition of stuffing for boars' heads, fish, and other kinds of animal food.

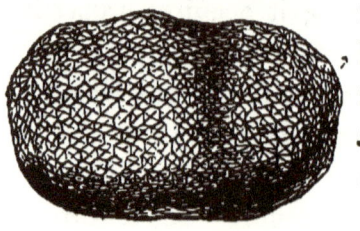

Fig. 7.—The Truffle.

The condiments I have already mentioned are all produced by the vegetable kingdom. But the power of producing both pleasant and unpleasant volatile and sapid products is not confined to plants. Most persons are acquainted with the perfumes known by the name of civet, musk, and ambergris, which are the produce of animal life. Each kind of animal has its own peculiar taste, and this is dependent on some of those products which I have mentioned so often as giving the great variety of our odours and flavours. Now in some cases animals have these flavours so strongly that we use them for flavouring those less favoured by nature. The lobster is used for making a sauce for fish with less flavour, so also the anchovy of Europe and the tamarind fish of the East. It was only the other day I received from my friend Dr. Gull a parcel of fish which had a strong smell of mouldy Stilton cheese. This fish, which is called the bummeloh, is caught in great abundance in the Indian Ocean, and is exported to all parts of the East. The Chinese are very fond of it;

they, nevertheless, call it koo-too, or dog's vomit. This word is the same as is used to express the abject obeisance required by the Chinese potentates on the introduction of strangers, and which has been so resolutely refused by our embassies.

But let us now turn to the spices. I have said we mostly eat these things with sugar; but the word spice means anything of which we take a little. A spice of a substance is a little of it, or a specimen, as we say in more pompous English. The substances of which I have now to speak differ from the last, in being mostly of foreign origin, and not only foreign, but tropical or sub-tropical. Well might our grandfathers call them spices, for little enough did they get of these things. But the ends of the earth have fallen to our lot, and every boy and girl at school can indulge in a taste for those spices of which the grandees of the land in the time of our rude forefathers knew nothing but through vague rumours of the luxuries of the wealthy East.

The first of these spices that I shall mention is cinnamon. This substance is the bark of a plant (*Laurus Cinnamomum*—Fig. 8) which is a native of the East Indies. It belongs to a family remarkable for yielding a volatile oil in various parts of their structure. The plants belonging to the genus *Laurus* yield not only cinnamon, but cassia and camphor, and the well-known bay of our gardens and shrubberies is the *Laurus nobilis*, the true Laurel of the ancients. It is a mistake to call the *Prunus Laurocerasus*, which is the English laurel, by that name, as it never occupied the position of honour attributed by the ancients to the bay.

The cinnamon of our shops is principally brought from Ceylon, where the cinnamon-plant, a small tree,

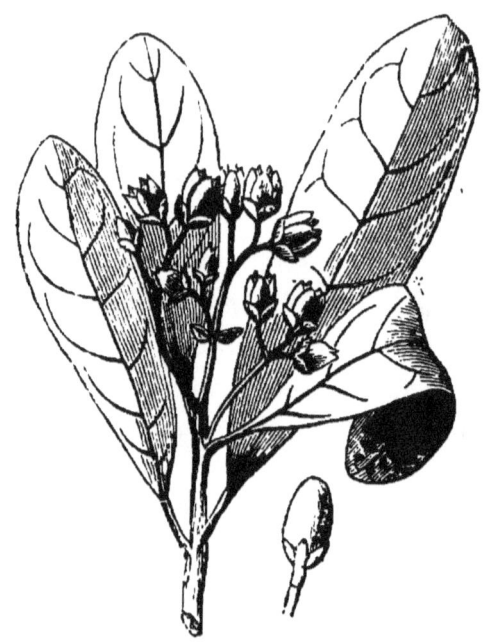

Fig. 8.—Cinnamon-tree.

is extensively cultivated. About 20,000 pounds are annually consumed in this country. This bark contains an oil which is distilled and sold under the name of oil of cinnamon. Chemically it is a very interesting substance, as it contains a base called cinnamyle, united with hydrogen, and is technically called a hyduret of cinnamyle. It has an agreeable odour and pleasant taste, and is extensively employed as an addition to various articles of food. It is a stimulant, and when taken assists in the digestion of the various kinds of food to which it is added. It is also employed in medicine, where stimulants, and what are called antispasmodics, are required.

Another species of Laurus yields the bark called cassia, which contains the same oil, but in less quantity, and mixed with a large proportion of tannic acid and other substances, which are less agreeable when added to articles of diet.

The same genus of plants yields camphor. Camphor, it is said, is procured from the roots of the cinnamon tree. Camphor is a concrete volatile oil, composed of the same constituents as the oil of cinnamon, and possessed of the same properties. Although best known in this country as a medicine, it is consumed in China as an article of luxury, and used as we take wine or spices. The Chinese do not, however, use the camphor obtained from the common camphor-tree (*Laurus Camphora*), which grows abundantly in Formosa and other islands on the Chinese coasts. They prefer the camphor of Japan and Borneo, which has a somewhat different flavour, and which is produced by a tree known by the name of *Dryabalanops Camphora*. This tree also grows in Sumatra, and is described as one of the noblest trees of the island. The camphor yielded by the young trees is liquid, but afterwards it becomes solid. It is seldom seen in this country, as the Chinese pay a high price for this camphor.

I might, perhaps, properly have spoken of cloves before cinnamon, as I find we import into this country no less than 200,000 pounds of cloves annually. This aromatic substance is the unopened flower of a plant called the *Caryophyllus aromaticus* (Fig. 9), which belongs to the myrtle tribe of plants. All the myrtle tribe, including our common myrtle, yield volatile oils in their fruits, flowers, or leaves. From this tribe we also obtain allspice, nutmegs, mace, and cajeput. The oil of cloves has the same general properties as that of cinnamon, and it is used under much the same circumstances. The *Pimento* berries or allspice, are the fruits of the *Eugenia Pimento*, a small tree growing in the West-Indian Islands. Four hundred thousand pounds of these berries are annually imported into Great Britain. They are extensively employed in the manufacture of sauces, which are eaten with steaks, chops, and other kinds of animal food. Their name, allspice, refers to the very compound flavour these berries possess.

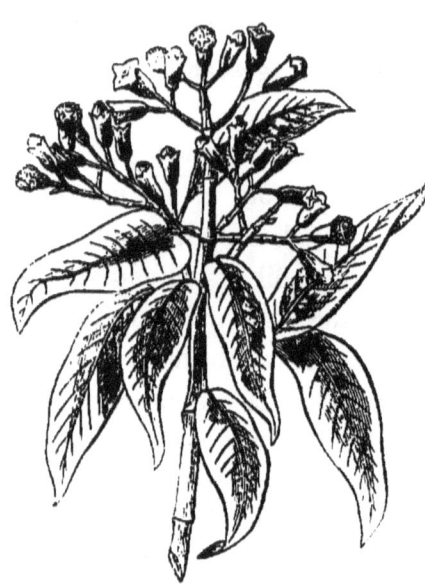

Fig. 9.—*Cloves.*

Nutmegs are the seeds of a plant belonging to the Laurel family, the *Myristica moschata*. These seeds contain an exceedingly grateful and pleasant oil, and when grated down, are employed to flavour cakes, custards, and negus. Outside the nutmeg seed is a curious organ called by botanists an *arillus*, which grows much larger in this than most seeds, and when separated it constitutes the commercial and dietetical article, mace. Mace, like nutmegs, contains a pleasant oil, and is added to sweet foods to give them a flavour. These oils are developed by tropical suns, and we obtain our nutmegs and mace from the Molucca Islands. The nutmeg-tree is also cultivated in Java, Borneo, Jamaica, and Cayenne.

Before leaving the laurel family, I will just remind you that the bay itself yields a fragrant oil both in its fruits and leaves, which are added to flavour various articles of food. Those who have read Soyer attentively —and what housewife who wished to make her home what it ought to be has not?—will remember how often the prescription occurs amongst his sauces of taking two bay-leaves, which of course must be removed before the sauce is served. I wish I could persuade some of my lady hearers, who spend so much time in thumping their pianos, in vain endeavouring to "discourse sweet sounds," to try their taste upon the manufacture of sauces. How many an uneaten dinner, which goes away to be thrown to the dogs, would be consumed; how often would the rich be thus lured on to take the food necessary for their restoration to health, which they now loathe and die for the want of. Fine ladies may think this a subject beneath them; foolish women may think they know quite enough about it; but the time may come when both alike will repent their pride and folly.

We must not pass over spices without speaking of ginger (*Zingiber officinale*), the most potent, the most useful, and most generally used of all spices. We count the consumption of ginger in Great Britain not by pounds but by hundredweights. Twenty thousand cwts. are annually consumed in Great Britain. What folly and madness, what waste and injury, must come of this consumption of condiments and spices, if certain of our philanthropic wiseacres are to be believed, who, combining the follies of teetotalism and vegetarianism with the delusions of homœopathy, denounce the addition of these substances to our diet. Ginger is used more largely on account of its comparative economy. It is added to cakes, and to ginger-bread, which is a popular article of diet in this country. It also finds its way into sauces, spiced wines, and a variety of the pleasant eatables found in the shop of the confectioner. The oil of ginger is deposited in the rootstock or underground stem of the ginger-plant. Similar oils are found in the same situation in other plants belonging to the same natural order as the ginger-plant. These are the Turmeric (*Curcuma longa*), the Zedoary (*Curcuma Zedoaria*), and the Galanga (*Alpinia Galanga*). These and other ginger-plants are cultivated in the East Indies. The ginger family (*Zingiberaceæ*) not only yield the plants I have mentioned, but another group whose fruits, containing seeds with an aromatic oil, are called cardamoms. These seeds are used as a medicine in this country, but as a condiment in other parts of the world. The Grains of Paradise, known of old to brewers' druggists, belong also to this group of plants.

Before taking leave of the spices, I must mention two products sold in the shops, and used both as condiments and spices. I mean "curry powder" and "mixed spices." Curry has been introduced into Europe from the East. In tropical climates, the inhabitants use much more extensively spices and condiments than we do. There are two reasons for this. In the first place, food containing these things is less liable to putrefy and decompose than when they are absent. They are antiseptics, and this antiseptic effect is, I believe, effected in the stomach. The effect of eating decomposing food is very disastrous in hot countries, and in our own country in hot weather. Hence one use of these warm aromatic oils. But there is another action of these oils, and that is their stimulant effect on the stomach. You will recollect what I said of the action of alcohol in this way. These oils act in the same manner, and as they produce their effects in smaller quantities, they can be taken without producing injury to the nervous system generally. This stimulant effect on the stomach seems most needed in hot countries, where the action of the heat on the skin causes an excessive activity on the part of its blood-vessels which needs to be counteracted by a powerful stimulus applied to the mucous membrane of the stomach. From this explanation, you will easily understand how many of these substances act in relieving pain in the stomach. Every child knows that a peppermint lozenge will frequently cure the pain brought on by eating an unripe apple.

Curry powder is composed of many condiments and spices. Thus we are told that genuine curry contains turmeric, cardamoms, ginger, allspice, cloves, black pepper, coriander, cayenne, fenegrick, and cumin. Mixed spice is a powder very popular amongst the housekeepers of England, and consists of ginger, allspice, cumin, and cloves.

This subject is a very wide one, and I might dwell on it further, but I must forbear. Nevertheless, there are two or three other things that I would speak of under the name of flavourers. We can hardly call oil of bitter almonds, vanilla, lemon-peel, lemon-juice, and fruit essences, spices or condiments, yet we add them to food to give it a flavour.

Although, as I have told you, the oil of bitter almonds can be made artificially, the oil as it exists in nature is better adapted for addition to food. This is done by the addition of those parts of plants which contain the oil. Thus, the bitter almond itself contains this oil, and is frequently used for giving a flavour to cakes. The oil is obtained separately from the almonds, and sold in the shops. It is a very curious substance, and does not appear to exist in the almond till water has been added. The way in which the oil is made is to take the paste of the bitter almonds, after the fixed oil is pressed out, and then to distil over the volatile oil. This product contains also hydrocyanic acid, which is removed by the action of iron, and the essential oil is redistilled.

This oil is produced in a very curious way by the decomposition of a substance in the almond-seed called amygdaline. The amygdaline is composed of carbon, hydrogen, oxygen, and nitrogen. The following diagram will show those who are learned in chemical symbols the nature of this change :—

1 of Hydrocyanic Acid	C_2	H	—	N
2 of Oil of Bitter Almonds ...	C_{28}	H_{12}	O_4	—
Sugar	C_6	H_7	O_7	—
2 of Tannic Acid	C_4	H_4	O_8	—
3 of Water	—	H_3	O_3	—
Amygdaline	C_{40}	H_{27}	O_{22}	N

From the fact that oil of bitter almonds itself is a

poison, and that hydrocyanic acid is a much more vigorous poison, it is a matter of the utmost importance that this flavour should be used with caution.

The leaves of the common laurel, or cherry laurel (*Prunus Laurocerasus*) also contain a similar oil to the oil of bitter almonds, and likewise hydrocyanic acid. Cherry laurel water has been known to destroy life, so that these leaves require to be used with caution. They are put into custards, and the milk and water with which cakes are made. Noyeau is made from peach kernels and bitter almonds, and the flavour of ratafia is obtained from the same source. The seeds of the peach, apricot, cherry, nectarine, and plum, all contain these products, and are used for flavouring food.

The fruit of an Orchidaceous plant known to botanists by the name of *Vanilla aromatica* (Fig. 10), yields in its tissues a delicious fragrance, which is highly esteemed both as a perfume and a flavourer of food. This plant is a native of the New World, and its flavour was first experienced by Europeans when Cortes led his band of Spanish brigands to the capital of Montezuma, where they found this sovereign smoking his pipe and sipping his chocolate flavoured with the fragrant vanilla. From the time that chocolate began to be consumed in Europe, a demand was made for vanilla, which is now

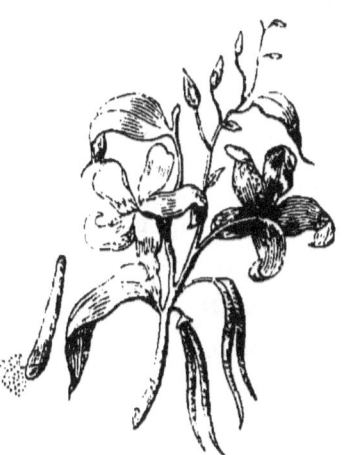

Fig. 10.—Vanilla.

not only used for flavouring cocoa, but puddings, cakes, custards, liqueurs, and other articles of food.

The fruit of the vanilla, when analyzed, has been found to contain a peculiar volatile oil, with which is mixed a certain quantity of benzoic acid. These substances give to it its peculiar fragrance.

Although we draw our supplies of vanilla almost entirely from Mexico, it appears not impossible to cultivate this plant even in the hothouses of Europe. Several years ago, when visiting the Continent, I saw plants of the vanilla growing in a hothouse in the botanic garden at Liége. They bore an abundance of fruit, and I was assured by Professor Morren, the superintendent of the garden, that they could be used for all the purposes to which foreign vanilla is applied. The consumption of vanilla in this country is about five or six hundredweights annually.

At the commencement of this lecture, I alluded to the manufacture of artificial fruit essences. Many of these, as apple oil, pear oil, grape oil, and pine-apple oil, are compounds of ethers and acids. Pear oil, or essence of Jargonelle pears, is a spirituous solution of the acetate of the oxide of amyle; apple oil is the same ether with valerianic acid; pine-apple oil is a compound of œnanthic ether with butyric acid. There are probably many others of these oils used. They are manufactured for the purpose of giving a flavour to low-priced confectionary.

To the same class of substances I may add the oils of lemon and orange peel. The rind of the fruit of all the orange tribe yields a volatile oil, contained in little depositories underneath the epidermis.

These oils are distilled and added to food, especially the oil of lemons. The recent and dried peels of these fruits are added to cakes, custards, puddings, and beverages, to give them a pleasant flavour. Preserved in sugar and dried, lemon and orange peel are eaten under the name of "chips," whilst the peel of orange, lemon, and citron, boiled in sugar, form the well-known "candied" peels.

This reminds me of a large class of substances which are employed to flavour sugar. The angelica is a plant belonging to the Umbelliferæ; the whole plant has a pleasant smell, and its stems are scraped and boiled in sugar, forming the candied angelica. The eryngoe, the sea holly (*Eryngium maritimum*), a despised plant on the sea-shore, is dug up, and its root, candied, is a sweetmeat for royal tables. But my time would fail me to tell of a tenth part of the roots, seeds, berries, and fruits, which, containing pleasant flavours, are done up into sugar sweetmeats, to please the appetite for variety. Sugar is a dull thing to eat from day to day, but, seasoned with these aromas from the vegetable kingdom, it becomes one of the most captivating of the indulgences that address themselves to the palate.

Here also I ought to allude to acids. I have always had some difficulty in classifying the organic acids which enter so largely into our food. In composition they resemble starch and sugar, and in consequence of this I have placed them, in my "Guide to the Food Collection" at Kensington, amongst the heat-giving foods. We have, however, no direct evidence that they are converted into carbonic acid and water. As articles of diet, they probably all exert the same influence on the system, and one of the great inducements to the taking of them seems to be their pleasant flavour. In certain states of the system, they are most agreeable to the palate, and there is a desire for them which has led man at all times and in all countries to use them. One of their uses undoubtedly is that they exert a solvent power on the mineral ingredients of our food, and thus assist in carrying them into the blood. This is the case with carbonic acid, which is so agreeable to us in the effervescence of soda water, Selters water, frothing beers, and sparkling wines. There is also reason to believe that in certain states of the system the organic acids may favour the development of the gastric juice in the stomach, and even assist by their decomposition, when in the blood, in oxidizing its contents. We know that however important may be the action of potash in scurvy, this action is vastly increased by the action of the citric acid with which it is combined in lemon-juice.

The most commonly used of the organic acids is vinegar, which is diluted acetic acid. Acetic acid is the hydrated oxide, the teroxide of an organic base called acetyle ($HO+O3+CH3$). It is usually obtained from the oxidation of alcohol, as I have before explained, but it may be also obtained by the destructive distillation of wood. It is then called pyroligneous acid. Vinegar obtained from the distillation of fermented malt or wine is, however, preferred by the public. It is a curious fact that although the vinegar-maker obtains his malt vinegar without colour, he is obliged to add burnt sugar to colour it in order to satisfy the public taste. This is a harmless addition, but it is one of those things which illustrate a feature in the adulteration of food generally, and that is, that a great deal of it is done to please the public taste.

The antiseptic and agreeable flavour of vinegar has led to its extensive use for preserving vegetable substances, which are eaten under the name of "pickles." These are generally agreeable additions to our diet, and vinegar taken in moderation is beneficial; but the practice of taking vinegar to the extent of destroying the digestive energy of the stomach, in order to get thin, is one of those dangerous experiments which folly sometimes pays for with its life.

Citric acid is found in many fruits, as the strawberry, the currant, and other acid fruits, but it is found in greatest purity and abundance in the fruits of the orange tribe (*Aurantiaceæ*). Lemon-juice and lime-juice are sold in the shops, and may be used for dietetical purposes. The slight flavour which the oil of the peel of the lemon gives to the juice renders it, for a variety of dietical purposes, preferable to vinegar. Lemon juice may be added to almost all kinds of stews and made dishes. It is a primary ingredient in sauces for chops, steaks, wild fowl, and game. A squeeze of lemon will improve the flavour of turtle, lamb, veal, and whitebait; it is a precious constituent of jellies; it is the distinguishing feature of lemonade; a boar's head should not be brought to table without a lemon in his mouth, and those who have drunk tea with only milk to tone it down, have a treat yet to come in the addition of a thin slice of lemon to a cup of genuine hyson. To those of you who would succeed in the art of pleasing the palate, let me recommend the profound study of the properties of a lemon.

It is a descent to speak of the other acids. Tartaric acid is found in the juice of the grape, and I have already spoken of its properties when telling you about wine. Like citric acid, it may be separated in the form of crystals, and when powdered, being cheaper than citric acid, it is used for making effervescing powders.

Malic acid is found in apples and pears, and gives the acidity to those fruits, and the wines made from them known under the name of cyder and perry. The poisonous oxalic acid is the flavouring ingredient that recommends sorrel (*Rumex acetosa*) and the wood-sorrel (*Oxalis acetosella*) as salad, and the leaf-stalks of rhubarb as a substitute for gooseberries and currants in the early season of the year.

All these acids, like oxalic acid, are poisonous in large doses, but we may learn from their beneficial action on the system, that many of these substances which, when taken in excess, destroy the system, may be taken in small quantities, not only with impunity, but with advantage.

But I must close this long lecture on matters of taste. I fear I have wearied you, but if I have impressed you with the importance of this subject, I shall have succeeded in my object, and I hope convinced you that Mr. Brooks gave a great practical hint to our cooks and housewives when he knowingly ejaculated, "It's the seasonin' as does it."

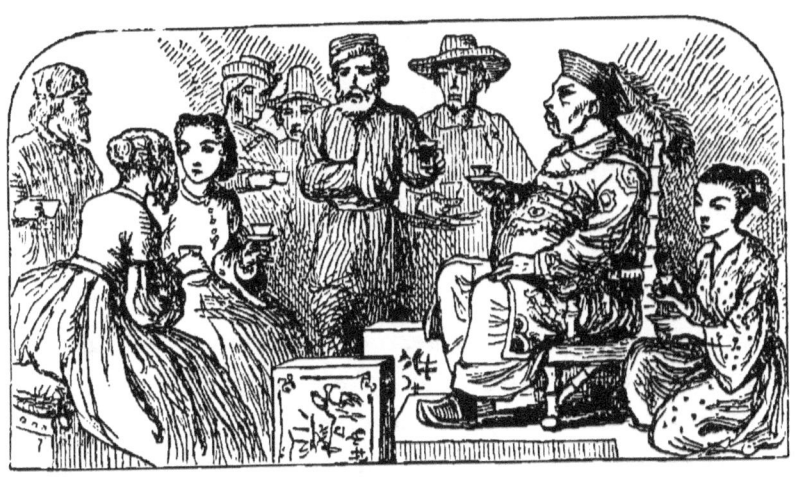

ON TEA AND COFFEE.

In these lectures, you may regard me as acting the part of your host. I began by giving you a cup of cold water, than which nothing is more provocative of appetite. I then placed before you the salt-cellar with its contents, and the various forms of plants we eat as salads, and popularly known as purifiers of the blood. Aware, however, that you could not be sustained on this diet, I introduced you to starch and sugar, and the philosophy of making puddings and eating sweetmeats. These, I explained to you, were heat-giving materials, but inferior even in that function to butter, fats, and oils. I then placed before you bread and meat, poultry, fish, and game, not denying you a glass of ale or wine, to stimulate your digestion, and give a relish to your food. In the present and succeeding lecture we will, if you please, repair to the drawing-room, and discuss the merits of tea, coffee, and chocolate, previous to taking a pipe of tobacco with the American Indian, and a dose of opium with the Chinese.

Tea, coffee, and chocolate belong to the same class of foods as alcohol and the volatile oils. The constituents they contain act on the nervous system, but they act in a different way. Alcohol and the condiments and spices, discussed in the last lecture, are stimulants of the nervous system; but tea and coffee are sedatives. The one is capable of destroying life by producing excessive action; the other destroys life by preventing action.

The way in which these substances act on the nervous system is still a mystery. One thing seems to be ascertained, and that is, that the active agent, whether we call it a food, a medicine, or a poison, must be brought in contact with the nervous matter on which it acts. Alcohol, on being brought in contact with a nerve, excites it to action; tea, on being brought in contact with the same nerve, calms and subdues its activity. Hence, alcohol and tea are natural antagonists. Physiologically antagonists in their action on the human nerves, they have been commercially and dietetically antagonists from the time the latter became known amongst the European nations.

The nations of antiquity — the Egyptians, Jews, Greeks, and Romans—knew nothing of tea. They all regarded alcohol as one of the most precious luxuries of food, and were no strangers to its seductions and destructive influences. The temptations of this powerful agent, and the want of a less stimulating and yet not less agreeable beverage, was one of the defects of their civilization. We miss from the sculptures of Nineveh, the paintings of Egypt, the statuary of Greece, and the furniture of Pompeii, those vessels which we have borrowed from the Chinese, and which are so characteristic of our civilization.

The strong spirituous draughts of the Celt, the Saxon, and the Norse, were inhaled from the polished skulls of slaughtered foemen; the sparkling and highly-tinted wines of the Mediterranean races were poured out of gold and silver tazzas and amphoras; or they stimulated appetite by shining through the transparent sides of crystal cups. These ostentatious utensils were unsuited to the modest character of tea or coffee; and China, which has the merit of supplying the civilized world with the finest of these invigorating infusions, has also presented us with appropriate vessels to contain it, with implements excelling in beauty and refinement anything of this kind that the world had before produced.

The Majolica ware of Southern Europe, though covered with a fine and durable glaze, and decorated with designs painted by the scholars of Giotto, Pietro Perugino, and Raphael, was disregarded when the novel and exquisite porcelain imported from China became known. The pure white body of this earthenware, formed of the yet unknown *kaolin* and *petuntze*, had a charm which, though unaided with artistic adjuncts, bore down all competition. The unpretending brown and semi-turbid "infusion of tea," held in these elegant *cyathides* and *cylices*, or cups and saucers, diffusing around its delicate aroma, soon surpassed, in the favour of the cultivated classes, the more exciting and showy freight of the sculptured bowl. For a time tea was sipped out of minute cups of eggshell porcelain by aristocratic lips only, and amongst elegant social groups, that would have satisfied the fastidious fancy of Watteau; but soon the fashion of tea-drinking descended to the lowest ranks, so that even in the time of Dr. Johnson, he was able to say, "no washerwoman sat down to her evening meal without tea from the East Indies, and sugar from the West."

Tea, coffee, and chocolate were unknown as articles of diet in Europe previous to the seventeenth century. The consumption of tea in the United Kingdom alone at the present time is 80,000,000 pounds annually; of coffee we consume 40,000,000 pounds; and of cocoa, 4,000,000 pounds in the year, making altogether about four pounds every year for each man, woman, and child in the country.

It is very natural that we should turn to the composition of these three things, and ask if there be anything they contain in common which can explain their action on the system, and the influence they have gained over the appetites of mankind? Have they, like wines, spirits, and beers, an active agent, which in each case is the basis of its actions and influence? The parts of these plants employed in diet are various. We obtain tea from the leaves of the plant, coffee from the roasted berries, and cocoa from the pounded seeds. Nor are their general properties less varied. Tea contains volatile oils and tannin; coffee contains empyreumatic oils and caffeic acid: whilst cocoa contains fifty per cent. of a fixed oil, solid at the temperature of our climate. But in each of these is found an active principle. It was first obtained from coffee, and called *caffeine;* then from tea, and called *theine;* and lastly from cocoa, and called *theobromine.* Now, the next interesting part of the history of these substances is that caffeine and theine are identical, and theobromine is so closely allied to these in composition, as to lead to the supposition that it must act on the system in the same way. I think, then, you must admit that the evidence is almost complete, from the result of chemical analysis, that their active principles are the agents which have rendered these articles of diet so popular throughout the world. But I have yet another piece of evidence to put in. The only plant used for infusion that could for a moment be put in competition with tea, coffee, and chocolate, is the Paraguay tea. This plant also contains an active principle, which was called *Paraguaine;* but, on being analysed, this substance is found to be identical with theine. It is in fact theine.

There is another instance of a plant containing theine, and this is in the case of the *Paulinia sorbilis,* the seeds of which are made into a bread by the Brazilian savages. This bread, called Guarana bread, is found to contain theine. It is pounded and mixed with water. and drunk by the Indians as an invigorating beverage

Added to these facts, we find that no leaves, seeds, or roots that do not contain theine, are used so extensively for infusions or decoctions by mankind. Under these circumstances, I think we may fairly claim for theine the same position in relation to these beverages that alcohol has in wines, spirits, and beer. It becomes, therefore, a matter of some interest to ascertain the precise action of this agent on the system.

I have no doubt in my own mind that the action of theine on the system is principally through the agency of the nerves. If given in sufficient doses to animals, it kills them. I have given it to frogs, and found that half a grain is sufficient to kill a full-grown frog. The animal is at first paralysed, and after some time becomes convulsed and dies. The death in this case is very similar to that which is observed from the action of hydrocyanic acid, hemlock, and other sedative poisons. Such poisons do not produce sleep or drowsiness at once, and it is only when insensibility comes on that any remarkable derangement of the functions of the brain is observed.

This action of the theine on the nervous system seems to me to account for the influence exerted on the system by tea and coffee. They exercise primarily a calmative influence, produce a sense of repose, which, without being depressing in the slightest degree, prevents a morbid activity of the nervous system. I cannot but think that the craving for tea and coffee which is frequently exhibited by strong men depends on this influence of the theine on the nervous system.

But the action of theine is not altogether dependent on its immediate influence on the nervous system. It has been shown by competent experimenters that it has the same kind of conservative action on the tissues that we found to take place with alcohol. It seems that any of those substances which exert an influence on the nervous system, whether that influence is sedative or stimulant, prevent the destruction of tissue.

As I have said before, this is not always a healthful or desirable action. When persons are growing stout, when the blood is getting corrupt from the introduction or retention of improper ingredients, it is frequently most desirable that every facility should be given for a change. It should also be recollected that all healthy life depends on the destruction of tissue, and that to prevent this is to retain old stuff instead of new, and to work with bad and imperfect materials when fresh and new ones might be obtained.

Besides this general action of theine, certain special actions have been attributed to it. Liebig at one time thought it substituted taurine, a compound procured from the bile, but he has probably abandoned this theory himself. Before leaving theine I would call your attention to its chemical composition, by which you will see that it closely resembles kreatinine, a substance I have before spoken of as contained in the flesh or muscles of animals. It also resembles another compound, which is called glycocoll, and which exists in gelatine, the substance from which we make jellies. It may be that theine exerts some action on the tissues, in virtue of this resemblance. If we compare the composition of theobromine, theine, and kreatinine, with certain active principles from plants with which we are acquainted, we shall find that, although they differ little in chemical compositions, some of them act as medicines whilst others act as frightful poisons. Take the following series, which gives the quantity of atoms of each of their elements:—

	Carbon.	Nitrogen.	Hydrogen.	Oxygen.
Theobromine	7	2	4	2
Theine or Caffeine	8	2	5	2
Kreatinine	8	3	7	2
Glycocoll	8	2	8	6
Kreatine	8	8	9	4
Quinine	20	1	12	2
Morphine	34	1	19	6
Atropine	34	1	23	6
Strychnine	46	2	26	4
Aconitine	60	1	47	14

Many of you will be reminded by this table of the composition of protein, which consists, according to its discoverer, Mulder, of carbon 40, nitrogen 5, hydrogen 31, oxygen 12. This substance, you will remember, lies at the foundation of albumen and fibrine, the materials of which our flesh is made, and you will thus see the close resemblance in composition between some of the most dangerous poisons and the materials of our nerves and muscles. It will probably be found eventually that those substances are most agreeable to the system as food which most nearly resemble the compounds that form the tissues of the body, whilst those act as poisons whose composition is most different from that of the tissues, on which the life of the body depends.

Having said thus much with regard to the action of theine on the system, and which applies equally to tea and coffee, I will now speak of these substances in detail; and first, of Tea.

That tea was first brought into Europe from China there seems to be no doubt; but the exact date of that event is involved in some obscurity. By some writers, the first introduction of tea into Europe is claimed for the Portuguese, who, as early as the year 1577, commenced a regular trade with China. Edmund Waller, in some complimentary lines to Catherine of Braganza, says—

> "Venus her myrtle, Phœbus has his bays,
> Tea both excels, which she vouchsafes to praise;
> The best of queens and best of herbs we owe
> To that bold nation which the way did show
> To the fair region where the sun doth rise,
> Whose rich productions we so justly prize."

One of the earliest literary references to tea, in a European language, is found in the writings of Giovanni Pietri Maffei, who, in his "Historiæ Indicæ," says, "The inhabitants of China, like those of Japan, extract from a herb called *Chia* a beverage which they drink warm, and which is extremely wholesome, being a remedy against phlegm, languor, and blearedness, and a promoter of longevity."* Father Alexander de Rhodes, who travelled in China in 1623, speaks of the use of tea by the Chinese, and of the fact of its having begun to be known in Europe. Olearius, who was in Persia in 1633, mentions the fact of tea being sold in the taverns and largely consumed by the Persians. There is also evidence about the same time that the Japanese were in the habit of consuming tea in the same way as the Chinese, and that tea was sold in England prior to the year 1657, at the rate of from six to ten pounds a pound.

The first coffee-shop was opened in London, in

* Quoted in article "Tea," in "Encyclopædia Britannica."

George-yard, Lombard-street, in 1652, by one Pasqua, a Greek. In 1660 an Act was passed levying a duty of eight-pence " on every gallon of coffee, chocolate, sherbet, and tea," made and sold. Mr. Pepys informs us in his Diary, under the date of " September 25th, 1661. I sent for a cup of tea (a Chinese drink), of which I had never drunk before." We should be glad now to know what he thought of it; but he does not say, and we are thankful for this short notice. In 1664 it is stated, that the East-India Company ventured to give an order for two pounds two ounces, as a present to his majesty. It was, perhaps, this identical two pounds of tea that, when served up at the royal table, appeared in the form of a dish of leaves, with pepper, salt, and melted butter, and was found so tough that nobody could eat it. Be that as it may, we find the East-India Company ordering 100 pounds of tea, in 1667; and the demand for it had increased to such an extent, that in 1678 they imported 4,713 pounds. From such small beginnings has the influence of this powerful drug increased, till its consumption employs a fleet of vessels to bring it to our shores, and the quantity consumed may be calculated by thousands of tons, while the revenue it produces by taxation is between five and six millions per annum.

The discovery of the value of tea as a dietetical agent has been very variously described. It was probably first used as medicine, and its pleasant aroma when drunk warm in infusion, and obvious soothing effect on the nervous system, led gradually to its extension from the domain of medicine to that of food. There may be, perhaps, two other good physiological reasons assigned for the extending use of this substance. In the first place, the waters of China are universally bad, and are only safe for drinking after they are boiled; they are also flat and tasteless: thus the demand for water in the system would be more pleasantly met by an agent like the infusion of tea. In the next place, the practice of taking warm drinks is a great economy when people live upon a scanty diet, and this added to the preservative effects of tea on the tissues, would lead to the use of tea. Before the introduction of tea or coffee into this country, our forefathers were in the habit of using various kinds of infusions, which were drunk warm, as we do tea and coffee. In this way sage was at one time extensively employed in this country, and its leaves were actually originally taken by the Dutch to China as an exchange for tea. Warm drinks are everywhere used by man, and the fact has great physiological interest. I am induced to think that the warmth saves the loss of heat to the stomach of raising the temperature of the liquid to that of the human body. Although when the body is full of food and in great integrity, this process of heating up the food in the stomach may not only not injure health, but become a source of comfort, as when ice and iced drinks are taken; yet it is very certain that when people are under-fed and there is any debility from disease, cold drinks and cold food act most injuriously. The youthful, vigorous, and healthy may undoubtedly enjoy cold or even iced food; but for the infant, the feeble, and the aged, warm drinks should be secured.

Very absurd stories are told about the early date of the introduction of tea amongst the Chinese, and which can only be believed by those who know nothing about China, and the history of its civilization. It was probably first generally used in China about the eighth or ninth century of the Christian era. The tea-plant is a native of China, and since its first use by the Chinese, it has been introduced into Japan, where it is cultivated to a very considerable extent.

The tea-plants are evergreen shrubs, having very much the same appearance and belonging to the same family as the plants which are so familiar to us under the name of Camellias. The leaves are not so shining, nor the flowers so large, as those of the camellia. The part of the plant which is used are the leaves, which are picked and dried at various periods of their growth, and are brought into the markets under the name of black and green teas. The different appearance of black and green teas and the different characters of the tea-plant led botanists to suppose that there were two species of tea-plant,—the *Thea Bohea*, the black-tea plant; and *Thea viridis*, the green-tea plant. It turns out, however, that the black and green teas of commerce do not depend on different plants, but on the way in which they are prepared, and that green tea can be made from the black-tea plant, and black tea from the green-tea plant. It does not, however, necessarily follow, as some people suppose, that therefore there are not two species of tea-plant. But this really is a matter of very

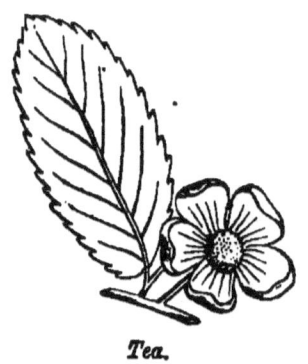

Tea.

little importance, although, from the earnestness with which this question has been discussed, you might really imagine that the whole supply of tea to the world depended on the answer.

One of the most interesting points in the history of the tea-plant has been its recent discovery in Hindostan. If you will take a map of Asia, you will see that the same character of country prevails from Shanghai to Nepaul, and that it would not be an extravagant inference that the plants of China should be found in the northern provinces of India. This had been suspected by more than one botanist, and in 1823 Major Bruce confirmed their suspicions, and brought specimens of the true tea-plant from Assam. Doubts, to be sure, had been thrown out as to whether this is the true tea-plant, or a new species; but whether that be the case or not, it makes very good tea. The discovery of this plant in Assam has led to very extensive efforts for the growth and manufacture of tea in the British East Indies, efforts which I am happy to say are being crowned with success. It would, indeed, be a reproach to England if, after having had this magnificent country placed in her hands, she should do little or nothing by her wealth and intelligence in developing its mighty resources. Great as is our national demand for tea, it would appear that the districts of India capable of supplying it are greater than our consumption. Its production, however, mainly depends on the price of labour. The tea-plant was early introduced into the New World, and grows luxuriantly, even without culture, at the present moment in the Brazils; but it requires Chinese poverty and Chinese patience to dry the leaves for general use: hence its failure in America. Recent experiments have been made to grow the tea-plant in South Carolina, and although the tree has flourished and the tea has promised well, the high price of labour has caused its failure.

The preparation of the tea for use is one that is carried on by the Chinese with great care and delicacy. Although many of the processes to which the tea is submitted appear perfectly unnecessary, and the excessive attention to little points a mere piece of Celestial refinement, yet the experience of a London washerwoman will at once indicate whether the tea she drinks has been prepared according to Chinese fashion or not. Hence the necessity of introducing Chinese labour where tea for European consumption is manufactured. The Assam tea was hardly a saleable article till manufactured by Chinese labourers. In the other plantations of India, as at Kumaon, where Chinese labour has been imported, and the native Chinese tea-plant introduced, the tea produced is so good, that little or none of it finds its way to England at all. The palates of our countrywomen at Calcutta, Madras, and Bombay are much too sensitive to the good things of this life to allow us to get much Kumaon tea.

I need not detain you long on the subject of the culture and the preparation of the tea. At the same time, there can be no doubt that many of those properties of tea which have rendered it so great a favourite as a beverage throughout the world are dependent on the wonderful care bestowed by the Chinese on its culture and preparation. The wild plants do not yield tea equal in quality or flavour to those of the cultivated plants.

The soils in which the tea-plants grow best are described as ferruginous clays and sandstones. It would appear that it flourishes in soils containing a little iron, and, as we shall subsequently see, there are small quantities of iron in the ashes of tea-leaves. The plants are grown from seeds, the best of which are selected, and from six to ten seeds are placed in holes dibbled in the earth. In all districts of China, the leaves are gathered from the plants at different periods of growth. The plants begin to be picked in their second year's growth. The first picking of leaves commences in April, and subsequent pickings are carried on till the beginning of September. The first picking consists principally of the young buds, and in each subsequent picking the leaves are larger and more expanded.

From the fact that the first picked leaves of the season are employed for the manufacture of the highest priced teas, both black and green, we may conclude that the theine is in larger proportion to the rest of the tissues of the leaf at this season than at any other.

The leaves, having been gathered, are always submitted to a process of *sorting*, which consists merely in separating the larger from the smaller, the coarser from the fine leaves. They are then *dried* in the open air, and during the drying they are submitted to various processes, but more particularly to tossing in the air. The Chinaman takes a handful of the leaves and throws them up into the air, and they are thus dried most effectually. It is at this stage of the process that a different plan is pursued according as it is wished to manufacture *green* or *black* tea. After drying, the leaves are *roasted* in hot uncovered pans, and from the exposure to the air in this process *green tea* results. This is called the *dry* way; but if during this process the pans are covered, the moisture evaporated continues in the pans, and a kind of fermentation takes place amongst the leaves, which is attended with an alteration in the colour of the leaves, and the tea is called black tea. This is called the *wet* way.

After the process of roasting, the leaves are again submitted to certain manual processes, by which the leaves are twisted in the hands, and made to assume the curled appearance so characteristic of tea. After this process the leaves are again dried and roasted, and afterwards packed in chests to be sold to the tea merchants. Even after the tea has been sold it is submitted to processes of separating and mixing. The leaves are sifted, so that the larger are separated from the smaller, and these are now sold under various names to the foreign purchaser.

The teas sold to the English and American merchants in China are known by various names, according as they are green or black. These names either express the quality of the tea, or the name of the district from whence it was brought. Thus green teas, according to their fineness or the period of their picking, are called Young Hyson, Gunpowder, Hyson, Hyson-skin, and Twankay; while the black teas are called Pekoe, Souchong, Congou, and Bohea. These names have some significance in the tea-markets of China and Europe; but in the retail sale of tea in this country, the original qualities and samples of tea are not preserved. Each considerable dealer buys his teas and mixes them, and sells them under his own particular names.

Teas are to be seen in China which never find their way into the European markets. In the Great Exhibition of 1851, teas were exhibited which fetch a price of from fifty to sixty shillings a pound in China. These, with many other examples of tea, are to be seen in the Food Collection at the South Kensington Museum. There is a peculiar tea called " Old Men's Eyebrows," which consists of tea formed into elongated rolls, looking very like delicate cigars made up in bundles. This tea is employed for making presents. Tea is also done up in little square packets, which seem to have undergone a slight degree of compression whilst preparing. Such tea was preferred by Commissioner Yeh, and some of it from his private stock, when prisoner at Calcutta, will be found in the South Kensington Food Collection. There also may be seen the brick tea, which seems to be a coarse kind of tea, which has been compressed during preparation. It is easily transported, and is much used by the Maotchu Tartars, and is also manufactured by the Japanese. In fact, I ought to have mentioned before, that the tea-plant is almost as generally planted in Japan as in China, and that the population of that country is equally addicted to its use. Most persons will remember the accounts recently brought to this country of the consumption of tea by the Japanese.

Although the natural flavour of the tea is very agreeable and refreshing, the Chinese use a variety of agents to increase its flavour or *bouquet*. These things are not at all employed for the purposes of fraud, and various flowers are cultivated for the purpose of adding them to the tea. Species of the *Camellia*, a genus belonging to the same order as the tea, yield fragrant scents, which are added to tea. These odours are, however, not appreciated in England, and highly-scented teas are not commonly seen in Europe at all.

Having said this much with regard to the culture and qualities of tea, let me now draw your attention to its special composition. According to recent analysis, a pound of tea contains the following ingredients:—

	OZ.	GRAINS.
Water	0	350
Theine	0	210
Caseine	2	175
Aromatic Oil	0	52
Gum	2	385
Sugar	0	211
Fat	0	280
Tannic Acid	4	87
Woody Fibre	3	87
Mineral Matter	0	350

Now I will just go over these ingredients, and point out to you their action on the system. It will be convenient for us to follow our usual classification, and speak of the water, the salts, the heat-giving and the flesh-forming substances, and, last of all, the medicinal or auxiliary food-materials of tea. I need say little or nothing about the water here, as in the dried leaves of tea it forms a very inconspicuous ingredient compared with the large quantities of water in which we find them infused before they are employed as food. In fact, the early use of tea and other substances which we inf in water may be traced to two causes—first, to improve the quality of water; and, secondly, to render it more palatable when warm.

Sugar is added to tea in this country to render it more palatable. Another reason why man adds various flavouring substances to water, is his instinctive tendency to take his food warm. In all parts of the world man not only cooks his food, but prefers it warm. This is not only the case with solid food, but also with liquid food; and whatever may be the quality of the liquid food, whether it be the liquor in which meat is boiled, the milk from the cow, or coffee, tea, or chocolate, he is in the habit of taking it warm. He has undoubtedly made selections of such substances as tea, coffee, or chocolate; but the more general condition which has led to their use is the innate tendency to partake of warm drinks in preference to cold. This subject is a highly interesting one, and I may allude to it again before I finish these lectures.

I now come to speak of the salts of the tea. You see they are in very considerable quantities, as compared with the saline matter of other kinds of food, and, as some of them are soluble, it becomes a matter of interest to know what they are. I am enabled to give you a list of these ingredients, as an analysis of the ashes of tea, by Lehmann, has been published by Baron Liebig, in the last edition of his "Familiar Letters on Chemistry."

Potash	47·45
Lime	1·24
Magnesia	6·84
Peroxide of Iron	3·29

Phosphoric Acid	9·88
Sulphuric Acid	8·72
Silicic Acid	2·31
Carbonic Acid	10·09
Oxide of Manganese	0·71
Chloride of Sodium	3·62
Soda	5·03
Charcoal and Sand	1·09

Now the point of interest about this analysis is not only that most of the ingredients form soluble compounds, but that they belong to a group of salts which are most important to the human system. Thus we find here potash, phosphoric acid, and iron, all of them substances required by the system for the performance of its functions and the construction of its tissues. Liebig very properly remarks on the composition of these ashes, that "We have, therefore, in tea a beverage which contains the active constituents of the most powerful mineral springs; and, however small the amount of iron may be which we daily take in this form, it cannot be destitute of influence on the vital processes."

The next groups of constituents are the heat-giving, but these I need hardly tell you are very unimportant compounds of the tea. They consist of small quantities of fat and sugar, and, in order that you may judge how much of these things is likely to get into the tea, I may tell you that a tea-spoonful of tea weighs about fifty grains, and as this is supposed to be enough to make a single individual all the tea he requires at a meal, you will see that in two cups of tea you would get about a grain and a half of sugar and two grains of fat. It is questionable whether you get the latter out of the tea at all. Then as we add sugar and milk to our tea, these things from the tea itself are of little or no consequence.

The same may be said of the flesh-forming constituents of tea. All vegetable matter contains, to a greater or less extent, nitrogenous constituents, and the quantity of caseine in tea, therefore, is not a matter of surprise. As the leaves are dried you get a larger quantity than you would from the fresh leaves of plants. In fifty grains of tea we should have about seven grains of cheese or casein, and as probably only a very small quantity of this is dissolved, the nutritive value of tea, as dependent on its casein, need not be discussed.

The gum and the woody fibre belong to the accessary groups of food. The gum is taken up probably by the water used in making tea, and would appear from its easy solubility in larger quantities in the first cup; but not being convertible into either heat-giving or flesh-forming matter, it can exert little or no influence in the action of tea in the system. The woody fibre, being insoluble and indigestible, of course can exert no influence.

I now come to the most important constituents of the tea. They belong to the group of medicinal foods. They are the very essence of the tea, and without which it would never have been consumed by mankind. These are the theine, the volatile oil, and the tannic acid.

Now I have told you all about theine, so that I need not dwell on its properties here. You should recollect, however, that it is readily soluble in hot water, and that the great proportion of the theine will be taken up by the water first poured on the tea. Perhaps I may press this matter on those who preside at the tea-table. In a large party it is very unfair to pour out the whole of the superior tea before adding a second quantity of water, as in this case the tea from the second watering contains little or no theine, and, what is worse, little or none of the flavouring volatile oil. The fact is, the beverage from the second mash is a mere apology for tea, and contains neither the active principle nor the flavour of tea. If this were a little thought over, arrangements might be made by which at our tea-drinkings and more fashionable *soirées* and evening parties, we might more frequently get hot tea instead of spoiled warm water, to which sugar and milk are added to render it tolerable.

The quantity of theine in a cup of tea will of course vary in proportion to the relative quantity of tea and water used, but the proportion varies, I calculate, in a cup of tea from the first brewing, from half a grain to one grain.

The aromatic oil of the tea, although small in quantity, is, in one sense, the most important constituent of tea. The pleasant scent of the tea, the flavour that addresses itself to the palate depends on this oil. I am not aware of any special chemical researches having been made on the composition of this oil. It does not appear to be present in the fresh or unprepared tea-leaf, but to be formed during the process of preparation. It is also much less developed in black than in green tea, and, indeed, it may be questioned whether the two processes by which these teas are prepared do not develop different oils. It is very certain, that whilst green and black tea contain the same quantities of other constituents, they act very differently on the nervous system. I have known many persons who could drink with impunity black tea, who are made ill and sleepless by very small quantities of green tea. At the same time, this oil does not generally disagree, and many persons can take green tea with impunity. But in estimating the action of tea, there can be no doubt we must always take into effect the oil which is so abundant in the green tea.

The effects of the oil of tea on the system closely approach those of Digitalis, or foxglove. When foxglove is given, there is great anxiety, with palpitation of the heart, and unless given in poisonous doses, inability to sleep. These are the same symptoms as persons complain of who take too much green tea, or who are remarkably susceptible of its action. The effect of the theine is to act as a sedative generally on the nervous system, and the oil of tea probably directs this action more particularly to the heart, and this accounts for the anxiety and nervousness felt by persons taking green tea.

It may occasionally happen that persons become alarmingly ill from taking green tea, and it is well to know that stimulants are the great antagonists of the action of this agent. A wine-glassful of brandy, with or without hot or cold water, is a potent remedy. The spirits of sal-volatile or any form of ammonia may be given with advantage.

The last of the substances found in tea which I shall mention is tannic acid. Tannic acid, or tannin, has been regarded as a very powerful medicine, and you will be surprised, perhaps, to see that above a quarter of the tea-leaves consist of tannic acid. We have no tannic acid in coffee or chocolate, so that tannic acid may be regarded as one of the distinguishing features of tea. Tannic acid has a remarkable affinity for certain organic substances. It is on this account that it is the great agent in the process of tanning. It forms with gelatine an insoluble compound, and this constitutes leather.* There is considerable variety in the composition and properties of the substances known as tannic acid, but they all form an insoluble compound with gelatine. They also render albumen insoluble, and otherwise act upon the compounds which are most common in our food. It is, therefore, a fair subject of inquiry, as to how the tannic acid of the tea acts as an article of diet.

The action of tannic acid on the tissues is seen in the effect produced on the numerous membranes of the mouth when it is introduced. A white floculent precipitate is formed with the mucus and saliva, and this hangs about the mouth, looking as if the person was afflicted with thrush,—an impression is produced on the nerves of taste similar to that which is produced by an acid. There is, however, no sour flavour, but the mouth is, as it were, "drawn up." This is what is called an astringent effect. Such an action in a slight degree is not unpleasant, and occurs with all acid articles of diet, and also when we take tea into the mouth. This effect is

---

* See "Leather," in Dr. Lankester's Course of Lectures on the Uses of Animals.

more obvious when the tea has neither sugar nor milk. It is apparently this action upon the mucous membrane of his mouth which is relished by the Hindoo in the chewing of the betel-nut, which contains tannic acid. This astringent or "drawing-up" effect is not imaginary, for we find tannic acid is one of the most powerful styptics we possess. A little applied to a bleeding part will arrest the hæmorrhage. Iuternally it is administered with the same object in view, and in losses of blood from the various surfaces of the body tannic acid is one of the most effectual remedies that can be employed.

Now, as tannic acid is soluble in hot water, tea must contain a very considerable quantity, at least two or three grains of this substance in every cup of the first brewing. It cannot be supposed but that the effect of this agent is very considerable. The two most remarkable points of its action are its effects upon the food in the stomach, and its effects as an astringent. I have so often seen dyspepsia removed by persons giving up the practice of taking tea at breakfast, that I have no doubt that the tannic acid of the tea renders the food taken with it more difficult of digestion. Of course, this would only occur in the case of persons in whom the digestive function was already impaired. Such persons may frequently take tea with advantage on an empty stomach.

I have often found myself, and observed it in others, that what we called tea dinners, produced a considerable amount of indigestion. As the action of the tannic acid in precipitating the compounds of the food is greater when taken with than without animal food, the objection is greater to taking tea with meals of animal food than merely with bread and butter.

The practice of taking tea, provided the theine and oil do not disagree, two or three hours after dinner, seems unobjectionable. At this time the food has proceeded too far in the process of digestion to be seriously interfered with by the tannic acid of the tea. The water of the tea supplies a quantity of liquid which, if taken earlier, would have interfered with digestion, whilst the theine counteracts the stimulating effect of the wine or beer taken at dinner. I know, however, that tea is extensively taken in this country at the evening meal after a middle-day dinner, and that, as it is the last meal taken in the day, solid food is consumed. I would here repeat my conviction that such a meal is always likely to be more healthily digested the less animal food that is consumed at it.

Nor is the astringent effect of the tannic acid to be lost sight of. The natural secretion of the mucous membrane of the stomach and bowels is diminished, and where there is a tendency to inaction of the bowels, it may be increased by tea. I need not, however, go further medically into this subject. I have only wished to say so much as would enable you to judge of the proper use of tea as an ordinary article of diet.

And now I come to the weighty and important matter of how to make tea. I have shown you of what tea is composed, and I have dwelt on the chemical, physical, and vital properties of its constituents. From my remarks you will have gathered that the two most important constituents of tea are the theine and the volatile oil: the one acting on the nervous system, the other giving flavour to the tea, and also having a share in the effect of the tea. The only other thing that can be said to exert any influence on the system at all is the tannic acid, and whether we get more or less of that is a matter of not much importance. Therefore, the question to consider in making tea is, how to get the largest quantity of theine and retain the greatest amount of the volatile oil. Now this object is not to be attained by boiling the tea, as we do coffee, and making a decoction, nor by allowing the theine and oil to exude into cold water, as in the case of beef-tea; but the two objects are to be attained by exposing the tea-leaves to the action of boiling water. Boiling water takes up a larger quantity of theine than water at a lower point: at the same time it gives intensity to the volatility of the oil of the tea without dissipating it.

Now this process seems a very simple thing, but you will find it is not so easy of accomplishment. When the kettle comes up from the kitchen before it is poured on the tea in the parlour, you may be sure the water does not boil. When the urn ceases to throw out steam the water does not boil. In nine cases out of ten, when the kettle is taken off the fire it ceases to boil. If you pour boiling water into a cold tea-pot it ceases to boil. If you pour it on cold tea it ceases to boil. The fact is, unless you heat your tea-pot to the boiling point, tea and all, before you put in the water, the tea will not be exposed to boiling water at all.

A good plan to secure the heating of the tea and pot, before the water is poured in, is to put it for a few minutes on the side of the fire-place, or expose it to the flame of a spirit-lamp. Putting boiling water into the tea-pot before putting in the tea, previously putting the tea in a cup on the hob, is another good plan.

I have invented a tea-pot, with a double cover, into the interstices of which boiling water may be poured, so that the whole is heated up to nearly the boiling point before tea or water is put into the pot. This answers very well, but it makes the tea-pot heavy, and I have never been able to induce a tea-pot manufacturer to invest his capital in the manufacture of my "double envelope tea-pot."

The late M. Soyer, to whom we English are so much indebted for popularising the art of cookery amongst us, recommended that the tea should be ground before being submitted to infusion. This is, undoubtedly, an economical mode of making tea: by it you extract every particle of theine, but then you get more of the tannic acid and the other constituents than you care to have. It makes the tea coarse. It is like new rough Port as compared with Steinberger or Johannisberger wines. When, however, the object is to supply large parties, and to make tea go the furthest way, this is a good plan. M. Loysell has invented an apparatus in which he makes both tea and coffee, and the tea is treated like coffee. It is powdered and submitted to the boiling water at a pressure, and in this way all the soluble compounds of the tea are effectually removed. In making tea for large assemblies I understand this process gives a better cup of tea all round than that secured by any other plan.

It is, however, in the preparation of this "cup, which cheers but not inebriates," for the household that we are all most interested. There is hardly any point in this process that is indifferent. Without being chemists, the Chinese are very particular as to the water they employ in the making of tea. We know from chemical investigation that some water will take up a great deal more soluble matter than others, and as a rule, soft waters are better for making soups, decoctions, and infusions than hard waters. In order to facilitate the action of hard water on tea some persons use soda, and it is true that a certain quantity of the compounds of the tea, especially the colouring matter, are thus rendered soluble which would not be so without the soda. But I question very much whether the tea, as far as its theine and volatile oil are concerned, is any the better for this process. There is no doubt that soft water, such as they get at Manchester, Liverpool, and Glasgow, is the water which makes the best and most economical tea.

Even the material and colour of your tea-pot is not a matter of indifference. Tea-pots that retain the heat are better than those that let it go. A rough black tea-pot is one of the best radiators of heat that could be invented. Hence, black earthenware tea-pots should not be used. While glazed earthenware or porcelain are much better; but better still are brightly polished silver tea-pots, for they radiate heat much less than any other material.

The tea thus made is an infusion of theine and tannic acid combined with the salts of the tea and the volatile oils which give it flavour. In England, before drinking it, we add sugar and milk, or cream. They modify to some extent the flavour of the tea, and probably its action. Sugar is a heat-giver as well as cream, whilst its caseine is a flesh-former; so that it should be remembered, in taking a cup of tea we are actually consuming one of the most compound of our foods, an article of diet which represents every group of our daily food. The Chinese do not thus adulterate their tea, and prefer, as also do our washerwomen, to take their tea *pur et simple*. The Russians add sugar, but either squeeze in a little lemon-juice or add a slice of lemon. This, I can assure you, is no despicable addition. When the stomach is already clogged with food, as is the case after dinner, or when thirst is best allayed by acids, then the addition of lemon or its juice is most palatable and pleasant. I have before spoken of the excellent action of lemon-juice on the system, at those seasons of the year when fruit is scarce, and fresh vegetables not easy to be obtained. I have no doubt that the addition of lemon-juice to tea would have a most beneficial effect on the health. At the same time, I do not flatter myself that any of you will try it; we are all too much the slaves of inveterate habit to allow reason to exercise any influence over our accustomed practice, and had our grandmothers chosen to add vinegar or pepper to their tea, instead of sugar and milk, we should have adhered to the practice, pitying all those whose tastes or judgment had led them to adopt any other way of drinking their tea.

I have not exhausted my subject, and in the next lecture, when I come to speak of the other beverages of which we partake after infusing in boiling or hot water, shall perhaps have an opportunity of adding a few more words on the subject of tea.

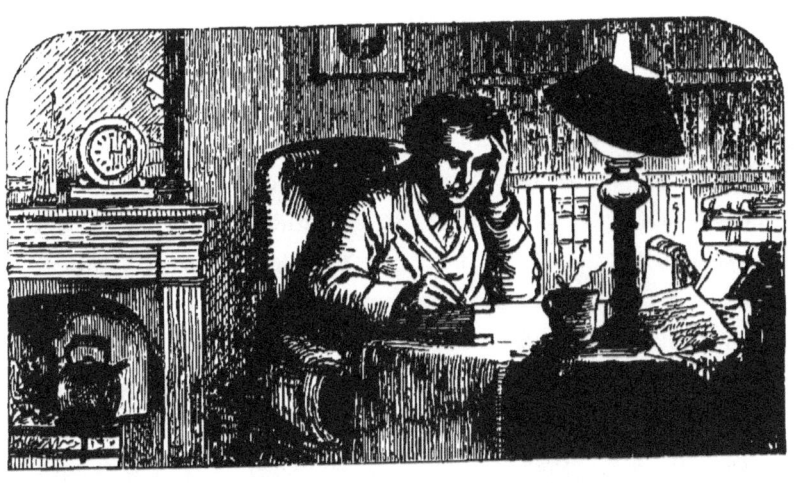

ON TEA AND COFFEE.
(CONTINUED.)

THE practice of taking warm beverages is almost universal amongst mankind. The inhabitants of the tropical forests of Africa, as well as the natives of Lapland and Kamschatka, are equally addicted to the practice of drinking warm infusions. The Egyptians and Jews, the Greeks and the Romans, all partook of heated beverages of some kind or other. Not only are fluids taken heated, but solid food cooked by heat is preferred warm. Long before the introduction of tea and coffee into this country, warmed beverages were popular, and an infusion or decoction called salep was sold hot in the streets of London. It is perhaps worth while, before speaking of coffee and chocolate, to remind you of the nature of this salep. The substance sold in the shops under this name is procured from the roots of several species of Orchidaceous plants. Some of these are natives of this country, as *Orchis Morio, Orchis mascula,* and *Orchis maculata.* They have all large tuberous roots, which yield, on boiling in water, a mucilaginous substance. This is one of the modifications of starch, and is called by chemists bassorin. There is also accompanying this undoubtedly some nutritious matter, which will account for the general use of salep amongst the natives of the East at the present day. When the roots are ready for use they are dug up and dipped in warm water, by which process a fine brown skin which covers them, something like the skin of a potato, is easily removed by means of a coarse cloth or brush; they are next arranged on a tin plate, and heated in an oven for ten minutes, which gives them a semi-transparent or horn-like appearance. They are then withdrawn from the oven, and, after exposure to the air for a few days, they are ready for use. When put into cold water they swell up and form a kind of mucilage. One part of powdered salep in forty-eight parts of boiling water forms a thick mucilaginous liquid. It is this liquid, flavoured with sugar and sassafras chips, that was sold in the streets of London before coffee was introduced. I do not know that it can be procured anywhere now; but I have met with persons who recollect having seen this beverage sold at stalls in the streets of London, as coffee is now. Dr. Percival, a physician in London, wrote a book, as late as 1773, on the preparation, culture, and uses of the orchis-root, in which he refers to the abundance of orchis plants in some parts of this country, and recommends them as an economical article of diet. I cannot, however, from any experience of my own, speak of the value of the orchis-root in diet. There is one remark I would make, and that is, that the beverages drunk before the introduction of tea and coffee seemed free from any agent capable of acting on the nervous system in the same way as theine. In fact, although the modern warm beverages contain so generally this principle, it would appear that the heat which they contain is, after all, their universal recommendation.

The cause of this preference for heated food is, perhaps, worth a moment's inquiry. It has been observed, where persons have taken cold food for a length of time, that they have become depressed, and their stomach disordered. The fact is, when we take food considerably lower than 98°, the temperature of the human body, it abstracts heat from the stomach and surrounding tissues; and unless the system has the power of manufacturing an additional quantity of heat to supply that which has been lost by raising the temperature of the food, a general depression of the vital powers will take place. We know that persons are sometimes made very ill, and even killed, by taking, in an exhausted state, a draught of cold water or an ice. This is, perhaps, sufficient to indicate the fact, that in taking warm foods and drinks, we are sparing the system the effort of producing a quantity of heat, which can only be done by the destruction of a certain quantity of tissue by the process of oxidation. There is no doubt, that where vigorous oxidation goes on in the body, and a rapid metamorphosis of tissue takes place, there the body will exhibit the greatest amount of power, provided this takes place within the limits of health. But the human body may be exposed to too much oxidation—there may be a more rapid combustion of tissue than there are processes of renewal, and under these circumstances the body will suffer. It is on this ground, I believe, that warm food and drinks are found so acceptable to mankind. When the body needs food or drink, it is usually in an exhausted state; and as cold food makes an immediate demand on the system for heat before it can itself supply the materials for combustion, the body is taxed to supply heat at a moment when it is least fitted for it—hence the instinctive preference for warm food. This is much more the case with liquid than with solid food, and as the former contains generally little nutritive or heat-giving matter, it acts all the more injuriously on the system when taken cold.

These facts will explain a great many of the peculiarities of our diet. It shows us why it is that we take our tea and coffee warm at breakfast, after the long abstinence from food during the night. It explains how it is that many persons cannot drink cold water when they first rise in the morning. It throws light on the practice of eating hot soup at the beginning of the principal meal. It accounts for so large a number of teetotallers substituting warm weak tea or coffee at their meals for cold water. It seems to me to be, in fact, the explanation of the universal preference for warm food amongst mankind where it can be procured.

I know there is a contrary taste for taking ices and iced drinks. But this I suspect is more an acquired than a natural taste, and is rather the luxury of the over-fed and the indolent than the instinctive tendency of the race. In fact, ice in this country is only thought of at any time, after the stomach has been well fortified by previous eating and drinking to resist its depressing action. In the summer season, when the temperature of the atmosphere approaches that of the human body, the taking of iced drinks is more largely indulged in, and it can be done with the greater impunity, as under such circumstances the heat-giving faculty of the system is little taxed by the withdrawal of heat for the surface of the body. Not to prolong my remarks on this subject, I would say what clothing is to the external surface of the body, warm food is to its internal surface, and that just as the skin is invigorated by the occasional application of cold, so the mucous membrane of the mouth and stomach may be momentarily pleasantly stimulated by the application of cold; but the continuous application of cold to either surfaces is a circumstance to be guarded against, as likely to be productive of injurious consequences.

But I must now invite your attention to the subject of Coffee. It is a very curious fact, that tea and coffee should have been introduced into Europe about the same time. - Coffee, however, came to us from quite a different district of the world from that which presented us with tea. The coffee-plant is a native of Abyssinia, from whence it appears to have been originally introduced into Persia and Arabia. It is known to have been used as an article of diet in Persia as early as 875; whilst the credit of its introduction into Arabia Felix is given to Megalleddin, Mufti of Aden. It seems to have been especially acceptable to a Mohammedan population, who by their religion were interdicted the consumption of fermented beverages. It was not till

1554 that it was publicly sold in Constantinople. Although attempts were made to stop its sale by the Syrian government, on the ground of its intoxicating properties, it made its way in spite of all opposition. It was not till the seventeenth century that it found its way into Europe. Several notices of it, however, were found amongst European writers before that time. Prosper Alpinus, a Venetian traveller, who visited Egypt in 1580, mentions it in his writings. Burton, an English writer, in his "Anatomy of Melancholy," published in 1621, says, "The Turks have a drink called coffee (for they use no wine), so named, of a berry as black as soot and as bitter, which they sip up as warm as they can suffer, because they find by experience that that kind of drink so used helpeth digestion and procureth alacrity."

Coffee was first sold in London in 1652. It soon became a favourite beverage in London, and coffee-shops were directed to be licensed by the magistrates at Quarter Sessions. They, however, became the resort of the soberer classes of people, who spent their time in talking politics, and were at one time regarded with suspicion by the Government. As the establishment of coffee-shops seems to have exercised a remarkable influence on the habits of the people of England, perhaps I may be excused for quoting the following passage from Lord Macaulay's "History of England." Speaking of the use of coffee-shops, he says,—

"The first of these establishments had been set up in the time of the Commonwealth, by a Turkey merchant who had acquired among the Mahometans a taste for their favourite beverage. The convenience of being able to make appointments in any part of the town, and of being able to pass, evenings socially at a very small charge, was so great that the fashion spread fast. Every man of the upper or middle class went daily to his coffee-house, to learn the news and to discuss it. Every coffee-house had one or more orators, to whose eloquence the crowd listened with admiration, and who soon became, what the journalists of our own time have been called, a Fourth Estate of the realm. The Court had long seen with uneasiness the growth of this new power in the State. An attempt had been made during Danby's administration to close the coffee-houses. But men of all parties missed their usual place of resort so much that there was a universal outcry. The Government did not venture, in opposition to a feeling so strong and general, to enforce a regulation of which the legality might well be questioned. Since that time ten years had elapsed, and during those years the number and influence of the coffee-houses had been constantly increasing. Foreigners remarked that the coffee-house was that which especially distinguished London from all other cities; that the coffee-house was the Londoners' home, and those who wished to find a gentleman, commonly asked, not whether he lived in Fleet Street or Chancery Lane, but whether he frequented the Grecian or the Rainbow. Nobody was excluded from these places who laid down his penny at the bar. There were houses near St. James's Park, where fops congregated, their heads and shoulders covered with black or flaxen wigs not less ample than those which are now worn by the Chancellor and by the Speaker of the House of Commons. The wig came from Paris, and so did the rest of the fine gentleman's ornaments. His embroidered coat, his fringed gloves, and the lapel which held up his pantaloons. The conversation was in that dialect which, long after it had ceased to be spoken in the fashionable circles, continued in the mouth of Lord Foppington to excite the mirth of theatres. The atmosphere was like that of a perfumer's shop. Tobacco in any other form than that of richly-scented snuff was held in abomination. If any clown, ignorant of the usages of the house, called for a pipe, the sneers of the whole assembly and the short answers of the waiters soon convinced him that he had better go somewhere else. Nor indeed would he have had far to go. For, in general, the coffee-rooms reeked with tobacco like a guard-room; and strangers sometimes expressed their surprise that so many people should leave their own firesides to sit in the midst of eternal fog and stench. Nowhere was the smoking more constant than at Will's. That celebrated house, situated between Covent Garden and Bow

Street, was sacred to Polite Letters. There the talk was about poetical justice and the unities of place and time. There was a faction for Perrault and the moderns, and a faction for Boileau and the ancients. One group debated whether 'Paradise Lost' ought not to have been in rhyme. To another an envious poetaster demonstrated that 'Venice Preserved' ought to have been hooted from the stage. Under no roof was a greater variety to be seen—earls in stars and garters, clergymen in cassocks and bands, pert templars, sheepish lads from the universities, translators, and index-makers in ragged coats of frieze. The great press was to get near the chair where John Dryden sat. In winter that chair was always in the warmest nook by the fire, in summer it stood in the balcony. To bow to him and to hear his opinion of Racine's last tragedy, or Bossu's treatise on epic poetry, was thought a privilege. A pinch from his snuff-box was an honour sufficient to turn the head of a young enthusiast. There were coffee-houses where the first medical men might be consulted. Doctor John Ratcliffe, who in the year 1685 rose to the largest practice in London, came daily, at the hour when the Exchange was full, from his house in Bow Street, then a fashionable part of the capital, to Garraway's, and was to be found surrounded by surgeons and apothecaries at a particular table. There were Puritan coffee-houses where no oath was heard, and where lank-haired men discussed election and reprobation through their noses; Jew coffee-houses, where dark-eyed money-changers from Venice and from Amsterdam greeted each other; and Popish coffee-houses, where, as good Protestants believed, Jesuits planned over their cups another great fire, and cast silver bullets to shoot the king."

The opposition met with by coffee and tea was not at all confined to the Governments of the world. Dr. Lettsom, who gave one of the best accounts of tea in the last century, was not wholly free from prejudices against it, and attributed the increase of intoxication to the use of tea. He says the practice of drinking stimulants is often owing " to the weakness and debility of the system brought on by the daily habit of drinking tea; the trembling hand seeks a temporary relief in some cordial in order to refresh and excite again the enfeebled system, whereby such persons almost necessarily fall into a habit of intemperance." The same charges were brought against coffee; but the older people grew the better able they were to judge for themselves of the effect of tea upon their system. Dr. Johnson confessed himself "a hardened and shameless tea-drinker, who for twenty years diluted his meals with only the infusion of this fascinating plant; whose kettle had scarcely time to cool; who with tea amused the evening, with tea solaced the midnight, and with tea welcomed the morning."

The plant which produces Coffee belongs to the same natural order of plants as the Cinchonas do, which yield quinine. It is called *Cinchonaceæ*, or the coffee tribe. The coffee plant which yields the greatest amount of the coffee of commerce is the *Coffea Arabica*. The genus Coffea is more particularly known in the order by the nature of its fruit, which is a red succulent berry, surmounted by the calyx and corolla, and which contains two cells lined with a cartilaginous membrane of the texture of parchment, and in each of these cells there is a single seed, curved at the back, and deeply furrowed in front. If you examine a coffee-seed, you can easily observe this structure, and the drawing (Fig. 1) will give you a good idea of the fruit.

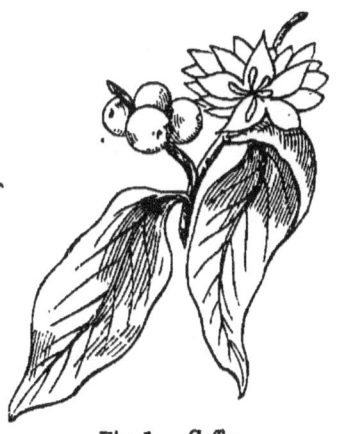

Fig. 1.—*Coffee.*

Coffea Arabica is an evergreen shrub, or small tree,

with oval, shining, wavy, sharp-pointed leaves, two or three inches in length. The flowers are white and fragrant, with fine cleft petals, which are united together into a tube, forming what is called a monopetalous corolla. The anthers of the stamens project beyond the flowers. As the inferior pistil becomes connected with the fruit, the calyx, corolla, and stamens fall off, and the berry first becomes red and then purple. This plant still grows wild in the mountainous districts of Abyssinia, but the demand for its seeds has caused it to be cultivated wherever it will ripen its leaves. The Dutch were the first to carry the plant from Arabia to Batavia, and from Batavia it was carried to Amsterdam. Here the plant flourished in the Botanic Gardens, and a plant was presented by the magistrates of that city to Louis XIV. This was planted in the Jardin du Roi, where it grew, and is said to have furnished the stock of all the French coffee plantations in Martinique. The coffee plant will not grow in any part of the world where the minimum temperature is below 55° Fahrenheit. At the same time it requires shade, and when planted in the plains of Arabia it is always surrounded with large-trees, which shelter it from the direct rays of the sun, and prevent its fruit ripening too rapidly. It is cultivated now in all quarters of the globe, and we derive our supplies in this country from very various sources. It comes to us from the Brazils, Venezuela, South Africa, the French and British West Indies, Cuba, St. Domingo, Java, Manilla, Arabia, the East Indies, and Ceylon.

Other species of Coffee yield seeds containing the same qualities as the *Coffea Arabica*. Thus, in Silhet and Nepaul a species is cultivated which is called *Coffea Benghalensis*. On the coast of Mozambique there is a species found called by botanists *Coffea Mozambica*, and in the Mauritius a species grows called *Coffea Mauritiana*. The seeds of the last species are said to be so acrid as to produce poisonous effects. Whether these are really independent species or merely varieties of *Coffea Arabica*, it is very difficult to say. Any one, of course, can give an opinion on the subject, and those who know least about the difficulty of determining the real nature of a species will hold the most decided opinions on the subject.

The coffee-plant is either propagated by cuttings or by seeds. The plants bear fruit at the end of three years, and are frequently in a condition to bear picking three times in a year. The trees continue to produce for twenty years. They seldom attain a height of more than fifteen or twenty feet. The seeds vary much in size; those which come from Yeman in Arabia, and which yield what is called Mocha coffee, are the smallest which are brought into the market. The next best coffee to the Mocha is the Java; then follows the Ceylon, the Martinique, and Batavia. Coffees of inferior quality are brought from the British West Indies.

The berries when ripe are collected and prepared in different ways. In Arabia they shake the trees and collect the fruit in cloths, which they expose to the sun and air to dry. When dried, they crush them with a heavy roller, and break the parchment envelopes, and separate the seeds by winnowing.

In our own West India plantations a different mode of preparing the seeds is adopted. A mill is used consisting of two wooden cylinders, furnished with iron plates. The berries are put into a hopper, and the beans eventually fall on a sieve, which allows the pulp to pass through and retains the seeds. The seeds are now soaked in water, then dried, and the parchment removed by the action of a vertical wheel. The parchment is then separated by a winnowing-machine. The seeds are immediately transferred to bags, by which the greenish colour they possess is preserved.

Before considering the method of preparing coffee for use, let us examine its composition. I present you here with the composition of the unroasted coffee berry, as given in my "Guide to the Food Collection at the South Kensington Museum." The calculation for the pound has been made after an analysis by Payen in the 100 parts. One pound of unroasted coffee contains:—

	OZ.	GRAINS.
Water	1	407
Sugar	1	17
Fat	1	402
Caseine	2	35
Caffeine or Theine	0	122
Aromatic Oil	0	1$\frac{1}{3}$
Caffeic Acid with Potash	0	280
Gum	1	192
Woody Fibre	5	262
Saline Matter	1	31

In reading over these analyses let me remind you that there are 437 grains in an ounce. Now there are only three things here that need remark, and they are the caffeine, the oil, and the salts. The heat-giving substances—the sugar and the fat—are in too small quantities to need comment. I may say of the caseine as of the same constituent in tea. It is probably not taken up at all; so with the accessaries gum and woody fibre. If we were in the habit of eating the coffee grounds, as the Turks are, then the consideration of these things might be of some importance. The caffeic acid has been dwelt upon by some writers. It appears to be a modification of tannic acid, but it has neither the power of forming black salts with iron nor of precipitating a solution of gelatine. Then it is in much smaller quantities than tannic acid in tea, so that should it turn out to have the composition of tannic acid, it cannot be regarded as possessing anything like the importance of that agent in tea. I think, for good or for evil, we may leave it out of our consideration altogether. We must also remember that it undergoes decomposition during the process of roasting.

The caffeine of the coffee is identical with the theine of tea. I need not, therefore, dwell on its properties. It is, however, an interesting fact worthy of a moment's consideration that the coffee plant should produce a compound which closely resembles the quinine and cinchonine of other members of the Cinchona family. If we were in doubt as to the effects of caffeine on the system, we might appeal to the known action of quinine, as illustrative of its action. If there is one fact better proved than another in the history of medicine, it is that quinine has the power of arresting intermittent fever or ague. This is so well known that no tyro in medicine would think of treating a case of ague without quinine. Now it so happens that there are certain cases of ague which will not yield to quinine, and these cases have been known to yield to theine. The composition of these substances is as follows:—

	Carbon.	Hydrogen.	Nitrogen.	Oxygen.	Water.
Theine	16	10	4	4	2
Quinine	20	12	1	2	3

We can hardly doubt that each of them is capable of acting on the nervous system, and that what is true of the action of quinine is also of theine or caffeine.

The aromatic oil mentioned in the analysis is the substance which gives the peculiar flavour to coffee. Although given in the analysis of unroasted coffee, it does not appear to be developed till after it has been submitted to this process. The nature of this oil is but imperfectly understood. It appears to be much more fully developed in coffee-seeds which have been kept for some time before they are roasted; at the same time, such is the importance attached to this oil in giving aroma to coffee, that the late Professor Johnston estimated, that if it could be manufactured it would be worth one hundred pounds an ounce. From some experiments by Professor Lehmann it appears that this oil produces on the system much the same effect as the caffeine itself. He distilled roasted coffee with water, and found that this oil could thus be procured separate from the other constituents of coffee. As the result of his experiments, he found that the oil produced the same results as caffeine in retarding the waste of the tissues of the body; that it produced an agreeable excitement and gentle perspiration, and that in its exhilarating action upon the brain it affected the imagination less than the reasoning powers.

When over-doses of the oil were taken, he found it produced violent perspiration, with sleeplessness and symptoms of congestion. These symptoms are somewhat different from those produced by the oil from green tea; at the same time, there can be no doubt that they assist the action of theine generally in the same way, and the fact that green tea and coffee produce the same effect on the system is thus explained.

But besides this aromatic oil, there are produced during the roasting certain compounds which give a peculiar bitter taste to coffee. These compounds have not been carefully investigated, and will probably be found to arise from the destruction of the woody fibre and Caffeic acid of the seed. These compounds are given up to the water in greater or lesser quantities, according to the degree of roasting to which the coffee has been submitted, and the kind of water used for making it. Thus, coffee roasted to a reddish-brown colour is said to yield 25 per cent. of its bulk to boiling water, whilst chestnut-brown coffee yields only 19 per cent. Waters containing alkali are found to take up more of the soluble matter than those without. Thus it has been recommended to add carbonate of soda to coffee in the proportion of forty grains to the pound of coffee. We know nothing, however, of the action of these soluble bitter matters on the system, and the taking them must be regarded as a matter of taste.

The saline matters, or ashes of coffee, deserve a moment's notice. They are nearly one-third greater than those of tea, and they contain a larger quantity of potash and phosphoric acid. These, as we have seen in one of the previous lectures, are important constituents of our food, and the habitual use of them must exercise an important influence on the system. It has been observed, that those who drink coffee are not liable to gout, and if this be true, it is not altogether improbable that the saline constituents of the coffee may be the agents which act thus favourably on the system. From what we know of the action of these saline substances, especially potash and phosphoric acid, there can be little doubt that they are capable of exercising a beneficial influence in certain states of the system.

I must now say a few words with regard to the preparation of coffee. You know that the seeds, or beans, as they are called, are brought raw into this country, and the first process they are submitted to is that of roasting. This is mostly done by those who sell the coffee. At the same time, it is a process on which the flavour and pleasantness of the coffee very much depend. If the seeds are roasted too little, the oil and empyreumatic products are not developed; whilst, if done too much, they are destroyed. The coffee-beans, when roasted, may have three degrees of shade; they may be reddish-brown, chesnut-brown, and dark brown, and where a full-flavoured coffee is preferred, perhaps the darkest is the best. When the coffee is roasted, it should not be kept long before it is ground and used. It is usually ground in a proper mill, or it may be powdered in a mortar; but whatever machine is employed for this purpose, it should not be used for anything else, as coffee has a peculiar tendency to absorb other odours, and thus to acquire a flavour not its own.

When ground, it should be used as soon as possible

for in this state it rapidly gives off its volatile oil. Many devices have been employed to keep coffee after it has been ground, and where this must be done, there is nothing more efficient than a clean stoppered bottle. It is, however, frequently sold in tin or lead packages; but these do not keep it so well as a bottle.

The greatest art, however, of all is, the making the coffee. Time would fail me were I to attempt to tell you of all the methods that have been employed and the instruments that have been invented for the making of coffee. The most common practice, however, of making this beverage, establishes a difference between it and tea. Everywhere tea is used as an infusion, whilst coffee is employed as a decoction. It seems to be very generally admitted, that coffee should be boiled before it is drunk. A common plan is to put the powdered coffee into hot water, in a coffee-pot, and to let it boil for two or three minutes, and then to let it stand by the side of the fire for some little time. The particles of ground coffee are often suspended in this liquid, and a process of clearing is required. This is effected sometimes by isinglass or white of egg; but this is not necessary, and the pouring a cupful out and returning it will produce the desired effect. Coffee-pots are sold with muslin bags, metallic sieves, and other contrivances, to produce the clearing. Coffee is, however, exposed to the danger of losing its aroma by boiling, and sometimes boiling water alone is added to it as in making tea. A coffee-pot has been recently invented by M. Loysell, in which the coffee is exposed to boiling water at a considerable pressure, and a very agreeable coffee is produced in this way. One great secret of making good coffee is, to put enough of the prepared powder. One ounce and a quarter to the pint of water is the least that should be allowed. The *café noir*, or black coffee of the French, contains a larger proportion than this. *Café au lait* consists of strong coffee, to which an equal quantity of hot milk is added. In the making of coffee, as in the making of tea, it should be remembered that the qualities of the coffee are not rendered to water at a lower temperature than the boiling point. It would also appear that coffee will bear boiling, which tea will not.

I must now add a few words on substitutes for coffee. At first sight it would not appear to be unnatural to expect to find in the vegetable world many things which might be used instead of either tea or coffee. And if we regard the general constituents of tea or coffee, this is certainly the case. But when we find that all substances which have been tried are deficient in the active principle—caffeine or theine—we then have a reason for their failure. As well might we expect to find a substitute for wine without alcohol as a substitute for tea or coffee without theine, or some analogous principle. The proposed substitutes for coffee have been very numerous, and the result of roasting these things has been the production of substances which, when prepared in the same way as coffee, have led to the hope that a substitute had been found. The failure of all of them has, however, clearly shown that they were destitute of the agent that addressed itself to the nervous system, and gave to coffee and tea their hold on the appetites of humanity. I have here a list of substances which have been thus used :—

Iris Seeds,
Broom Seeds,
Fenugrec Seeds,
Spanish Acorns,
Chick Peas,
Rice,
Carrot Root,
Parsnip Root,

Acorns,
Beans,
Lupin Seeds,
Chicory Root,
Dandelion,
Beetroot,
Wheat,
Fruits of the Goosegrass.

To these might, undoubtedly, be added many more. In some parts of the world, where coffee is difficult to be had or expensive, they are extensively employed. But you recollect what I said of the necessity of warm beverages. Many of these things are known only in this country as a means of adulterating coffee. There is one of these things, however, which has been so frequently associated with coffee in this country, although I do not think it is drunk to any extent alone, that I ought to mention it. I refer to chicory, or succory root. The plant which yields this root is a native of our own chalk soils, and is known by its pretty blue flowers, which appear in the autumn of the year: it is the Cichorium Intybus of botanists, and is the type of a great division of Compositous plants, known by their milky juice, and to which the dandelion and lettuce belong. It does not, however, contain caffeine; the part of the plant used is the root, and when this is roasted and ground, and boiled, it yields a drink not unlike coffee. From being recommended as a substitute for coffee it came to be used for adulterating it, and then a curious fact was elicited: many persons preferred coffee with chicory in it; and there seems to be no doubt that chicory does take from coffee a part of that roughness which renders it disagreeable to the taste of some individuals. Be this as it may, the sale of chicory is now legalised; and although the addition of it to coffee is regarded as an adulteration, many persons purchase it for that purpose.

Chicory contains an empyreumatic oil, and a bitter principle similar to that found in coffee; it has also a sweetish taste, which probably contributes more than anything else to its modification of the flavour of coffee. On the continent of Europe it is used very extensively alone, and perhaps the influence of its empyreumatic oil on the system may be its recommendation. There is, however, one great objection to its use altogether, and that is the fact of its being adulterated with a variety of utterly worthless and tasteless vegetable matters.

I may refer here to substitutes for tea. It is not uncommon to hear reference made to Paraguay tea as a substitute for Chinese tea; but this is really a misnomer, as Paraguay tea is used extensively on its own merits, and is found to contain the same active principle as tea and coffee.

The Paraguay tea-plant is a native of the New World, and in some parts of South America it is used as extensively, for the purpose of making a hot infusion, as tea and coffee are in Asia and Europe. This plant belongs to the genus *Ilex*, plants belonging to the order *Aquifoliaceæ*, and which is remarkable for containing our indigenous holly, the *Ilex Aquifolium*. The Paraguay tea-plant, or Maté, as it is sometimes called, from the name of the little cup out of which it is drunk, is the *Ilex Paraguaensis*. It is a shrub attaining the size of an orange-tree. It thrives well in hothouses in this country, and may be seen growing in great vigour at the Royal Gardens at Kew. It has leaves three or four inches in length, quite smooth, of a bluntish wedge-shape, with large serratures at their edges. This plant grows wild in the forests of Paraguay and Brazils, but is not cultivated at all. The labour of collecting and preparing the leaves of this plant for use is entirely dependent upon the native Indians. The merchants of Chili and Buenos Ayres send various articles of merchandise up into the interior, which they exchange with the natives for this plant. A considerable trade is thus carried on, as it is calculated that upwards of 5,000,000 lbs. of the leaves of this plant are annually collected in Paraguay. Much less care is taken in the preparation of this tea than in preparing Chinese tea. The natives at certain seasons of the year penetrate the forest, and having selected a tree, they cut off its principal branches with a hatchet. When a sufficient number are cut down they are placed on hurdles. A wood fire is then made, over which, when the flames have ceased to ascend, the hurdles are placed. The branches are kept on the hurdles till they are dried. They are then removed from the fire, and a clean hard floor being made on some spot of ground, they are strewn upon it and beaten with sticks. The dried leaves and smaller branches are thus reduced to a coarse kind of powder, which is usually placed in bullocks' hides, which, when sewed up and dried, are ready for exportation. Some little selection, however, is made during the packing, and three sorts are known in the market; thus far resembling the same stages of proceeding in the collecting of Chinese tea. The kinds known in the South American markets are Caa-Cuys, which consists of the young leaf-buds; the Caa-Miri, which is the leaf separated from its midrib and secondary ribs; and the Caa-Guaza, or Yerva de Palos of the Spaniards, which consists of the leaf, leaf-stalks, and young branches, all mixed together.

The method of preparing this tea is very simple; it is, nevertheless, peculiar. A cup, which is called a maté, is employed, which frequently consists of a gourd, but is sometimes made of silver or other materials. Into this cup is introduced a long tube, called a bombilla, at the end of which is a bowl pierced with holes, or a round piece of basket-work, the object of which is to allow the fluid to be sucked up without the solid particles passing into the mouth. A small quantity of the yerva is then placed in the cup covering the bowl of the tube, and boiling water is poured upon it. A little sugar is frequently added, and when cold enough, the liquid is sucked up through the tube. The beverage thus formed has a slightly aromatic smell, but very much less than either tea or coffee, and is slightly bitter to the taste.

The most curious point about the history of this plant is, that the active principle, which was first called paraguaine, is found to be identical with theine and caffeine. The effects attributed to the action of the Paraguay tea on the system are precisely the same as those of tea and coffee. Probably from knowing less of its action in Europe, we hear less of its evil effects than of even those of tea and coffee; but we are not to conclude from this that it is at all probable that Paraguay tea is preferable as an article of diet to tea or coffee. The great reason of its not coming into the British market is, that it has to pay the same duty as tea. At the same time, I have known English persons who have contracted so great a love for this beverage at Buenos Ayres, that they regularly consume it, now that they live again in England, and willingly pay the duty for their favourite beverage.

It certainly is worth while considering whether the theine could not be obtained and made use of independently of the constituents of this plant. I have recently had some theine lozenges made by Messrs. Savory and Moore, of Bond-street, and I find them to possess all the refreshing qualities of tea. I think if such lozenges were made pleasant and sold cheap, that they might have an extensive sale, and be made the means of consuming some of the theine which annually perishes in the forests of Paraguay.

The other constituents of the maté are the volatile oil and an astringent principle. The volatile oil, which is evidently in much less quantity than in tea and coffee, appears to be developed by roasting. The astringent and slightly bitter principle is probably some form of tannic acid. It is on this account perhaps that it is used in the Brazils by dyers. I cannot tell you the exact quantity of this astringent matter there is in Paraguay tea, but from its flavour I should judge that there is quite as much as in Chinese tea. I can find no analysis of the salts of Paraguay tea. They probably contain iron, as the infused tea when exposed to the air becomes of an almost inky colour.

From what I have said about this Paraguay tea, you will come to the conclusion, I am sure, that it is a very valuable plant, and that it would probably repay attention to its culture and propagation. If it were not that the Government is perpetually putting its finger into our food, now into our sugar-basin, then into the pepper-box, and again into the tea-pot, it is probable we should have known long ago more about this plant, and have found it an article of diet much cheaper and more efficient than Chinese tea.

I find that other species of Ilex, as *Ilex Gonghona*, have been used in the same way as the Paraguay tea; but whether this possesses theine, I am not able to say. Our common holly, the *Ilex Aquifolium*, yields a crystallisable principle called Ilicine, which is very bitter, and is said to be an excellent remedy, like quinine, in ague. There can be no doubt of the beneficial action of these principles on the system, and it is well worth further study and experiment as to how far they may be possessed by native and readily-accessible plants. Unfortunately, the system of taxing food is so deeply rooted in all European systems of government, that the people are frequently prevented from consuming the less expensive products of their own soil, because a revenue is raised on the productions of foreign countries. It is quite possible that some of our native plants may contain theine, or some active principle so nearly allied as to act in the same way, and this can only be discovered by use. A compound made of native plants was formerly sold in this country under the name of " British Herb tea," but its manufacture and sale were prohibited by the Government.

Whilst speaking of substitutes for tea, I ought to mention that one of the most promising of them is coffee-leaves. It appears that in the islands of the Eastern Archipelago the leaves of the coffee-plant are dried and prepared in the same way as those of tea, and used in infusion for drinking. At the Great Exhibition, in 1851, Dr. Gardner exhibited some prepared coffee-leaves, and stated that he had succeeded in obtaining from them a considerable amount of theine. The quantity of theine in coffee-leaves appears to be greater than either in Chinese tea or coffee. Mr. Ward, a gentleman who lived for some time in Sumatra, gave some years ago an account, in the *Pharmaceutical Journal*, of the action of the infusion of coffee-leaves on the natives and himself. His account of its effects agrees very closely with what we know of the action of tea.

The Sumatrans prefer the tea from coffee-leaves to the beverage made from coffee-seeds. Mr. Ward himself employed it habitually, and found from it all the comfort and advantage of tea. One great recommendation of the coffee-leaf is, that it will grow in soils and under circumstances that will not develop the coffee-seed. The coffee-leaves are sold in Sumatra, at the price of about three halfpence a pound, and might be packed, of good quality for the European market, at the rate of twopence a pound. Specimens of the dried coffee-leaves with the theine obtained from them are to be seen in the food collection of the South Kensington Museum. I am sure it would be worth while to try the coffee-leaf on an extensive scale, if it be thought desirable to render available for the great bulk of the community a very important article of diet.

There is yet one other plant containing theine, which is employed by man as an article of diet, and which we may yet again hear of as supplying food. The plant to which I allude is the *Paullinia sorbilis*, or Guarana plant. It belongs to the same family of plants as the horse-chestnut. It grows on the river Tapagos, on some of the head waters of the Orinoco, and elsewhere in the great valley of the Amazon. The fruit of this tree is gathered when ripe and roasted; after this process the seeds are removed and powdered between stones or mallets, and then made into a thick paste with water. The paste is moulded into cakes, which are baked by the heat of the sun. These cakes will keep good for any length of time. When used they are scraped, and a table-spoonful is added to a pint of boiling water. It is sold all through the Brazils, and is used as a medicine in ague, dysentery, and other diseases. It appears to differ but little in composition from tea and coffee, except that it contains a larger quantity of fat or oil, and in this respect it resembles cocoa or chocolate. According to the analysis of Dr. Stenhouse, guarana is richer in theine than any other of the substances of which I have spoken to you. The following are the per-centages as given by Dr. Stenhouse:—

Guarana	5·07	per cent. of Theine.
Good Black Tea	2·13	,, ,,
Coffee	1·0	,, ,,
Coffee Leaves	1·26	,, ,,
Paraguay Tea	1·20	,, ,,

The plants which are infused and used as warm drinks where Chinese tea has not been introduced, and which do not contain theine, are hardly worth dwelling on. They possess no properties which would lead us for one moment to suppose that they could ever take the place of tea or coffee, or exercise so beneficial an influence on the nervous system. The various agents which have been thus employed have been reduced by Professor Johnstone to a tabular form, and I present you these in the accompanying diagram.

SUBSTITUTES FOR CHINESE TEA.

NAME OF THE PLANT.	NATURAL ORDER.	WHERE COLLECTED AND USED.	NAME GIVEN TO IT.
Hydrangea Thunbergii	Hydrangeaceæ	Japan	Amatsja, or Tea of Heaven
Sageretia theezans	Rhamnaceæ	China	
Ocymum album	Labiatæ	India	Toolsie Tea
Catha edulis	Celastraceæ	Abyssinia	Khat or Chaat
Glaphyria nitida	Myrtaceæ	Bencoolen (flowers used)	Tea Plant and Tree of Long Life
Correa alba	Rutaceæ	New Holland	
Acæna sanguisorba	Sanguisorbaceæ	Ditto	Tea Plants and Tasmanian Tea
Leptospermum scoparium and L. thea	Myrtaceæ	Ditto	
Melaleuca scoparia and M. genistifolia	Myrtaceæ	Ditto	
Myrtus ugni	Myrtaceæ	Chili	Substitutes for Paraguay Tea
Psoralea glandulosa	Leguminosæ	Ditto	Ditto
Alstonia theæformis	Styraceæ	New Granada	Sante Fé Tea
Capraria bifolia	Scrophulariaceæ	Central America	(?)
Lantana pseudothea	Verbenaceæ	Brazil	Capitaõ da matto
Chenopodium ambrosioides	Chenopodiaceæ	Mexico and Columbia	Mexican Tea
Viburnum cassinoides	Caprifoliaceæ	North America	Appalachian Tea
Prinos glaber	Aquifoliaceæ	Ditto	New Jersey Tea (medicinal)
Ceanothus Americanus	Rhamnaceæ	Ditto	Mountain Tea
Gaultheria procumbens	Ericaceæ	Ditto	Labrador, or James's Tea
Ledum palustre			
Ledum latifolium	Ericaceæ	Ditto	Oswego Tea
Monarda didyma			
M. purpurea	Labiatæ	Ditto	Bourbon, or Faham Tea
Angræcum fragrans	Orchidaceæ	Mauritius	(?)
Micromeria theæsioensis	Labiatæ	France	Brazilian Tea
Stachytarpheta jamaicensis	Verbenaceæ	Austria	Sloe and Strawberry Tea, one of our best substitutes for Chinese Tea
Prunus spinosa, ⅓ mixed with ⅔ Fragaria collins or F. vesca	Drupaceæ / Rosaceæ	Northern Europe	
Salvia officinalis	Labiatæ	Ditto	Sage Tea

There is one other substance that has a claim to be considered amongst these neurotic beverages, and that is Cocoa. Nevertheless, cocoa differs so much in its mode of preparation, that we might almost regard it as a kind of soup. As cocoa is generally prepared, we take it thick, and consume all it has to offer us. I place it amongst the medicinal foods, because it contains an alkaloid. Nevertheless, it contains more fat, and as much flesh-forming matter as beef; and on looking at it from this point of view, one feels the difficulty of classifying food; and the necessity of weighing well all the constituents of food, if it is to be administered wisely and well. The things you buy in the shops under the name of cocoa and chocolate are the produce of the seeds of a plant known to botanists under the name of *Theobroma Cacao.* This plant is a native of the New World. The Spaniards, who so cruelly conquered and took possession of Mexico, were the first Europeans who became acquainted with cocoa. Prescott, the American historian, in that splendid picture which he draws of the magnificence and state of Montezuma, the emperor of Mexico, says—

"The emperor took no other beverage than *chocolate*, a potation of chocolate flavoured with Vanilla and other spices, and so prepared as to be reduced to a froth of the consistency of honey, which gradually dissolved in the mouth. This beverage (if so it could be called) was served in golden goblets, with spoons of the same metal, or of tortoise-shell finely wrought."

The golden vessels excited the cupidity of the Spaniard, but the new drink was despised. A Spanish traveller, after the conquest of Mexico, describes the cocoa-nut tree, but speaks of its seeds as an article of diet with infinite contempt, and says that chocolate was a drink "fitter for a pig than for a man." It was left for Linnæus to name the plant; and with a much finer judgment of the good things of this world, declared that so far from its being food fit for pigs, regarded it as worthy the regard of gods, and named it *Theobroma*, the food of gods. Several species of this genus yield seeds from which cocoa may be obtained; but the *Theobroma Cacao* is the species from which the cocoa is obtained in Mexico, and the plant which is cultivated in many parts of the world on account of the commercial value of the seeds. The cocoa plant is a tree with large single leaves and small flowers, which grow on flower stalks direct from the stem. (Fig. 2.) The flower is succeeded by a large capsular fruit, about the size of a common vegetable marrow, and in it are contained from twenty-five to thirty seeds. They are about the size of an almond, and are covered with a thin skin or husk of a light reddish brown colour. These seeds, with the husks on, are brought into this country. In Mexico they are used as money, six of these seeds being worth about a halfpenny.

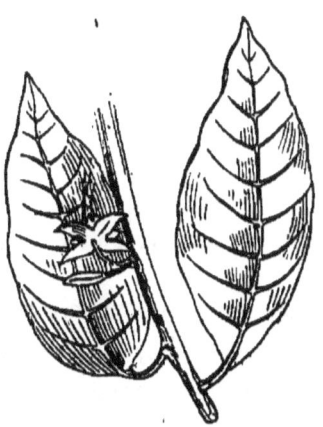

Fig. 2.—*Cocoa Plant*.

When brought into this country the seeds are prepared in various ways. They are heated and ground down in a mill, and a coarse kind of paste is formed, which is called *cocoa paste;* or it is rubbed into a coarse powder, and called granulated cocoa; or it is cut into slips, and called flaked cocoa. The husks are more or less removed in these preparations. Again the seeds are submitted to heat, the husks removed and the kernel somewhat broken: they are sold under the name of *cocoa-nibs*. Lastly, the husks are removed, the nuts are reduced to a paste, and various flavouring agents are added, as vanilla, and the cakes thus prepared are called chocolate.

The composition of one pound of these seeds in the form of cocoa-paste, is as follows:—

	OZ.	GRAINS.
Water	0	350
Albumen and Gluten	3	85
Theobromine	0	140
Butter	8	0
Gum	0	426
Starch	1	53
Woody Fibre	0	280
Colouring Matter	0	140
Mineral Matter	0	280

If we compare this composition for one moment with tea and coffee, we shall see that the flesh-forming and heat-giving elements of food are greatly in the ascendant. The albumen and gluten are in larger proportions than in bread, or oats, or barley. There is no doubt, then, that when these seeds are eaten entire, or in the form of paste, that they constitute a highly nutritive article of diet.

Again, let us look at the fat. Here we have half the paste consisting of pure fat, and acting on the system as any other kind of fatty matter: so that, in estimating the value of cocoa as an article of diet, we must not estimate its medicinal action alone, but the influence of its heat-giving and flesh-forming matters.

The alkaloid it contains, and which is called *theobromine*, is, nevertheless, an interesting substance. It differs from theine in containing a larger quantity of nitrogen. It is, however, a curious fact, that recently theobromine has been converted artificially into theine; it is, therefore, not at all improbable that theobromine may be converted in the human body into theine, and act in the same way upon the nervous system.

Cocoa is prepared in various ways. The paste or powder is boiled with water, and sugar and milk are added according to taste. In this way, however, it can hardly be regarded as a substitute for tea and coffee; it is, in fact, a substitute for all other kinds of food, and when taken with some form of bread, little or nothing else need be added at a meal. The same may be said of chocolate, which only differs from cocoa in the more careful manner in which it is prepared, and the flavouring substances which are added to it. Chocolate may be mixed with water and milk, and taken in the same manner as cocoa. When a sufficient quantity of sugar is added, it is made into a variety of articles of confectionary, in the preparation of which our French neighbours so greatly excel us.

One of the delusions practised on the public is to call certain preparations of cocoa "homœopathic;" but analysis shows that these preparations, neither in their quality nor the proportions in which they may be taken, differ at all from ordinary cocoa.

The cocoa seeds roasted, and sold under the name of

"nibs," may be infused in boiling water in the same way as tea-leaves; and under these circumstances a beverage is obtained which in many respects resembles tea and coffee, as the albumen and fat are not taken up in this way.

The husks of the cocoa seeds which are separated in some of these preparations are not lost. They are said to contain a noticeable quantity of theobromine, and also the flavouring aromatic oil of the cocoa. They are sold for making a beverage which is not unlike tea or coffee in its action on the system.

I must now conclude my notice of this group of substances, which have gradually come to be used in such enormous quantities by mankind in the form of warm beverages. Whatever may have been the influence of a heated liquid in leading to their first use, I think you cannot but see that the principle they contain which addresses itself to the nervous system is the agent which has determined their special selection. It would, therefore, be unwise in the highest degree to neglect the study of these important agents. From what we already know, they are evidently potent for good and for evil, and it is only by a careful study of their action on the human body that we can expect to secure the one or prevent the other.

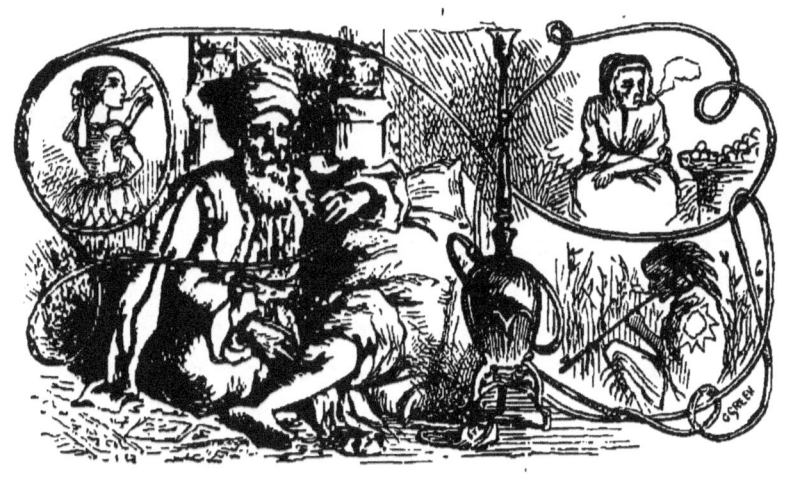

ON TOBACCO.

In this lecture I propose to make some remarks on those substances indulged in by man, known by the name of narcotics, and more particularly on tobacco. In approaching this subject, I am reminded of the connection that exists between food and medicine, and medicine and poisons. The more one investigates the relation of food to the human system, the greater must be the conviction that food is not only capable of maintaining healthy life, but, by proper modification, can be made the means of curing disease. Our life is so essentially dependent on food, that we may increase its activity by increase of food, and decrease it by decrease of food, and change its character by change of food. Diseases manifest themselves in an increase, or decrease, or a change of vital action. It must be evident, therefore, that in the management of food we have the great means for the cure and removal of disease.

In the classification of food which I gave you at the commencement of these lectures, I showed you that certain substances which we habitually take as food act in the same way as medicines; hence I called them medicinal foods. Such substances are alcohol, the volatile oils, and the theinal principles. These are themselves powerful medicinal agents, or belong to groups of substances which yield them. From a medicine to a poison there is but a step, and that is not one of kind, but of degree. The alcohol that invigorates the stomach and cheers the social meal, recalls to life the frame exhausted with febrile poison, but kills when taken to excess. The oxalic acid of our spring tart is a pleasant febrifuge in fever, but poisonous when swallowed by the ounce. Common salt is one of the great necessaries of life, but in drachm doses acts as an emetic, and may be accumulated in the system till it destroys life. Such, then, is the connection between food, medicine, and poison, that all our food may be made medicinal and all our medicines may become poisons.

I need not remind you how such a view as this lays the axe at the root of all pretensions to cure disease by remedies that can exert no influence on the system. If you are eating and drinking, and men tell you they are curing your diseases with infinitesimal doses, don't believe them. Your food is exercising a far more powerful effect on your system than their remedies. The only remedies that can be rationally employed as medicines are those which act as food on the system. If they are capable of increasing or decreasing the vital actions of your bodies, then they may or may not do you good, according to the skill with which they are administered; but away with the folly and imposture that would lead you to believe that the natural actions of your bodies are influenced by agents whose existence cannot be detected by the senses. I know nothing more degrading in the intellectual history of the past, with its witchcraft, charms, amulets, royal touches, and holy waters, than the belief of certain portions of the medical profession and the public in the abracadabra of "similia similibus curantur," and the efficacy of infinitesimal doses. You must excuse these expressions, I speak strongly because I feel warmly. I am ever ready to make allowance for the opinions and practice of my medical brethren. The rational treatment of disease involves problems of the highest complexity, in endeavouring to understand which, two minds, equally anxious to reach the truth, may yet arrive at different conclusions. But such conclusions, arrived at by the painful road in which truth ever leads her votaries, are very different from the ready-made hypothesis which is adopted to get rid of the difficulties of inquiry, and which is acted on regardless of the sacrifice of human life, so long as the selfish object for which it was adopted is attained.

The substances, then, to which I wish now to draw your attention, are more particularly known as poisons. In proportion as our food becomes dangerous to human life so does it appear to exercise a fascinating influence. Our life is distinguished by its nervous activity. We feel, we think, we are conscious, we enjoy only as the nervous system acts. It is on this system that the pleasant poisons of which I have now to speak act. Poisons, or at any rate our food-poisons, act on the nervous system in various ways. They may stimulate the nervous system, and we call them stimulants: such foods are alcohol and the volatile oils. On the other hand, they may depress the nervous system, and we call them sedatives: such an action we found tea and coffee to exert. I would not, however, lead you to suppose that all stimulants of the nervous system are pleasant in their action. Such is not the case with strychnia, which, far short of acting as poison, stimulates the motor nerves to very unpleasant and sometimes painful activity. So with sedatives. However pleasant may be the sedative action of tea and coffee, few persons could be found to enjoy hydrocyanic acid or Digitalis. You must not, therefore, misunderstand me, it is not because all foods may act as medicines, and medicines poisons, that, therefore, all poisons may be used as foods. Nevertheless, the addiction of some people to taking medicine is so remarkable that I should not wonder at some clever writer starting the theory that all physic may be food. The Turks indulge in corrosive sublimate; the Styrians in arsenic. Quack pills, containing gamboge, jalap, calomel, and other drugs, are consumed, to the utter destruction of health, in this country by ton loads every year. I know of nothing so virulent and nasty that has not its defenders or victims.

Now I am not going to speak of the stimulant or sedative group of our poisonous foods to-night, but of a group to which the term narcotic has been more particularly applied. When a medicine attacks more particularly the brain we call it a narcotic. Our stimulants and sedatives are narcotics at last, as you know by the action of alcohol on the brain. But some of these things seem to attack the brain at once, and such are tobacco and opium and henbane. They act also as stimulants and sedatives. So that you see that these things all act generally on the nervous system; but that some prefer exerting their greatest action on the sympathetic nerves, others on the spinal nerves; this on one part of the brain, and that on another (see diagram). We cannot explain all this, but it is interesting for us to know the fact.

Of the two agents of this class most largely used by mankind, the one—tobacco—is called an intoxicating narcotic, whilst the other—opium—is a soporific narcotic. I shall have little time to speak at all of the latter, and my remarks must be chiefly devoted to tobacco. The plant which yields this substance belongs to the genus Nicotiana, a name given to it in honour of Jean Nicot, a French ambassador at the court of Portugal, who first introduced this plant into France. Belonging to this genus are several species which yield, at the present day, the tobacco of commerce. These plants belong to the natural order *Solanaceæ*, a family which yields us not only tobacco, but stramonium, deadly nightshade, henbane Cayenne pepper, tomatoes, winter cherries, vegetable eggs, smoking cane, potatoes, Quito oranges, and mandrakes. At first sight this looks like an incongruous family, but still you will see certain common properties running through the whole order. All contain, more or less, substances that act on the nervous system, and thus increase from the mild poison of the solanums till we arrive at the deadly principles of the atropas, the henbanes, and the tobaccos.

Although there seems little doubt that smoking was introduced from the New world into the Old, yet the material for the practice was not found wanting, for at least two species of Nicotiana, the *N. rustica* and *N. Persica*, are indigenous to Asia. It is, however, to the American plant, the *Nicotiana Tabacum* (Fig. 1), to which I would more particularly confine your attention. This plant is an annual, and great care is taken in its culture in the countries where it grows. Its stem rises five or six feet in height, branching at the top. The leaves are sesile, very large, and ovate or lanceolate in form. They are of a pale-green colour, and are sticky when taken hold of. The flowers appear in bunches at the end of the stem or branches. The corolla is funnel-shaped, yellowish, of a dull-red colour at their edges. The seeds are numerous and contained in an ovate two-celled capsule, which is surrounded by the calyx.

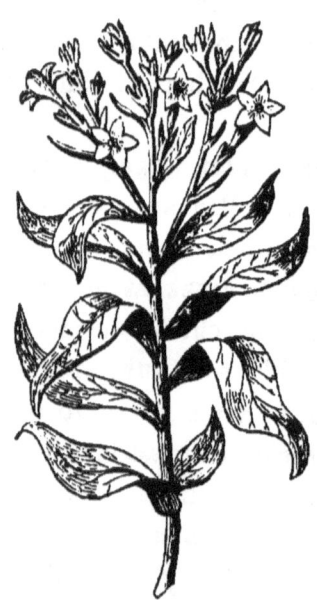

Fig. 1.—*Virginia Tobacco.*

The tobacco-plant grows readily in this country in almost any good garden-soil. The seeds should be sown in March or April, and in July or August the flowers will appear, and at this time it may be cut down and dried for use. It is, however, a native of tropical and subtropical regions, and, like other plants under the same circumstances, it fails to yield its peculiar products in perfection. When first introduced into Europe, it was grown with the potato in the British islands. Sir Walter Raleigh cultivated it in his garden at Youghal; it was also grown in France, Germany, Spain, Portugal, and other parts of Europe. It is now only grown in gardens in Great Britain. Although its first cultivation for sale in England was prohibited, the reason now is very different from what it was at first. Our rulers then thought it would injure the people to allow them to grow it, now they think it would injure the revenue to allow them to do so. Those who smoke need not regret this, as European tobacco is very inferior in all the properties for which tobacco is consumed, compared with that which comes from the warmer countries of the world.

The best tobacco in the world comes at the present day from Cuba, where it was originally discovered. It is, however, cultivated extensively in the United States, in Virginia, Maryland, Ohio, and Kentucky. Even Canada produces a decent tobacco. South America sends also its tobacco into the markets of Europe, known by the name of Kanaster. It is grown extensively in the northern and western provinces of India, and ·in the islands of the Eastern archipelago. A famous tobacco is brought from Manilla. From Persia is brought the delicate "Shiraz tobacco," procured from *Nicotiana Persica*, whilst the aristocratic

Latakia is produced in Turkey by the *Nicotiana rustica*.

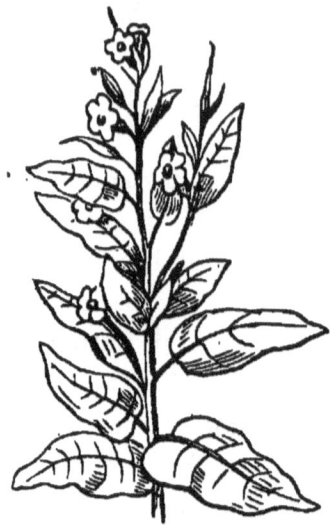

Fig. 2.—Syrian Tobacco.

(Fig. 2). In Africa and Egypt, the American species flourish, and France is supplied with the principal part of her tobacco from Algeria. Even the Cape of Good Hope sends its cigars to England, and for weak smokers the inferior tobaccos of Germany, Holland, and other parts of Europe, find their way here. In the Food collection at South Kensington will also be found tobaccos from Japan, Siam, and China.

For smoking, tobacco undergoes little or no preparation. At the proper season of the year, the plant is cut down, and the leaves are packed together and dried under cover. At first they undergo a process of change, which is known technically by the term "sweating," and perhaps the constituents of the plant are modified at this stage. Chemically, however, nothing is known on this point. After a month's drying, the tobacco is said to be "in case," that is, it is now ready for being sorted and packed. The leaves, which resemble each other, are tied up in bundles, and they are put into boxes or casks. The latter are used in Virginia, and each contains from 1,000 to 1,200 lbs. of tobacco. The qualities of the tobacco differ even from the same district, and in the markets they go by various names. Thus in America ship's tobacco is manufactured from the *strong* Virginian leaf, whilst the *fine* Virginia leaf is prepared for chewing. One sort is prepared for making Cavendish, whilst another is used for *cut* and *shag* tobaccos.

Tobacco is brought into this country either in the form of the leaf, or as manufactured. Manufactured tobaccos pay a much higher duty than the leaf tobacco; hence, those who prefer the foreign manufacture, as cigars, cheroots, or cigarettes, Cavendish, Latakia, Turkey, or Shiraz tobaccos, have to pay a much higher price for them than if they patronized the British manufacturer. Unless persons are well acquainted with foreign tobaccos, they had better at once make up their minds to the consumption of that which is British made.

In manufacturing the tobacco, the first thing done is to open the hogsheads or bales in which the leaves have been packed. The leaves are pulled apart, and if the mid-rib or centre rib of the leaf has not been removed it is now cut out; not, however, thrown away. The largest and strongest leaves are used as covers for pigtail tobacco; the other leaves are spread on the floor and moistened with water. This is all the English manufacturer is allowed to do; on the Continent, however, the manufacturer adds salt and sugar and other things to the water, which is necessary to the manufacture at this stage. These additions give various qualities to the tobacco, and some may even improve it; but under present circumstances the principle is bad, as it gives the fraudulent manufacturer an opportunity of adding substances which give no flavour to the tobacco, but increase considerably its weight. In this country the penalty is very heavy for using any substance in the adulteration of tobacco; nevertheless, the high duty presents a great temptation, and if during the moistening process nothing is added to the water, there are frequently other leaves substituted for those of the tobacco. These, however, can be easily detected, not so much from their chemical composition as from their microscopic structure. If you examine the leaves of tobacco under the microscope you will find them covered with very peculiarly shaped hairs. They are club-shaped. None of the leaves which are used for adulteration have these hairs, and the presence of other shaped hairs or the absence of the club-shaped ones in a leaf are sure signs of adulteration.

The presence of sugar or salt or nitre can of course only be detected by chemical operations. Sugar is found naturally in the tobacco leaf; but when it is found in excess, it must be looked upon as a fraud.

After the leaves have been properly moistened, they are arranged according to the ultimate form they are to assume. If they are to be cut into tobacco, they are laid one on the top of another, and pressed, and placed under a cutting-machine, which, acting in the same manner as a chaff-cutting engine, cuts the tobacco leaf into strips. The cut tobacco is shaken out by the hands, and afterwards dried, and, according to the leaf used, is called "Virginia shag," "Maryland returns," "Kanaster," "Turkey," or any other recognizable name. "Bird's eye" is produced from the same leaf as "shag;" but the mid-rib is allowed to remain in the leaf, and, on being cut, leaves those little white bits which have acquired for it its fanciful name.

Every country where tobacco is grown manufactures its own cigars, and these are frequently sold in shops in England. The British manufacturer, however, generally prefers West Indian, Havannah, or European tobacco for making cigars. These cigars are sold at varying prices, according to the value of the tobacco. The price paid for British-made cigars in the shops is from 10s. to 16s. a pound. The price for foreign cigars is from 25s. to 40s. a pound; and as I am speaking of the price of tobacco, I may say that shag and other coarse tobaccos manufactured in this country are sold from 4s. to 5s. a pound, while foreign manufactured tobacco costs from 14s. to 18s. a pound.

In making cigars the mid-rib of the leaf is removed altogether, whilst the perfect leaves are used for making the outside wrappers and the imperfect ones for the inside of the cigar. Cheroots are elongated cones which are cut in two. The cheroot is often preferred to the cigar on account of its allowing a freer access of air to the tobacco, and burning more quickly and with less accumulation of oil at the smoked end. Cigars can of course be made of any size; at the same time, a common size is usually adhered to in particular manufactories, so that the size at once indicates the maker of the cigar.

The prepared leaf of the tobacco-plant, when not made into cigars, is called tobacco, whether its destination be mastication or smoking. Thus there are uncut tobaccos known by the names of "Pigtail," "Negro-head," and "Cavendish." Pigtail, which is a long string of tobacco, is made by sorting the leaves one within the other, in such a way, that when a wheel to which the tobacco is first fastened, is turned, the tobacco is drawn into a long cord. This cord is made up into balls, which are called rolls, casks, hanks, cakes, or negro-heads, according to the form or shape they assume. This tobacco is used both for chewing and smoking. It is cut up when used for smoking. Such tobacco is generally stronger than any other form, as from its method of manufacture the volatile narcotic principles are prevented from escaping.

Of course, with an article consumed to such an enormous extent as tobacco, the varieties of forms which its manufactured produce presents are very great. I have only mentioned those which are perhaps familiar to those who never ventured on smoking even a cigarette. This reminds me that this term is applied to a small cigar extemporaneously manufactured. A little tobacco is taken and rolled up in a piece of paper, and the cigarette is produced.

Tobacco is usually smoked from a pipe. Whatever doubt may attach to the statement, that smoking came from the New World, there seems to be no doubt that the pipe was invented in America. Many of the native tribes of North America celebrated their great national solemnities with the pipe. This pipe, called the calumet, was adorned on such occasions with the coloured feathers of birds, with beads and gems, and other ornaments. The bowl was made of a red stone resembling porphyry, and the stem was six feet in length. A pipe-bearer first held it to the sun, then to the different points of the compass, after which it was handed to the principal chief, who, after smoking himself, presented it to the assembled conclave. The forms which this instrument assumes at the present day are almost infinite. Almost every solid material which can be chiselled or moulded have been employed to make the bowl, whilst the stem has been made of a still greater number of substances. Whatever presents itself naturally in the form of a tube, or that can be converted into one, has been thus employed. The end of the tube which is placed in the mouth frequently differs in material from the stem itself, and amber, costly gems, ivory, and other materials, have been used for this purpose. Sometimes between the bowl and the stem a vessel of water is inserted, so that the smoke is purified by this kind of washing, and this is a favourite form of the nargheli of the Turks. But I need not discourse to you on pipes, as a peep into the window of any one of the 1,800 tobacconists' shops in London will give you an idea of their variety. Suffice it to say, they have been made of the most costly materials, have had bestowed on them the most elaborate workmanship, and their form, size, and character, are frequently characteristic of the races of men who use them.

The honour of introducing the pipe into England is disputed. You have all heard the story of Sir Walter Raleigh, whose servant, having observed him smoking, thought he was on fire, and threw a pail of water over his head. It appears, however, that Sir Francis Drake and his companions had become smokers, and brought the practice to England before Sir Walter ever laid his eyes on the New World. This was as early as 1560. Whole fields of tobacco were cultivated in Portugal before 1584, the assumed date of the exploit of Raleigh's servant; at any rate, at the latter end of the sixteenth century, the practice of smoking was becoming so general in Europe, that fears were entertained lest the populations that smoked would degenerate into a barbarous state. It was at the beginning of the seventeenth century that tobacco-smoking spread over the East. So thoroughly oriental has this practice become, and so essentially a part of the habits of the great Asiatic nations, that many writers have professed themselves sceptics as to its recent introduction amongst them.

It was not on account of its favourable reception by the rulers and governments of the world that tobacco found its way to the remotest corners of the earth. Everywhere persecution awaited it. It was excommunicated by the Pope. The sultans and priests of Turkey and Persia denounced smoking as a sin against their religion. In Russia the practice was punished by the bastinado for the first offence, by cutting off the nose for the second, and by decapitation for the third. In Transylvania the punishment for growing tobacco was a confiscation of all property. In the canton of Berne an eleventh commandment was added to the decalogue—"Thou shalt not smoke." Good Queen Bess, perhaps out of regard to her favoured Raleigh, rather winked at than approved the practice, only interdicting its use in churches. She even condescended to banter Sir Walter about it; and he induced her to lay him a wager that he could not tell the weight of the smoke he sent out from his pipe. He performed before her majesty a chemical experiment, which, if it had not won the wager, is worthy of being recorded as a proof that he possessed the genius that might have laid the foundation of modern chemical science. He took the tobacco he was about to smoke, and having weighed it, he put it in his pipe; having smoked the tobacco, he weighed the ashes, and proved to her majesty's satisfaction that the difference between the two must be the weight of the smoke. What a subject for an historical painter. The queen paid her lost wager, saying she had often heard of those " who had turned their gold into smoke; but Raleigh was the first who had turned his smoke into gold." But a philosopher was soon to sit upon the throne of England; one who judged men and nature not according to the tendencies of the vulgar rabble, but by the high standard of a royal intellect. His majesty not only passed laws to forbid smoking, but fulminated " a counterblaste to tobacco," which, as it is the type of most of the counterblasts since issued, I may be excused for quoting a specimen.

" Surely," saith our monarch, " smoke becomes a kitchen farre better than a dining chamber; and yet it makes a kitchen oftentimes in the inward parts of men; soyling and infecting them with an unctuous and oyley kind of soote as hath been found in some great tobacco takers, that after their death were opened. Now my good countrymen let us (I pray you) consider what honour or policie can move us to imitate the barbarous and beastlie manners of the wild, godless, and slavish Indians, especially in so vile and filthy a custom. Shall we that disdain to imitate the manner of our neighbour France (having the style of the greate Christian kingdome), and that cannot endure the spirit of the Spaniards (their king being now comparable in largenesse of dominions to the greatest emperor of Turkey); shall we, I say, that have been so long civill and wealthy in peace, famous and invincible in war—fortunate in both—we that have been able to aid any of our neighbours (but never deafened their ears with any of our supplications for assistance); shall we, I say, without blushing, abase ourselve˙ so far as to imitate these beastlie Indians, slaves to the Spaniards, the refuse of the worlde, and as yet aliens from the holy covenant of God? Why do we not as well imitate them in walking naked as they do, in preferring glasses, feathers, and toys, to gold and precious stones as they do? Yea, why do we not deny God, and adore the devils as they do? Have you not, then, reasons to forbear this filthie noveltie, so basely grounded, so foolishly received, and so grosslie mistaken in the right use thereof? In your abuse thereof sinning against God, harming yourselves both in person and goods and raking also, thereby the marks and notes of vanitie upon you, by the custom thereof, making yourselves to be wondered at by all forreine civill nations, and by all strangers that come among you to be scorned and contemned. A custom loathsome to the eye, hateful to the nose, harmfull to the braine, dangerous to the lungs, and in the blacke stinking fume thereof, nearest resembling the horrible Stygian smoake of the pit that is bottomless."

But tobacco is not only smoked, it is also chewed, and distinguished above all other substances in being stuffed up the nose. The practice of chewing is not confined to tobacco, nor was it introduced from the New World. Throughout the nations of Asia the practice of chewing the betel-nut is prevalent. This nut is the fruit of a palm, the *Areca Catechu*, and contains in its albumen a quantity of tannic acid. The seed is cut with a knife, and the shavings mixed with long pepper and lime, and introduced into the mouth as a masticatory. Narcotic effects are ascribed to these agents. The practice of chewing the one thing would probably pave the way for the other. But chewing does not appear to have been practised in Europe till the introduction of tobacco. The effect of this very disagreeable use of tobacco is the same on the system as smoking, the only difference arising from the absence of an empyreumatic oil, which is produced by burning the tobacco. All forms of tobacco may be chewed, but those who have acquired this habit generally prefer the woven and pressed tobacco, as pigtail and negrohead.

A third method of employing tobacco is snuffing. The practice of introducing irritating substances up the nose for the purpose of producing sneezing is as old as Hippocrates, but I am not aware that it was ever regarded as an indulgence till the introduction of tobacco. The preparation of the tobacco for snuffing is much more elaborate than for smoking. According to the quality of the snuff, the entire leaf or the ribs and mid-ribs of the leaves alone are employed. These are sprinkled with water and laid in heaps; they thus become heated, and a kind of fermentation takes place, which produces a considerable change in the composition and qualities of the tobacco. The leaves, after having been subjected to this process, are dried and powdered. They are then put into close boxes and undergo a second time a process of heating and fermentation. This gives to the snuff its agreeable pungent odour. In this process some of those ethers are probably developed which give flavour and odour to so many other things. Snuffs are either moist or dry. The moist snuffs are called rappees, and are frequently scented by the addition of various kinds of perfumes. The "high-dried" snuffs, such as those which are called Scotch, Irish, and Welsh, are exposed to heat in shallow metal trays or pans before a brisk fire, and strongly heated. During this process a large quantity of ammonia is evolved.

Although the general effects of tobacco are to a certain extent produced by snuffing, there is no doubt that the pleasure of the snuff-taker is more local than that of the chewer or smoker. At the same time snuff can be consumed to an injurious extent, and like all other forms of narcotic it may be easily abused. There is one use of snuff that is so local and peculiar that I ought to allude to it here. I mean the practice of "dipping," patronized by the ladies of some parts of America. This form of taking snuff is practised in North and South Carolina, in Georgia, Alabama, Florida, and Eastern Tenessee. It consists in rubbing a stick, wetted at the end and dipped in snuff, about the interior of the mouth and within the interstices of the teeth. Sometimes the mouth is filled with the delicious powder, which the dipper moistens and sucks with the same pleasure as the male chewer sucks his quid.

Other substances are both occasionally chewed and snuffed as substitutes for tobacco, but only in exceptional instances. The practice of snuffing, I ought to add, is liable to a dangerous action in the system, which is not the case with smoking and chewing. This arises from the introduction, by accident or design, of substances more injurious to health than an excess of tobacco. Thus, snuff is frequently packed in lead packages, and the snuff, acting on the lead, gets into it a sufficient quantity to act poisonously in the system. I have been consulted by persons with all the symptoms of lead poisoning, who have got rid of them when they have left off their snuff. I may add that this is only the case with the moist snuffs, and that the lovers of high-dried Welsh and Lundy Foot need not be alarmed. But then there is the retailer, the fraudulent fellow who wants to get more out of everybody than fair profits and short weight will enable him. He adds all sorts of things to snuff; and not being instructed in toxicology, he sometimes adds poisons. The oxides of lead, mercury, antimony, and other poisonous metals, have been found in snuff.

But I must now say something to you on the action of tobacco. In order to do this, we must first ascertain what are the chemical constituents of the tobacco leaf, and of tobacco smoke; for we shall find the smoke differs somewhat from the tobacco itself. I present you here with the analysis of a pound of tobacco—shag tobacco:—

	Oz.	Grs.
Nicotina	0	419
Concrete volatile oil	0	7
Chlorophyle	1	46
Gum	1	222
Starch	0	279
Albumen and gluten	0	349
Sugar	0	139
Salts	2	245
Water	1	402

It is very evident that, with the exception of the two first, none of these constituents can exercise much influence on the system, even when the tobacco is taken in the form of a quid. I might, perhaps, be allowed to draw your attention to the ashes, which exist in unusually large quantities. The soluble salts amongst them would be swallowed if the tobacco was chewed, and might act on the system in the same way as the other saline constituents of plants. They are also interesting as explaining how it is that the cultivator of the soil finds tobacco an exceedingly exhausting crop.

It is also worthy of note that the nitrates are abundant in the salts, and perhaps account for the ready way in which tobacco burns.

In smoking, of course the volatile products of the above analysis are alone taken into the mouth, and the following are the ingredients which various observers have detected in tobacco smoke:—

Nicotine.	Empyreumatic Resin.
Empyreumatic Oil.	Acetic Acid.
Butyric Acid.	Carbonic Oxide.
Carbonic Acid.	Carburetted Hydrogen.
Ammonia.	Water.
Paraffine.	

Sir Walter Raleigh would have been astounded could he have known the villanous products liberated from his experimental pipe. King James must have had an inkling of its composition when he denounced it as a " black, stinking fume," resembling " the horrible Stygian smoake of the pit that is bottomlesse." Butyric acid is the stinking product of rancid butter. Carbonic oxide is the poison of charcoal stoves. Carburetted hydrogen and paraffine are products of coal gas. We can hardly discover the tobacco in the smoke, but there is the nicotine; and although we do not find the concrete oil, we find the empyreumatic oil, and these are the three things alone of which we need take any notice in our inquiry. In fact, those who smoke need not to regard the concrete oil of the tobacco at all, as it appears to be dissipated or changed into the empyreumatic oil. So that we must seek for the influence of tobacco in its nicotine and empyreumatic oil.

Nicotine is an alkaloid, like quinine or morphine, and

is found in the tobacco combined with acids. It can be separated from these acids and obtained in its pure form, when it presents itself not as a solid, like other alkaloids, but as a colourless liquid. It has a most offensive, suffocating odour, and an acrid, burning taste. By exposure to the air it becomes brown, and this is the colour it generally presents when kept. It boils and is decomposed at a temperature of 482°; but as it passes into a vapour before it reaches this point, it is not decomposed in the process of combustion, to which it is exposed in smoking. It is an active poison, and a very small quantity destroys life. I have known two distinguished chemists who have within the last few years destroyed themselves by its agency. It was the poison employed by Count Bocarmé for the murder of his brother-in-law, and whose trial at Mons, a few years ago, will be remembered.

The quantity of nicotine contained in different kinds of tobacco varies from 2 to 8 per cent. Virginia and Kentucky leaves, from which shag and bird's-eye tobaccos are manufactured, contain 6 per cent.; Maryland leaves, from which returns are made, contain 2 per cent.; and Havannah cigars contain less than 2 per cent. It is clear that if the effect of the nicotine is alone sought to be attained, that it is much more economical to purchase shag or bird's-eye than returns or real Havannah cigars. But amongst those who indulge in tobacco, as with those who affect wine and tea, there are other qualities sought for besides the mere action on the nervous system. The palate must be gratified, and there are bouquets in tobaccos and cigars as there are in wines and teas flavours, for which those who have cultivated a taste for them will pay a higher price than for the quantity of the active principle which renders these articles of consumption desirable.

Of the empyreumatic oil there is less chemically known than of nicotine. It is, however, easily obtained by passing tobacco smoke through water. It is this oil which collects in the tubes of pipes, and which renders them so offensive to all but the most inveterate smokers. It has an oleaginous appearance, and is of a yellow colour when pure. It is acrid to the taste, producing a sensation of heat in the mouth. One drop placed on the tongue of a cat has been known to produce death. The Hottentots use it to kill snakes. It has been supposed to be the "juice of cursed hebenon" referred to by Shakspeare, in the play of "Hamlet," as a "leperous distilment." But, in this instance Shakspeare follows the old story on which his play was founded, and the "juice of cursed hebenon" was rather

"The mixture rank of midnight weeds collected
With Hecate's ban, thrice blasted, thrice infected,"

than any natural production. No poison that we know of at the present day would answer to the Ghost's description of a poison,

"Whose effect
Holds such an enmity with blood of man,
That, swift as quicksilver, it courses through
The natural gates and alleys of the body;
And with a sudden vigour it doth posset
And curd, like eager droppings into milk,
The thin and wholesome blood: so did it mine;
And a most instant tetter bark'd about,
Most lazar-like, with vile and loathsome crust,
All my smooth body."

Both nicotine and the distilled oil act on the nervous system, yet with a difference: nicotine paralyses the heart, which the oil does not. It paralyses the heart by its action on the brain. This was shown by Sir Benjamin Brodie, who found that, although the heart of a dog was paralyzed by tobacco when its head was on, the heart went on beating if its head was cut off. On the other hand, the oil seems to address itself more to the spinal cord and the motor nerves. The respiratory muscles cease to act, the lungs become congested, and convulsions and coma terminate life, whilst the heart still beats. The two together seem to leave no part of the nervous system unattacked; whilst nicotine seizes on the citadel, the distilled oil attacks the outposts, and the whole man—body and mind—is brought under their influence.

What man is there who has reached the age of twenty who has not experienced the effects of these agents? First, the sneezing and coughing, indicative of the objection of the respiratory nerves; then the sensation of heat and dryness in the throat, and presently the sense of nausea; then a tendency to sigh, followed by a general uneasiness,—a wish to get home if out, or to go to bed if at home. Perhaps the heart has palpitated; but, at any rate, the eyes have become dim, the nicotine has forced its way to the base of the brain; at last there is giddiness, and now the pipe or cigar is laid down and dropped from the hand. If the determination to smoke has not been very energetic, water is asked for, and perhaps brandy-and-water is supplied, and a speedy recovery has taken place; but where the will has been at work in spite of all premonitory symptoms, the novice may become insensible, and a fainting fit be the result. Such are the results of a first smoke: a sure proof, one would have thought, that tobacco ought not to be indulged in. But even this state has its fascinations. In those first moments, before any painful effects were experienced, the poison had spread its snares. In that languor there was a sense of relief, and in that giddiness there was a dreamy pleasure, which even as you smoked became more real, whilst the agonies of the first trial became ever less, and thus many of you have become confirmed smokers. I can defend you on no other ground than that it gives you pleasure. I cannot say that it does you any positive good; and I have looked in vain for proofs of its destructive influence on health. The late Dr. Pereira states, in his book on "Materia Medica," that he is not acquainted with any well-ascertained ill-effects resulting from the habitual practice of smoking. Dr. Christison says the same. Duchatelet examined statistically into the health of the workmen in the French snuff and tobacco manufactories, amounting to 4,000 in number, and could not discover that they were less healthy than other artisans. Dr. Prout gave it as his opinion that excessive tobacco smoking interfered with the healthy qualities of the blood. Many medical writers have recorded cases in which excessive smoking has produced symptoms of illness, which have disappeared when the smoking has been given up.

But with regard to the effects of the moderate use of tobacco, I am sorry to say that I have nothing decidedly against it to tell you. The opinions of medical men are really not worth quoting, unless backed by something like evidence. It is not because a man dies of apoplexy, or paralysis, or fever, or any other disease, after smoking tobacco, that we are to conclude he died in consequence of it. My allopathic brethren, as they are called, are very ready to laugh at the absurd conclusion of the homœopathist, who, because his patient gets well after a homœopathic dose, concludes that he gets well on account of it; but they should be careful not to fall into the same error with regard to tobacco.

If you will not, therefore, give up this habit of smoking, from motives of economy, from a sense of its unseemliness, from its making your breath smell, and your clothes filthy, from its polluting your hands and your house, and driving women and men from you who do not smoke, I dare not, as a physiologist or a statist, tell you, that there exists any proof of its injurious influence when used in moderation. I know how difficult it is to define that word moderation; and yet, in my heart I believe that every one of you has an internal monitor that will guide you to the true explanation of it in your own case. The first symptoms of giddiness, of sickness, of palpitation, of weariness, of indolence, of uneasiness, whilst smoking, should induce you to lay it aside. These are the physiological indications of its disagreement, which, if you neglect, you may find increase upon you, and seriously embarrass your health.

The action of tobacco is much stronger on children and young persons than on adults. The fatal cases of poisoning by smoking or the application of tobacco on abraded surfaces have been chiefly in children and lads from fourteen to seventeen years of age. I think this should serve as a warning to parents and those engaged in the education of youth, to prevent the practice of smoking amongst boys. In more than one case where I have been consulted, I have been led to suspect that smoking has produced a state of the nervous system, which resulted in attacks of palpitation from slight causes.

In certain diseased conditions of the system I have found tobacco most injurious. There is a state of the nervous system which frequently comes on as the result of dyspepsia amongst the overworked men of London, which is accompanied with a slow pulse, and tobacco seems to act as a poison. In such cases, it needs to be carefully avoided. In some diseases of the heart, it acts injuriously when taken to excess; whilst in others I have found it to have an exceedingly beneficial action. Generally where there is depression or lethargy, or a tendency to inactivity of the muscular system, or the mental powers, there tobacco would appear to act injuriously. Its effects in such states may be judged of by the fact, that many persons who can smoke with impunity after a meal, or whilst drinking alcohol, are utterly unable to do so before a meal, or without some form of alcoholic beverage.

The modifying effect produced on the system by tobacco after large potations of alcohol is a subject of some interest. A distinguished medical writer has stated his conviction, that the man who both drinks and smokes is less liable to injure himself than the man who smokes or drinks alone. We have no means of testing this theory upon a scale sufficiently large to answer for its truth; but from what I have said of the action of alcohol and nicotine, you will see that the one agent is the antagonist of the other in its action on the nervous system. The one is a stimulant, the other is a sedative. Nevertheless, they both stimulate, and they both act as sedatives; but the tobacco acts as a sedative in small doses, and the alcohol in large. The quiet intoxication, which is the last result of alcohol, is one of the immediate effects of tobacco; and this may in some measure account for its supplanting alcohol; for we find, that just in proportion as tobacco has increased in consumption, alcohol has diminished. However much this may be regretted by those who dislike the practice of tobacco-smoking, it must be a source of gratification to all those who wish well to their race. Whatever may be the evils, real or imaginary, of the abuse of tobacco, they are as nothing compared with the terrible effects of alcohol. If tobacco and alcohol were tried before any competent tribunal for all the evils they have inflicted on society, I believe, that if alcohol were condemned to be hanged, tobacco ought to get off with a month's imprisonment.

I have hardly left myself time to dwell upon another narcotic agent which is consumed largely by mankind. I mean Opium. This substance is the produce of the poppy-plant, *Papaver somniferum* (Fig. 3), which, although it grows in this country, is a native

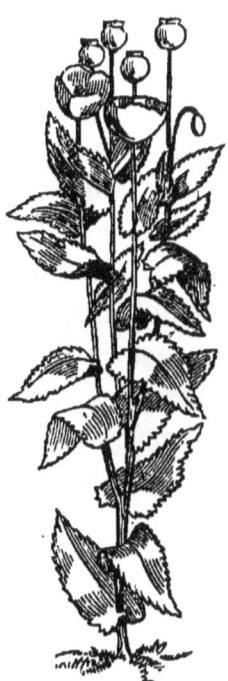

Fig. 3.—Poppy.

of Syria, from whence it has found its way to other parts of the world. The Poppy tribe of plants yield a milky juice. This juice is collected from the opium poppy, and the dried juice is the substance known by the name of opium. This substance has from the earliest times been known as a powerful narcotic agent acting on the brain, and producing a tendency to sleep. It has been on this account used in medicine, and perhaps to no other agent does man owe so deep a debt for the alleviation of his pain and sorrow in disease as this. It would be altogether impossible for me here to speak of the medicinal properties of opium. It must suffice you for me to say that, whilst its primary action seems to be to subdue the activity of the brain and to produce sleep, it acts generally on the nervous system. The sympathetic nerves, the nerves of motion and sensation, the spinal cord, are all alive to its action, and where the object in the treatment of disease is to subdue the activity of any of these portions of the nervous system, there opium is employed. It was hardly to be expected that an agent possessing so much power over the human system should escape the strong tendency of mankind to employ as luxuries all agents affecting pleasurably the nervous system. Gradually has the use of opium spread. Turkey first set the example, and the practice has wound its way throughout the East, till it has become the besetting sin of the Chinese. The practice of opium-eating is exceptional in Europe, but much larger quantities of it are consumed than could be accounted for by its medicinal use, and there is no doubt it is taken to a certain extent upon the same principle as alcohol, tea, and tobacco. The effects of opium-eating, though not so disastrous as those of tippling, are nevertheless much more destructive than those of smoking. The action of the opium is less exciting than that of alcohol, but more pleasant than that of tobacco, while its subsequent effects are less dangerous than those of alcohol and greater than those of tobacco. It is on this account that it becomes a matter of serious consideration for those who would put down both drinking alcohol and smoking tobacco, as to whether it might not lead to the equally objectionable practice—eating opium.

Opium when analyzed chemically is found to be a very compound body. Its narcotic properties, or its soporific properties, are now known to depend on an active principle called morphine. This principle is often separated and used in medicine instead of opium.

Other narcotic agents are employed by the inhabitants of various parts. Thus, throughout Asia and Africa, the Hemp plant, the *Cannabis sativa* (Fig. 4), is cultivated, and in these regions yield a resinous principle which produces a kind of inebriating effect. The narcotic properties of this plant were known to the ancient Egyptians and

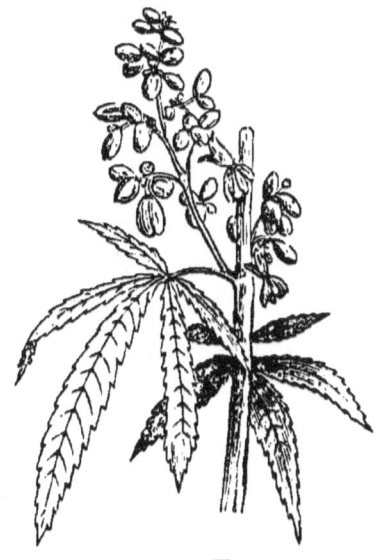

Fig. 4.—Hemp.

Greeks. It is known in the countries where it is used by various names. In Syria it is called haschisch, and it may be news to some of you to know that our word assassins is supposed to have come from this word. The story is that during the wars of the Crusaders, the soldiers of the Saracen army, when delirious with their favourite drug, were in the habit of rushing down upon the camp of the Christians at night, plundering and murdering, in spite of the danger to themselves. They were known by the name of hashasheens: hence our word.

Other narcotics of interest, on account of their employment as intoxicants, are the Coca of South America and the Amanita of Lapland. I have before alluded to the latter. The coca grows wild in the woods of Bolivia and Peru. It was cultivated by the natives of Peru when they were discovered by Pizarro and his band of Spaniards, and to this day it is the solace and the support of the Indian in his native mountains. He is never seen without his leather pouch to hold the leaves of the coca plant. The leaf is generally chewed, but it is sometimes infused and made into tea. Wondrous effects are attributed to this poison by those who take it, and certainly the statement of travellers of the power of endurance of hunger and labour under the influence of this strange drug are sufficiently noteworthy to render a further investigation of its properties desirable.

Another narcotic remarkable for its application as a poison and an inebriant, is the Thorn-apple—*Datura stramonium* (Fig. 5.) It grows wild in this country, and its leaves are gathered and dried, and smoked by those who suffer from asthma. In Russia the seeds were formerly employed to increase the intoxicating effects of beer. They are used in India for the purpose of being added surreptitiously to the food of travellers,

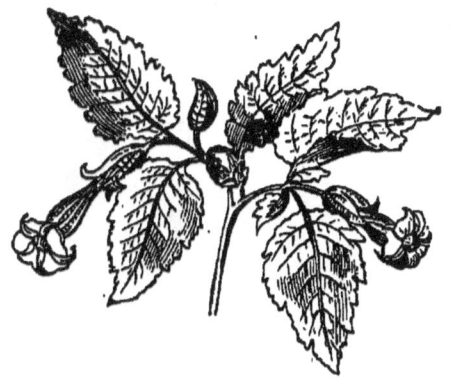

Fig. 5.—Thorn Apple.

and producing a state of intoxication, in which the victim is robbed. Under the name of "Jamestown weed," Dr. Beverly, in his "History of Virginia," gives a curious account of the action of this plant on some soldiers who ate it as a salad :—

"The effect," he says, "was a very pleasant comedy, for they turned natural fools upon it for several days. One would blow up a feather into the air; another would dart straws at it with much fury; another, stark naked, was seen sitting in a corner, like a monkey, grinning and making mouths; a fourth would fondly kiss and paw his companions and sneer in their faces with a countenance more antic than any in a Dutch droll. In this frantic condition they were confined lest in their folly they should destroy themselves. A thousand simple tricks they played, but after eleven days they returned to themselves again, not remembering anything that had passed."

Another of our native weeds deserves notice on

account of its narcotic properties, and that is the Deadly Nightshade — *Atropa Belladonna*. (Fig. 6.) Its rich

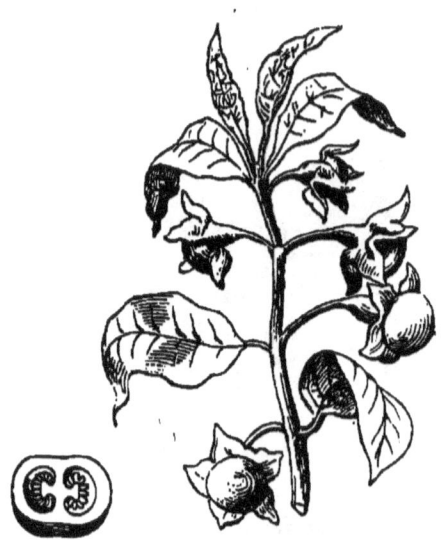

Fig. 6.—Deadly Nightshade.

black berries often tempt children to take them, when they are seized with a delirium, which often ends in death. The Henbane (*Hyoscyanus niger*) is also one of our own narcotic poisons, producing, as the result of its being smoked, a peculiar kind of delirium, with other effects, on the nervous system. The beautiful Foxglove (*Digitalis purpurea*) also contains a principle acting on the nervous system in a similar way to nicotine. But I must leave these native "sisters of sleep."* The whole subject of poisons is worthy of popular study, as I hope I have convinced you, from the short notice I have given of those which we use as a part of our daily food.

* For much interesting information on these subjects, the reader may consult "The Seven Sisters of Sleep," by M. W. Cooke.

In the remarks I have made in this lecture, I know that there are some persons in this audience, and some for whom I entertain the highest respect, who could have wished me to adopt a very different line of treatment to that which I have thought it right to pursue. To them I would say, that the way I should treat this subject has not been a less serious matter of consideration with me than their own views on it. I have not dared to regard the pleasure of partaking of these narcotics as altogether vicious, when I consider how largely they contribute to the solace and enjoyment of my fellow creatures. I hope I have said nothing that could by any straining be interpreted into countenancing a use of these things, which would interfere with the healthy development either of the mind or the body. One of the objects I have had in view in the delivery of these lectures has been, to bring before you the wonderful laws by which God upholds your daily life. To be sure I have chiefly spoken of the materials which God uses from day to day in the maintenance of that glorious "temple" which He has given you to dwell in, a temple in which He himself has condescended to dwell, but, I trust, that in the fulfilment of this humble purpose, however imperfectly it may have been performed, that I have never forgotten the apostolic rule for the guide of Christian men, that " whether, therefore, ye eat or drink, or whatsoever ye do, do all to the glory of God."

ROBERT HARDWICKE, PRINTER, 192, PICCADILLY.

A CATALOGUE

OF WORKS OF

NATURAL HISTORY, SCIENCE,

ART, AND GENERAL LITERATURE,

PUBLISHED BY

Hardwicke & Bogue.

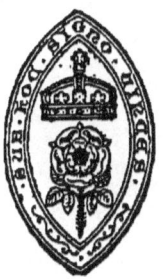

192, PICCADILLY, W.

HARDWICKE'S SCIENCE GOSSIP:

An Illustrated Medium of Interchange and Gossip for Students and Lovers of Nature.

Edited by J. E. TAYLOR, F.L.S., F.G.S., &c.

Contains the fullest Information respecting Animals, Aquaria, Bees, Beetles, Birds, Butterflies, Ferns, Fish, Fossils, Fungi, Lichens, Microscopes, Mosses, Reptiles, Rocks, Seaweeds, Wildflowers.

Monthly, price 4d.; Annual Subscription, 5s. (including Postage).

Twelve Volumes are now published, bound in cloth, price 5s. each.

THE MONTHLY
MICROSCOPICAL JOURNAL:

Transactions of the Royal Microscopical Society, and Record of Histological Research.

Edited by HENRY LAWSON, M.D., F.R.M.S.,
Assistant Physician to, and Lecturer on Histology in, St. Mary's Hospital.

Published monthly, price 1s. 6d. Annual subscription (including postage), 19s.

Sixteen Volumes are now ready, bound in cloth, price 10s. 6d. each.

THE
POPULAR SCIENCE REVIEW:

A Quarterly Summary of Scientific Progress and Miscellany of Entertaining and Instructive Articles on Scientific Subjects by the Best Writers of the Day.

Edited by W. S. DALLAS, F.L.S.,
Assistant Secretary of the Geological Society.

In addition to Articles which are of abiding interest, the POPULAR SCIENCE REVIEW contains a Complete Record of Progress in every Department of Science, including

ASTRONOMY.	GEOGRAPHY.	MICROSCOPY.
BOTANY.	GEOLOGY.	PHOTOGRAPHY.
CHEMISTRY.	MECHANICS.	PHYSICS.
ETHNOLOGY.	METALLURGY.	ZOOLOGY.

SCIENCES applied to the ARTS, MANUFACTURES, & AGRICULTURE.

Published Quarterly, price 2s. 6d.; sent Post-free to any part of the United Kingdom for 10s. 10d. per annum.

The early numbers having been reprinted, Volumes I. to XV. may be had, bound in cloth, price 12s. each.

London: HARDWICKE & BOGUE, 192, Piccadilly, W.

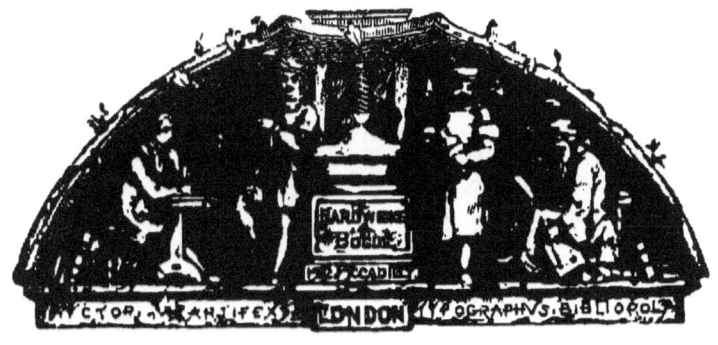

ACROSTICS.—One Hundred Double Acrostics. Edited by "Myself." 16mo, cloth gilt, 2s. 6d.

ANSTED, D. T., M.A., F.R.S.
THE APPLICATIONS of GEOLOGY to the ARTS AND MANUFACTURES. Six Lectures delivered before the Society of Arts. Illustrated. Fcap. 8vo, cloth, 4s.

ARMITAGE, T. R., M.D.
EDUCATION and EMPLOYMENT of the BLIND: What it has been, is, and ought to be. Demy 8vo, 2s. 6d.

BALL, E.
INVENTIVE DRAWING: A Practical Development of Elementary Design. 4to, bds., 6s.

BARKER, S., M.D.
MANAGEMENT OF CHILDREN in Health and Disease: A Book for Mothers. Demy 8vo, 6s.

BARNARD, H.
ORAL TRAINING LESSONS IN NATURAL SCIENCE AND GENERAL KNOWLEDGE: Embracing the subjects of Astronomy, Anatomy, Physiology, Chemistry, Mathematics, Geography. Crown 8vo, 2s. 6d.

BELCHER, REV. HENRY, M.A.
DEGREES AND "DEGREES"; or, The Traffic in Theological, Medical, and other "Diplomas" Exposed. Demy 8vo, 1s. 6d.

BENSON, J. W.
TIME and TIME TELLERS: A Book about Watches and Clocks. With many Woodcuts. Crown 8vo, cloth, 2s. 6d.

BIRKS, PROFESSOR, Camb.
THE UNCERTAINTIES of MODERN PHYSICAL SCIENCE; being the Annual Address of the Victoria Institute, or Philosophical Society of Great Britain, for the Year 1876. 8vo, 6d.

BLINCOURT, A. de, B.E.L.
FRENCH GENDERS: An Easy Method of Distinguishing them at Sight. 8vo, 6d.

BONER, CHARLES.
IN THE PLAIN AND ON THE MOUNTAIN: A Guide for Pedestrians and Mountain Tourists, With Illustrations of Dress requisites, &c. Fcap. 8vo, cloth, 2s.

BOOK of KNOTS. Illustrated by 172 Examples, showing the manner of Making every Knot, Tie, and Splice, by "Tom Bowling." Second Edition. Crown 8vo, cloth, 2s. 6d.

BOTANY SIMPLIFIED ON THE NATURAL SYSTEM. Crown 8vo, cloth, 1s.

BRIOT, M.C.
ELEMENTS OF ARITHMETIC. Translated by J. SPEAR. Crown 8vo, cloth, 4s.

BURBIDGE, F. W.
COOL ORCHIDS, AND HOW TO GROW THEM. With Descriptive List of all the best Species in Cultivation. Illustrated with numerous Woodcuts and Coloured Figures of 13 Varieties. Crown 8vo, cloth, 6s.

BUSHNAN, J. S., M.D., F.R.S.
INTRODUCTION TO ICHTHYOLOGY. With 33 Coloured Plates. Fcap. 8vo, cloth, 4s. 6d.

CAPEL, C. C.
TROUT CULTURE. A Practical Treatise on Spawning, Hatching, and Rearing Trout. Fcap. 8vo, cloth, 2s. 6d.

CARPENTER, ALFRED, M.D.
HINTS on HOUSE DRAINAGE. Second Edition, with Appendix. 8vo, sewed, 1s.

CARRINGTON, B., M.D., F.R.S.
BRITISH HEPATICÆ. Containing Descriptions and Figures of the Native Species of Jungermannia, Marchantia, and Anthoceros. Imp. 8vo, sewed, Parts 1 to 4, each 2s. 6d. plain; 3s. 6d. coloured. To be Completed in about 12 Parts.

CASH, JAMES.
WHERE THERE'S A WILL THERE'S A WAY; or, Science in the Cottage; being Memoirs of Naturalists in Humble Life. Crown 8vo, cloth, 3s. 6d.

CHAMISSO, ADALBERT VON.
PETER SCHLEMIHL. Translated by Sir JOHN BOWRING, LL.D., &c. Illustrations on India paper by GEORGE CRUIKSHANK. Crown 8vo, cloth, 5s.

CHANGED CROSS (THE). Words by L. P. W. Illuminated by K. K. Dedicated to the Memory of those blessed ones who having, "through much tribulation," finished their course with joy, now rest from their labours; and to those also who are still running with patience the course set before them, "Looking to Jesus." Square 16mo, elegantly printed, with Illuminated Crosses and Border Lines, 6s. See also "*Crown of Life.*"

CHANGED CROSS (THE). A Large Edition of the above work, printed in outline on best Plate Paper, for those persons who, being proficient in the art of Illumination, wish to illuminate the work according to their own tastes. Fcap. 4to, handsomely bound, cloth gilt, 6s.

COELEBS. THE LAWS AND PRACTICE OF WHIST. Square 16mo, cloth, 2s. 6d.

COLLECTION CATALOGUE for NATURALISTS. A Ruled Book for keeping a permanent Record of Objects in any branch of Natural History, with Appendix for recording interesting particulars, and lettered pages for general Index. Strongly bound, 200 pages, 7s. 6d.; 300 pages, 10s.; and 2s. 6d. extra for every additional 100 pages. Working Catalogues, 1s. 6d. each.

COMPANION TO THE WRITING DESK. See "*How to Address Titled People.*"

CONCHOLOGY, Quarterly Journal of. Containing Original Communications, Descriptions of New Species, Bibliography, &c. Demy 8vo, Parts 1 to 9, each 6d. Part 10, 1s.

COOKE, M. C., M.A., LL.D.
A PLAIN and EASY ACCOUNT of THE BRITISH FUNGI. With especial reference to the Esculent and other Economic Species. Third Edition, revised. With Coloured Plates of 40 Species. Fcap. 8vo, cloth, 6s.

THE BRITISH REPTILES: A Plain and Easy Account of the Lizards, Snakes, Newts, Toads, Frogs, and Tortoises indigenous to Great Britain. Numerous Illustrations, Coloured by hand. Fcap. 8vo, cloth, 6s.

RUST, SMUT, MILDEW, AND MOULD. An Introduction to the Study of Microscopic Fungi. Illustrated with nearly 300 Coloured Figures. Second Edition, with Appendix of new Species. Fcap. 8vo, cloth, 6s.

COOKE, M. C., M.A., LL.D.
A MANUAL OF BOTANIC TERMS. New Edition, greatly enlarged, including the recent Teratological terms. Illustrated with more than 300 Woodcuts. Fcap. 8vo, cloth, 2s. 6d.

A MANUAL OF STRUCTURAL BOTANY. Revised Edition, with New Chemical Notation. Twentieth Thousand. Illustrated with 200 Woodcuts, 1s.

INDEX FUNGORUM BRITANNICORUM. A Complete List of Fungi found in the British Islands to the present date. 8vo, cloth, 2s. 6d.

CRESSWELL, C. N., of the Inner Temple.
WOMAN, AND HER WORK IN THE WORLD. Crown 8vo, cloth, 3s. 6d.

CROWN OF LIFE (THE). By M. Y. W. With elegantly Illuminated Borders from designs by ARTHUR ROBERTSON. Uniform with "*The Changed Cross.*" Fcap. 4to, cloth extra, 6s.

DANIEL, P. A.
SHAKESPEARE'S PLAYS, Notes on Conjectural Amendments of certain Passages in. Crown 8vo, 3s. 6d.

DARBY, W. A., M.A., F.R.A.S.
THE ASTRONOMICAL OBSERVER: A Handbook for the Observatory and the Common Telescope. Embraces 965 Nebulæ, Clusters, and Double Stars. Rl. 8vo, cloth, 7s. 6d.

DAVIES, THOMAS.
THE PREPARATION and MOUNTING of MICROSCOPIC OBJECTS. New Edition, greatly Enlarged and brought up to the Present Time by JOHN MATTHEWS, M.D., F.R.M.S., Vice-President of the Quekett Microscopical Society. Fcap. 8vo, cloth, 2s. 6d.

DICK, Capt. ST. JOHN.
FLIES AND FLY FISHING. Illustrated. Crown 8vo, cloth, 4s. 6d.

DUNCAN, JAMES, F.L.S.
INTRODUCTION TO ENTOMOLOGY. With 8 Coloured Plates. Fcap. 8vo, cloth, 4s. 6d.

BRITISH BUTTERFLIES: A complete description of the Larvæ and full-grown Insects of our Native Species. With Coloured Figures of Eighty Varieties. Fcap. 8vo, cloth, 4s. 6d.

DUNCAN, JAMES, F.L.S.

BRITISH MOTHS: A complete description of the Larvæ and full-grown Insects of our Native Species. With Coloured Figures. Fcap. 8vo, cloth, 4s. 6d.

BEETLES, BRITISH AND FOREIGN. Containing a full description of the more important species. With Coloured Figures of more than One Hundred Varieties. Fcap. 8vo, cloth, 4s. 6d.

NATURAL HISTORY of EXOTIC BUTTERFLIES. With 36 Coloured Plates. Fcap. 8vo, cloth, 4s. 6d.

NATURAL HISTORY OF EXOTIC MOTHS. With 34 Coloured Plates. Fcap. 8vo, cloth, 4s. 6d.

ECONOMIC PRODUCTS (Principal) **FROM THE VEGETABLE KINGDOM.** Arranged under their respective Natural Orders, with the names of the Plants and the parts used in each case. Demy 8vo, 1s. 6d.

ELEMENTARY SCIENCE SERIES. Intended for the Use of the People and for Self-instruction. Each volume is fully Illustrated. MECHANICS, 4d.; HYDRAULICS, 2d.; HYDROSTATICS, 2d.; OPTICS, 4d.; CHEMISTRY, 6d.; PNEUMATICS, 2d. The Six Volumes in One, cloth, 1s. 6d.

ELVIN, C. N., M.A.

A SYNOPSIS OF HERALDRY. With 400 Engravings. Crown 8vo, cloth, 3s.

EYTON, C.

NOTES ON THE GEOLOGY OF NORTH SHROPSHIRE. Fcap. 8vo, cloth, 3s. 6d.

FALCONER, HUGH, A.M., M.D.

PALÆONTOLOGICAL MEMOIRS OF. By CHARLES MURCHISON, M.D., F.R.S. Illustrated. Two Vols., demy, cloth, £2 2s.

FERN COLLECTOR'S ALBUM: A descriptive Folio for the reception of Natural Specimens; containing on the right-hand page a description of each Fern printed in Colours, the opposite page being left Blank for the Collector to affix the dried Specimen; forming, when filled, an elegant and complete collection of this interesting family of Plants. Size 11¾ in. by 8½ in., handsomely bound, price One Guinea.

FLEISCHMANN, A., M.R.C.S.

PLAIN AND PRACTICAL MEDICAL PRECEPTS. Second Edition, revised and enlarged. On a large sheet, 4d.

FRY, HERBERT.
  ROYAL GUIDE TO THE LONDON CHARITIES, 1876–7. Showing, in alphabetical order, their Name, Date of Foundation, Address, Objects, Annual Income, Chief Officials, &c. Crown 8vo, cloth, 1*s.* 6*d.*

  GUIDE TO THE LANGUAGE OF FLOWERS. With Coloured Illustrations. 32mo, cloth, 1*s.*

HAMILTON, R., M.D., F.R.S.
  THE NATURAL HISTORY OF BRITISH FISHES. With 72 Coloured Plates. Two Vols., fcap. 8vo, cloth, 9*s.*

  The **NATURAL HISTORY of SEALS, WALRUSES,** &c. With 30 Coloured Plates. Fcap. 8vo, cloth, 4*s.* 6*d.*

  THE NATURAL HISTORY OF WHALES and other Cetaceæ. With 32 Coloured Plates. Fcap. 8vo, cloth, 4*s.* 6*d.*

  HANDY BOOK OF LONDON. An Easy and Comprehensive Guide to Everything Worth Seeing and Hearing. Royal 32mo, cloth, price 1*s.* New Edition annually.

HEAPHY, THOMAS.
  THE LIKENESS OF CHRIST. Being an Enquiry into the verisimilitude of the received likeness of our Blessed Lord. Edited by WYKE BAYLISS, F.S.A. Illustrated with Twelve Photographs Coloured as Facsimiles, and Fifty Engravings on Wood from original Frescoes, Mosaics, Pateræ, and other Works of Art of the first Six Centuries. Handsomely bound in cloth gilt, atlas 4to. Price to Subscribers before issue, £3 3*s.*

HOOKER, Sir W. J., F.R.S., and J. G. BAKER, F.L.S.
  SYNOPSIS FILICUM; or, A Synopsis of all Known Ferns, including the Osmundaceæ, Schizæaceæ, Marratiaceæ, and Ophioglossaceæ (chiefly derived from the Kew Herbarium), accompanied by Figures representing the Essential Characters of each Genus. Second Edition, brought up to the Present Time. 8vo, cloth, £1 2*s.* 6*d.*, plain; £1 8*s.*, coloured.

HOWDEN, PETER, V.S.
  HORSE WARRANTY: A Plain and Comprehensive Guide to the Various Points to be noted, showing which are essential and which are unimportant. With Forms of Warranty. Fcap. 8vo, cloth, 3*s.* 6*d.*

HOW TO ADDRESS TITLED PEOPLE. With Explanations of A.R.A., B.C.L., C.P.S., D.F., E.I.C.S., F.R.S.E., G.C.M.G., H.A.C., I.H.S., J.P., K.C.H., L.A.H., M.R.A.S., N.S., O.S., P.C., Q.E.D., R.I.P., S.S.C., T.S., U.S., V.C., W.S., X.T., and other Abbreviations (over 500), Academical, Ecclesiastical, Legal, Literary, Masonic, Imperial, and Ancient. A Companion to the Writing-desk. Royal 32mo, 1s.

HOW TO CHOOSE A MICROSCOPE. By a Demonstrator. With 80 Illustrations. Demy 8vo, 1s.

HUNTER, J., late Hon. Sec. of the Brit. Bee-keepers' Association.
A MANUAL OF BEE-KEEPING. Containing Practical Information for Rational and Profitable Methods of Bee Management. Full Instructions on Stimulative Feeding, Ligurianizing and Queen-raising, with descriptions of the best Hives and Apiarian Appliances on all systems. With Illustrations. Second Edition. Fcap. 8vo, cloth, 3s. 6d.

IDYLS OF THE RINK. Illustrated by G. BOWERS and J. CARLISLE. Royal 16mo, cloth gilt, 2s. 6d.

"A series of capital parodies on well-known poems, all exceedingly clever."
—*Examiner.*

JARDINE, Sir W., F.L.S., F.R.S.
THE NATURAL HISTORY OF BRITISH BIRDS. With 120 Coloured Plates. 4 vols. Fcap. 8vo, cloth, 18s.

THE NATURAL HISTORY OF SUN BIRDS. With 30 Coloured Plates. Fcap. 8vo, cloth, 4s. 6d.

THE NATURAL HISTORY OF HUMMING BIRDS. With 64 Coloured Plates. 2 vols. Fcap. 8vo, cloth, 9s.

THE NATURAL HISTORY OF GAME BIRDS. With 30 Coloured Plates. Fcap. 8vo, cloth, 4s. 6d.

THE NATURAL HISTORY OF PHEASANTS, PEACOCKS, &c. With 29 Coloured Plates. Fcap. 8vo, cloth, 4s. 6d.

THE NATURAL HISTORY OF LIONS, TIGERS, &c. With 34 Coloured Plates. Fcap. 8vo, cloth, 4s. 6d.

THE NATURAL HISTORY of DEER, ANTELOPES, &c. With 33 Coloured Plates. Fcap. 8vo, cloth, 4s. 6d.

THE NATURAL HISTORY OF SHEEP, OXEN, &c. With 31 Coloured Plates. Fcap. 8vo, cloth, 4s. 6d.

THE NATURAL HISTORY OF MONKEYS. With 29 Coloured Plates. Fcap. 8vo, cloth, 4s. 6d.

THE NATURAL HISTORY OF BEES. With 32 Coloured Plates. Fcap. 8vo, cloth, 4s. 6d.

JARDINE, Sir W., F.L.S., F.R.S.
THE NATURAL HISTORY of the PERCH FAMILY.
With 34 Coloured Plates. Fcap. 8vo, cloth, 4s. 6d.

THE NATURAL HISTORY OF THICK-SKINNED QUADRUPEDS—Elephants, Rhinoceri, &c. With 30 Coloured Plates. Fcap. 8vo, cloth, 4s. 6d.

JESSE, GEO. R.
RESEARCHES INTO THE HISTORY OF THE BRITISH DOG. With Original Anecdotes and Illustrations of the Nature and Attributes of the Dog. With 33 Plates, designed and etched by the Author. Two Volumes, demy 8vo, £1 12s.; India Proofs, £3 3s.

JEWITT, LLEWELLYN, F.S.A.
HALF-HOURS AMONG ENGLISH ANTIQUITIES.
With numerous Illustrations. Crown 8vo, cloth, 5s.

JOHNSON, R. LOCKE, L.R.C.P., L.R.C.I., L.S.A., &c.
FOOD CHART, giving the Names, Classification, Composition, Elementary Value, rates of Digestibility, Adulterations, Tests, &c., of the Alimentary substances in general use. In wrapper, 4to, 2s. 6d. ; or on roller, varnished, 6s.

KEENE, JAMES, F.R.C.S.
DEFECTIVE HEARING: Its Curable Forms and Rational Treatment. Fourth Edition. Cr. 8vo, cloth, 2s. 6d.

KINAHAN, G. H.
THE HANDY BOOK OF ROCK NAMES. Fcap. 8vo, cloth, 4s.

LANKESTER, E., M.D., F.R.S., F.L.S.
OUR FOOD : A Course of Lectures delivered at the South Kensington Museum. Illustrated. New Edition. Crown 8vo, cloth, 4s.

THE USES OF ANIMALS in Relation to the Industry of Man: A Course of Lectures delivered at the South Kensington Museum. Illustrated. New Edition. Crown 8vo, cloth, 4s.

PRACTICAL PHYSIOLOGY: A School Manual of Health, for the Use of Classes and General Reading. Illustrated with numerous Woodcuts. Sixth Edition. Fcap. 8vo, cloth, 2s. 6d.

HALF-HOURS WITH THE MICROSCOPE: A Popular Guide to the Use of the Instrument. With 250 Illustrations. Twelfth Thousand, enlarged. Fcap. 8vo, cloth, plain 2s. 6d. ; coloured 4s.

LANKESTER, E., M.D., F.R.S., F.L.S.
SANITARY INSTRUCTIONS: A Series of Handbills for general Distribution.
1. Management of Infants.
2. Scarlet Fever, and the best Means of Preventing it.
3. Typhoid or Drain Fever, and its Prevention.
4. Small Pox, and its Prevention.
5. Cholera and Diarrhœa, and its Prevention.
6. Measles, and their Prevention.

Each, 1*d.*; per dozen, 6*d.*; per 100, 4*s.*; per 1,000, 30*s.*

LANKESTER, MRS.
TALKS ABOUT HEALTH: A Book for Boys and Girls; Being an Explanation of all the Processes by which Life is sustained. Illustrated. Small 8vo, cloth, 1*s.*

A PLAIN and EASY ACCOUNT of BRITISH FERNS. Together with their Classification, Arrangement of Genera, Structures, and Functions, Directions for Out-door and Indoor Cultivation, &c. Numerous Coloured Illustrations. Fcap. 8vo, cloth, 4*s.*

WILD FLOWERS WORTH NOTICE: A Selection of some of our Native Plants which are most attractive for their Beauty, Uses, or Associations. With Coloured Illustrations by J. E. SOWERBY. Fcap. 8vo, cloth, 4*s.*

LE HARDY, ESTHER.
THE HOME NURSE: A Manual for the Sick-room. Second Edition. Fcap. 8vo, cloth, 2*s.* 6*d.*

LEIGHTON, REV. W. A., B.A., F.L.S., F.B.S. Edin.
THE LICHEN-FLORA OF GREAT BRITAIN, IRELAND, AND THE CHANNEL ISLANDS. Second Edition. Fcap. 8vo, cloth, 16*s.*

LONDON CATALOGUE OF BRITISH PLANTS. Published under the direction of the London Botanical Exchange Club, adapted for marking Desiderata in Exchanges of Specimens; and for a Guide to Collectors, by showing the rarity or frequency of the several Species. Seventh Edition. 8vo, sewed, 6*d.*

LORD, J. KEAST.
AT HOME IN THE WILDERNESS: What to Do there and How to do it. A Handbook for Travellers and Emigrants. With numerous Illustrations of necessary Baggage, Tents, Tools, &c. &c. Second Edition. Crown 8vo, cloth, 5*s.*

MACGILLIVRAY, W., F.R.S.
NATURAL HISTORY OF BRITISH QUADRUPEDS. With 34 Coloured Plates. Fcap. 8vo, cloth, 4*s.* 6*d.*

MACKENZIE'S EDUCATIONAL SERIES.

Intended for Schools or Self-instruction.

MACKENZIE'S TABLES: Commercial, Arithmetical, Miscellaneous, and Artificers'. Calculations in Bricklaying, Carpentry, Lathing, Masonry, Paper-hanging, Paving, Painting, Plastering, Slating, Tiling, Well-sinking, Digging, &c. &c. Fractions and Decimals. Forms of Receipts and Bills. Calculations on Man, Steam, Railways, Power, Light, Wind, &c. Language and Alphabets. Calendar of the Church. Scripture Money, Principal Foreign Moneys and Measures. Geographical and Astronomical Tables, &c. &c. Complete, 2*d.* ; cloth, 6*d.*

MURRAY'S ENGLISH GRAMMAR. Complete, word for word with the Shilling Editions. 2*d.*

MAVOR'S SPELLING. With numerous Woodcuts. 4*d.*

WALKINGHAME'S ARITHMETIC. Same as the Half-crown Edition. 4*d.*

SHORT-HAND. With Phrases and Exercises, to gain facility in the use of all the characters, by which perfection may soon be attained. 2*d.*

PHRENOLOGY Explained and Exemplified. 2*d.*

BOOKKEEPING by Single Entry, with Explanations of Subsidiary Books: Being a useful System for the Wholesale and Retail Shopkeeper. 2*d.*

MAIN, REV. R., F.R.S., V.P.R.A.S. "Radcliffe Observer."

MODERN PHILOSOPHIC SCEPTICISMS EXAMINED. Demy 8vo, cloth, 2*s.* 6*d.*

MANGNALL'S HISTORICAL & MISCELLANEOUS QUESTIONS. New Edition, carefully revised and brought up to the Present Time. Well printed and strongly bound. 18mo, cloth boards, 1*s.*

MARTIN, W. C. L.

The **NATURAL HISTORY of HUMMING BIRDS.** With 14 Coloured Plates. Fcap. 8vo, cloth, 4*s.* 6*d.*

MICHOD, C. J., late Secretary of the London Athletic Club.

GOOD CONDITION: A Guide to Athletic Training, for Amateurs and Professionals. Small 8vo, cloth, 1*s.*

MICROSCOPICAL JOURNAL (THE). Transactions of the Royal Microscopical Society, and Record of Histological Research. Edited by HENRY LAWSON, M.D., F.R.M.S., Assistant Physician to, and Lecturer on Histology in, St. Mary's Hospital. Published Monthly. Demy 8vo, Illustrated, price 1*s.* 6*d.* Sixteen Volumes issued. Cloth, 10*s.* 6*d.* each.

MILTON, J. L., M.R.C.S.
THE STREAM OF LIFE ON OUR GLOBE: Its Archives, Traditions, and Laws, as revealed by Modern Discoveries in Geology and Palæontology. A Sketch in Untechnical Language of the Beginning and Growth of Life, and the Physiological Laws which govern its Progress and Operations. Second Edition. Crown 8vo, cloth, 6s.

MIVART, ST. GEORGE, F.R.S., V.P.Z.S., Lecturer on Zoology and Comparative Anatomy at St. Mary's Hospital.
MAN AND APES: An Exposition of Structural Resemblances and Differences bearing upon Questions of Affinity and Origin. With numerous Illustrations. Crown 8vo, cloth, 6s.

MONKHOVEN, D. VAN, Ph.D.
PHOTOGRAPHIC OPTICS, including the description of Lenses and Enlarging Apparatus. With 200 Woodcuts. Crown 8vo, cloth, 7s. 6d.

NAVE, JOHANN.
THE COLLECTOR'S HANDY-BOOK OF ALGÆ, DIATOMS, DESMIDS, FUNGI, LICHENS, MOSSES, &c. With Instructions for their Preparation and the Formation of an Herbarium. Translated and Edited by the Rev. W. W. SPICER, M.A. Illustrated with 114 Woodcuts. Fcap. 8vo, cloth, 2s. 6d.

NELSON, DAVID, M.D.
On the **BEING** and **ATTRIBUTES** of the **GODHEAD,** as evidenced by Creation. Demy 8vo, cloth, 10s. 6d.

NEWMAN, EDWARD, F.Z.S.
AN ILLUSTRATED NATURAL HISTORY OF BRITISH MOTHS. With Life-size Figures from Nature of each Species, and of the more striking Varieties; also full descriptions of both the Perfect Insect and the Caterpillar, together with Dates of Appearance and Localities where found. Super-royal 8vo, cloth gilt, 20s.

AN ILLUSTRATED NATURAL HISTORY OF BRITISH BUTTERFLIES. With Life-size Figures from Nature of each Species, and of the more striking Varieties, &c. &c. Super-royal 8vo, cloth, 7s. 6d.

The above Works may also be had in One Volume, cloth gilt, 25s.

NEWTON, JOSEPH, F.R.H.S.
THE LANDSCAPE GARDENER: A Practical Guide to the Laying-Out, Planting, and Arrangement of Villa Gardens, Town Squares, and Open Spaces, from a Quarter of an Acre to Four Acres. For the Use of Practical Gardeners, Amateurs, Architects, and Builders. With 24 Plans. Fcap. folio, cloth, 12s.

NOTES ON COLLECTING AND PRESERVING NATURAL HISTORY OBJECTS. Edited by J. E. TAYLOR, F.L.S., F.G.S., Editor of "Science Gossip." With numerous Illustrations. Crown 8vo, cloth, 3s. 6d.

Contents—Geological Specimens, by the Editor; Bones, by E. F. ELWIN; Birds' Eggs, by T. SOUTHWELL, F.Z.S.; Butterflies, by Dr. KNAGGS; Beetles, by E. C. RYE, F.Z.S.; Hymenoptera, by J. B. BRIDGMAN; Fresh-water Shells, by Prof. RALPH TATE, F.G.S.; Flowering Plants, by JAMES BRITTEN, F.L.S.; Trees and Shrubs, by Prof. BUCKMAN, F.G.S.; Mosses, by Dr. BRAITHWAITE, F.L.S.; Fungi, by W. G. SMITH, F.L.S.: Lichens, by Rev. J. CROMBIE; Seaweeds, by W. GRATTANN.

PHILLIPS, LAWRENCE B., F.R.A.S.

THE AUTOGRAPHIC ALBUM: A Collection of 470 Facsimiles of Holograph Writings of Royal, Noble, and Distinguished Men and Women of Various Nations, &c. Small 4to, cloth, 12s.

POPULAR SCIENCE REVIEW: A Quarterly Summary of Scientific Progress and Miscellany of Entertaining and Instructive Articles on Scientific Subjects, by the Best Writers of the Day. SECOND SERIES. Edited by W. S. DALLAS, F.L.S., F.G.S. With high-class Illustrations by first-rate Artists. The FIRST SERIES, edited by Dr. HENRY LAWSON, F.R.M.S., is Complete in 15 Volumes, fully Illustrated. Price in Parts, £7 12s. 6d.; in cloth gilt, £9 2s.; in half morocco, extra, £11 8s.

PROCTOR, RICHARD A., B.A.

HALF-HOURS WITH THE STARS: A Plain and Easy Guide to the Knowledge of the Constellations; showing, in 12 Maps, the position of the principal Star-groups, night after night throughout the Year, with Introduction and a separate Explanation of Each Map. Seventh Edition. Demy 4to, boards, 5s.

HALF-HOURS WITH THE TELESCOPE: A Popular Guide to the Use of the Telescope as a means of Amusement and Instruction. Fifth Edition, Illustrated. Fcap. 8vo, cloth, 2s. 6d.

QUEKETT MICROSCOPICAL CLUB, Journal of the. Published Quarterly. Demy 8vo, price 1s. Thirty-two Parts are now issued.

RANSONNETT, BARON EUGENE DE.

SKETCHES OF THE INHABITANTS, ANIMAL LIFE, and VEGETATION in the LOWLANDS and HIGH MOUNTAINS OF CEYLON, as well as the Submarine Scenery near the Coast, taken in a Diving Bell. Illustrated with 26 large Chromo-lithographs. Folio, cloth gilt, £2 10s.

READE, T. M., C.E., F.G.S.

THE MOON AND THE EARTH: Being the Presidential Address to the Liverpool Geological Society, 1875. Illustrated with Two Photographs. Demy 8vo, sewed, 1s.

ROBSON, JOHN E.

BOTANICAL LABELS for Labelling Herbaria, adapted to the names in the London Catalogue of Plants and the Manuals of Professor BABINGTON and Dr. HOOKER, with Extra Labels for all New Species and Varieties recorded in the recent volumes of "The Journal of Botany" and the Exchange Club Reports. In all 3,576 Labels, with Index. Demy 8vo, 5s.

ROOPER, GEORGE, Author of "Flood, Field, and Forest."

A MONTH IN MAYO. Comprising Characteristic Sketches (Sporting and Social) of Irish Life, with Miscellaneous Papers. Crown 8vo, cloth, 2s. 6d.

THAMES AND TWEED: A Book for Anglers. Second Edition. Crown 8vo, cloth, 1s. 6d.

THE FOX AT HOME, and other Tales. With Illustrations by G. BOWERS and J. CARLISLE. Crown 8vo, cloth, 5s.

ROSS, JAMES, M.D.

ON PROTOPLASM: Being an Examination of Dr. JAMES HUTCHINSON STIRLING's Criticism of Professor HUXLEY's Views. Crown 8vo, cloth, 3s. 6d.

ROSS-OF-BLADENSBERG, JOHN, Coldstream Guards.

ENGLAND'S MARITIME RIGHTS. A Pamphlet on the Declaration of Paris. Demy 8vo, 1s.

RUSSELL, C.

THE TANNIN PROCESS. Second Edition, with Appendix. Fcap. 8vo, cloth, 2s. 6d.

SCHAIBLE, CHARLES H., M.D., Ph.D.

FIRST HELP IN ACCIDENTS: Being a Surgical Guide in the absence, or before the arrival, of Medical Assistance, for the use of the Public. Fully Illustrated. 32mo, cloth, 1s.

SCHLEIDEN, J. M., M.D.

THE PRINCIPLES OF SCIENTIFIC BOTANY; or, Botany as an Inductive Science. Translated by Dr. LANKESTER. Numerous Woodcuts, and Six Steel Plates. Demy 8vo, cloth, 10s. 6d.

SCHMIDT, ADOLPH, assisted by *GRUNDLER, GRUNOW, JANECH, &c.*
  ATLAS OF THE DIATOMACEÆ. This magnificent work consists of Photographic Reproductions of the various forms of Diatomaceæ, on Folio Plates, with description (in German). Ten Parts are now ready. Price to Subscribers, for Twelve Parts, payable in advance, £3 12s. To be completed in about 25 parts.

SCHOMBURGK, R. H., M.D.
  THE NATURAL HISTORY OF THE FISHES OF BRITISH GUIANA. With 66 Coloured Plates. Two Vols. Fcap. 8vo, cloth, 9s.

  SCIENCE GOSSIP. A Monthly Medium of Interchange and Gossip for Students and Lovers of Nature. Edited by J. E. TAYLOR, F.L.S., F.G.S., &c. Price Fourpence, or by post Fivepence. 12 Volumes published, price 5s. each.

SELBY, P. J., F.R.S., F.L.S.
  THE NATURAL HISTORY OF PIGEONS. With 30 Coloured Plates. Fcap. 8vo, cloth, 4s. 6d.
  THE NATURAL HISTORY OF PARROTS. With 30 Coloured Plates. Fcap. 8vo, cloth, 4s. 6d.

SHARPE, W., M.D., Surgeon Army Medical Department.
  MAN A SPECIAL CREATION; or, The Preordained Evolution of Species. Crown 8vo, cloth, 6s.

SIMMONDS, P. L., Editor of the Journal of Applied Science.
  WASTE PRODUCTS AND UNDEVELOPED SUBSTANCES: A Synopsis of Progress made in their Economic Utilization during the last Quarter of a Century at Home and Abroad. Third Edition. Crown 8vo, cloth, 9s.

  SCIENCE AND COMMERCE: Their Influence on our Manufactures. A Series of Statistical Essays and Lectures describing the Progressive Discoveries of Science, the Advance of British Commerce, and the Activity of our Principal Manufactures in the Nineteenth Century. Fcap. 8vo, cl. 6s.

SMITH, DAVID, M.D.
  LECTURES ON PRESERVATION OF SIGHT. Crown 8vo, 2s. 6d.

SMITH, LIEUT. COL. C. H.
  THE NATURAL HISTORY OF DOGS. With 60 Coloured Plates. Two Vols. Fcap. 8vo, cloth, 9s.
  THE NATURAL HISTORY OF HORSES. With 35 Coloured Plates. Fcap. 8vo, cloth, 4s. 6d.

SMITH, LIEUT. COL. C. H.
THE NATURAL HISTORY OF MAMMALIA. With 30 Coloured Plates. Fcap. 8vo, cloth, 4*s.* 6*d.*

THE NATURAL HISTORY OF MAN. With 34 Plates. Fcap. 8vo, cloth, 4*s.* 6*d.*

SMITH, J., A.L.S., late Curator of the Royal Gardens, Kew.
FERNS, BRITISH AND FOREIGN: Their History, Organography, Classification, Nomenclature, and Culture; with Directions showing which are the best adapted for the Hothouse, Greenhouse, Open Air Fernery, or Wardian Case. With an Index of Genera, Species, and Synonyms. Third Edition, revised and greatly enlarged, with new Figures, &c. Crown 8vo, cloth, 7*s.* 6*d.*

SMITH, WORTHINGTON, F.L.S.
MUSHROOMS AND TOADSTOOLS: How to Distinguish easily the Difference between Edible and Poisonous Fungi. Two large Sheets, containing Figures of 29 Edible and 31 Poisonous Species, drawn the natural size, and Coloured from Living Specimens. With descriptive letterpress, 6*s.*; on canvas, in cloth case for pocket, 10*s.* 6*d.*; on canvas, on rollers and varnished, 10*s.* 6*d.* The letterpress may be had separately, with key-plates of figures, 1*s.*

SMOKER'S GUIDE (THE), PHILOSOPHER AND FRIEND. What to Smoke—What to Smoke With—and the Whole "What's What" of Tobacco, Historical, Botanical, Manufactural, Anecdotal, Social, Medical, &c. By a Veteran of Smokedom. Royal 32mo, cloth, 1*s.*

SOWERBY, J.
ENGLISH BOTANY. Containing a Description and Lifesize Drawing of every British Plant. Edited and brought up to the Present Standard of Scientific Knowledge, by T. BOSWELL SYME, LL.D., F.L.S., &c. With Popular Descriptions of the Uses, History, and Traditions of each Plant, by Mrs. LANKESTER. Complete in 11 Volumes, cloth, £22 8*s.*; half morocco, £24 12*s.*; whole morocco, £28 3*s.* 6*d.*

STABLES, W., M.D.
MEDICAL LIFE IN THE NAVY. Being the experiences of a Naval Surgeon described for non-professional readers. Fcap. 8vo, cloth, 2*s.* 6*d.*

STEVENSON, G. de ST. CLAIR.
ALSACE AND LORRAINE, Past, Present, and Future. With an Illustration by F. W. LAWSON. Demy 8vo, cloth, 4*s.*

SWAINSON, W., F.R.S., F.L.S.
THE NATURAL HISTORY OF THE BIRDS OF WESTERN AFRICA. With 64 Coloured Plates. 2 vols., fcap. 8vo, cloth, 9s.

THE NATURAL HISTORY OF FLYCATCHERS. With 31 Coloured Plates. Fcap. 8vo, cloth, 4s. 6d.

SYMONDS, Rev. W. S., *Rector of Pendock, Author of "Stones in the Valley,"* &c.
OLD BONES; or, Notes for Young Naturalists. With References to the Typical Specimens in the British Museum. Second Edition, much improved and enlarged. Numerous Illustrations. Fcap. 8vo, cloth, 2s. 6d.

TATE, *Professor* RALPH, F.G.S.
BRITISH MOLLUSKS; or, Slugs and Snails, Land and Fresh-water. A Plain and Easy Account of the Land and Fresh-water Mollusks of Great Britain, containing Descriptions, Figures, and a Familiar Account of the Habits of each Species. Numerous Illustrations, coloured by hand. Fcap. 8vo, cloth, 6s.

TAYLOR, Rev. ISAAC, M.A., *Author of "Etruscan Researches."*
THE ETRUSCAN LANGUAGE. Illustrated. Second Edition. Demy 8vo, sewed, 1s.

TAYLOR, J. E., F.L.S., F.G.S., *Editor of "Science Gossip."*
HALF-HOURS IN THE GREEN LANES. A Book for a Country Stroll. Illustrated with 300 Woodcuts. Third Edition. Crown 8vo, cloth, 4s.

HALF-HOURS AT THE SEA SIDE; or, Recreations with Marine Objects. Illustrated with 250 Woodcuts. Third Edition. Crown 8vo, cloth, 4s.

GEOLOGICAL STORIES: A Series of Autobiographies in Chronological Order. Numerous Illustrations. Third Edition. Crown 8vo, cloth, 4s.

THE AQUARIUM; its Inhabitants, Structure, and Management. With 238 Woodcuts. Crown 8vo, cloth extra, 6s. (*See also* NOTES ON COLLECTING AND PRESERVING NATURAL HISTORY OBJECTS.

TRIMEN, H., M.B. (Lond.), F.L.S., *and* DYER, W. T., B.A.
THE FLORA OF MIDDLESEX: A Topographical and Historical Account of the Plants found in the County. With Sketches of its Physical Geography and Climate, and of the Progress of Middlesex Botany during the last Three Centuries. With a Map of Botanical Districts. Crown 8vo, cloth, 12s. 6d.

TROTTER, M. E.

A METHOD OF TEACHING PLAIN NEEDLE-WORK IN SCHOOLS. Illustrated with Diagrams and Samplers. New Edition, revised and arranged according to Standards. Demy 8vo, cloth, 2s. 6d.

TURNER, M., and HARRIS, W.

A GUIDE to the INSTITUTIONS and CHARITIES for the BLIND in the United Kingdom. Together with Lists of Books and Appliances for their Use. A Catalogue of Books published upon the subject of the Blind, and a List of Foreign Institutions, &c. Demy 8vo, cloth, 3s.

UP THE RIVER from WESTMINSTER to WINDSOR: A Panorama in Pen and Ink. Illustrated with 81 Engravings and a Map of the Thames. Demy 8vo, 1s. 6d.

VINCENT, JOHN.

COUNTRY COTTAGES: A Series of Designs for an Improved Class of Dwellings for Agricultural Labourers. Folio, cloth, 12s.

WAITE, S. C.

GRACEFUL RIDING: A Pocket Manual for Equestrians. Illustrated. Fcap. 8vo, cloth, 2s. 6d.

WALFORD, E. M.A., Late Scholar of Balliol College, Oxford. Dedicated by Express Permission to H.R.H. the Prince of Wales.

THE COUNTY FAMILIES; or, Royal Manual of the Titled and Untitled Aristocracy of the Three Kingdoms. It contains a complete Peerage, Baronetage, Knightage, and Dictionary of the Landed Commoners of England, Scotland, Wales, and Ireland, and gives a Brief Notice of the Descent, Birth, Marriage, Education, and Appointments of each Person (in all about 11,000), his Heir Apparent or Presumptive, a Record of the Offices which he has held, together with his Town Address and Country Residences. 1,200 pages. Imp. 8vo, cloth gilt, £2 10s. Published annually.

THE SHILLING PEERAGE. Containing an Alphabetical List of the House of Lords, Dates of Creation, Lists of Scotch and Irish Peers, Addresses, &c. 32mo, cloth, 1s. Published annually.

THE SHILLING BARONETAGE. Containing an Alphabetical List of the Baronets of the United Kingdom, Short Biographical Notices, Dates of Creation, Addresses, &c. 32mo, cloth, 1s. Published annually.

THE SHILLING KNIGHTAGE. Containing an Alphabetical List of the Knights of the United Kingdom, Short Biographical Notices, Dates of Creation, Addresses, &c. 32mo, cloth, 1s. Published annually.

THE SHILLING HOUSE OF COMMONS. Containing a List of all the Members of the British Parliament, their Town and Country Addresses, &c. 32mo, cloth, 1s. Published annually.

THE COMPLETE PEERAGE, BARONETAGE, KNIGHTAGE, AND HOUSE OF COMMONS. In One Volume, 32mo, half-bound, with coloured edges, marking the divisions, 5s. Published annually.

WATERHOUSE, G. R.
THE NATURAL HISTORY OF MARSUPIALIA. With 34 Coloured Plates. Fcap. 8vo, cloth, 4s. 6d.

WHINFIELD, W. H.
ETHICS OF THE FUTURE. Demy 8vo, cloth, 12s.

WILSON'S AMERICAN ORNITHOLOGY; or, Natural History of the Birds of the United States; with the Continuation by Prince CHARLES LUCIAN BONAPARTE. New and Enlarged Edition, completed by the insertion of above One Hundred Birds omitted in the original Work, and by valuable Notes, and Life of the Author, by Sir WILLIAM JARDINE. Three Vols. demy 4to, with Portrait of WILSON, and 103 Plates, exhibiting nearly 400 figures, carefully Coloured by hand, half-Roxburghe, £6 6s.

WYNTER, ANDREW, M.D., M.R.C.P.
SUBTLE BRAINS AND LISSOM FINGERS: Being some of the Chisel Marks of our Industrial and Scientific Progress. Third Edition, and corrected by ANDREW STEINMETZ. Fcap. 8vo, cloth, 3s. 6d.

CURIOSITIES OF CIVILIZATION. Being Essays reprinted from the *Quarterly* and *Edinburgh Reviews*. Crown 8vo, cloth, 6s.

ZERFFI, G. G., Ph.D., F.R.S.L.
A MANUAL of the HISTORICAL DEVELOPMENT OF ART—Prehistoric, Ancient, Hebrew, Classic, Early Christian. With special reference to Architecture, Sculpture, Painting, and Ornamentation. Crown 8vo, cloth, 6s.

SPIRITUALISM AND ANIMAL MAGNETISM. A Treatise on Spiritual Manifestations, &c. &c., in which it is shown that these can, by careful study, be traced to natural causes. Third Edition. Crown 8vo, sewed, 1s.

www.ingramcontent.com/pod-product-compliance
Lightning Source LLC
Chambersburg PA
CBHW051242300426
44114CB00011B/856